# Clubfoot and Vertical Talus

Matthew B. Dobbs • Ashok N. Johari
Mitzi L. Williams

Editors

# Clubfoot and Vertical Talus

## Etiology and Clinical Management

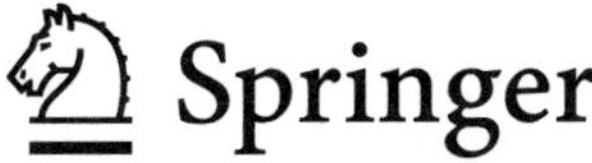 Springer

*Editors*
Matthew B. Dobbs
Paley Institute
St. Mary's Medical Center
West Palm Beach, FL, USA

Ashok N. Johari
Children's Orthopedic Centre
Mumbai, Maharashtra, India

Mitzi L. Williams
Podiatric Surgery/Orthopedics
Kaiser Permanente Oakland Medical Center
Oakland, CA, USA

ISBN 978-3-031-35885-2        ISBN 978-3-031-34788-7   (eBook)
https://doi.org/10.1007/978-3-031-34788-7



This Springer imprint is published by the registered company Springer Nature Switzerland AG
The registered company address is: Gewerbestrasse 11, 6330 Cham, Switzerland

*I dedicate this book to the children and their families whom I treat. I continue to be inspired by these families. I too dedicate this book to my three children Ellison, Thomas, and Kathleen whom I love unconditionally.*
*—Matthew B Dobbs MD, FACS*

# Preface

In the field of pediatric orthopedics, clubfoot has undergone an incredible paradigm shift in how we as physicians treat the condition in infancy as well as relapses in life. Years ago, families embarked on an extensive surgical journey; one filled with large grandiose incisions and scarring. Despite such many developed stiff, painful, and often undercorrected feet. The functional outcome scores were not what any physician would hope for in a young child. These results were studied and much like we learn from surgical outcomes we learned that with this condition a less invasive approach would be more beneficial.

Dr. Ignacio Ponseti, a pioneer in this less invasive approach and mentor to all he met, continued to practice and teach his beliefs. He believed with gentle manipulation and maintenance via serial casting that the results produced supple, corrected, and less painful feet. He learned from Dr. Kite's approach, which blocked the motion of the calcaneus beneath the talus, the precise maneuver that would result in a plantigrade foot. In 2006, what some do not realize is Dr. Matthew Dobbs strived to bring to light research highlighting poorer outcomes following posterior medial releases in young children. This study was complex in its design and was not accepted by all. This publication validates the effectiveness of the precise Ponseti method for treating clubfoot while also highlighting the emergence of another pioneering figure.

It is not always easy developing treatment pathways that initially may not be accepted by all and must gain eventual acceptance. Without question, Dr. Matthew Dobbs has obtained a unique position in the field of Pediatric Orthopedics. He has furthered our understanding of not only clubfoot but also vertical talus. He has paved the way in the field of genetics of lower limb deformities while serving all with compassion as Dr. Ponseti did for the world.

On any given day, Dr. Matthew Dobbs's clinic is filled with children who have traveled from all over the world to seek care. He leads the way in treatment of both the atypical and complex clubfoot subsets. Vertical talus families seek his expertise and commend him for his advances while carrying on the spirit of Dr. Ponseti. The Dobbs method in the treatment of vertical talus has spared many children from more involved surgeries just as the Ponseti method has done for clubfoot. Through research we continue to learn various casting maneuvers to treat all clubfoot subsets and recognize surgical execution now takes on an "a la carte" approach to care.

I have witnessed Dr. Dobbs in the office and have worked in numerous countries with him. He treats all children and families with dignity. Families continue to travel worldwide because of his second to none skills and compassion. Healthcare professionals seek his mentorship.

With pride I commend all authors in this book and would recommend Dr. Matthew Dobbs to any family navigating life with a child who has a lower extremity condition.

Respectfully,

Oakland, CA, USA                                                    Mitzi L. Williams

# Preface

This book has been a work in progress for several years. Each chapter has been developed with specific authors in mind while too presenting topics with compassion. As a pediatric orthopedic surgeon who treats numerous musculoskeletal conditions, I realize clubfoot and vertical talus are quite unique. Very few conditions lead to children being seen weekly for care at a time where many families are simply learning how to care for a young infant. There are many emotions demonstrated from families throughout this process. As a result, I feel a closeness to these families and an incredible desire to optimize the quality of life for every child.

With pleasure I have dedicated my life to the treatment of children with clubfoot, vertical talus, and cerebral palsy. My work in genetics leads to a large population of children with vertical talus seeking care. Much like my mentor, Dr. Ignacio Ponseti, who developed the Ponseti method which changed clubfoot treatment, I channeled a less invasive approach and developed the Dobbs method to treat vertical talus. These methods along with advanced treatment modalities in the world of clubfoot and vertical talus are described in this book.

Writing this book has given me pause in my own life. It has allowed me to reflect on my strengths and hopes for where care should be directed in the years to come. I commend all authors in this book for their dedication to treating children.

Sincerely,

West Palm Beach, FL, USA                                                    Matthew B. Dobbs

# Contents

# Chapter 1
# Etiology and Pathogenesis of Clubfoot and Vertical Talus

Christina A. Gurnett, Mitzi L. Williams, and Matthew B. Dobbs

Clubfoot, also called talipes equinovarus, is one of the most common congenital foot malformations. The clubfoot abnormality occurs in approximately 1 in 1000 of all live births [1]. The incidence is much higher in Maori (7/1000) and Hawaiians (6.8/1000), and Australian Aboriginals where it occurs in up to 1 in 300 births [2, 3]. Clubfoot is more than twice as common in males as females. Two-thirds of patients with clubfoot have bilateral involvement, in the remaining unilateral cases, there is a slight propensity toward right-sided abnormalities. While other limb birth defects such as metatarsus adductus can be directly related to maternal factors, such as in utero-compression or positioning, clubfoot is rarely associated with these factors and, as such, does not improve without manipulation.

## Environmental Factors

As a relatively common human malformation, epidemiological studies and birth defects registries have been widely utilized to determine the potential effects of maternal in utero environmental exposures on risk of clubfoot (Table 1.1). Environmental influence on clubfoot risk is strongest for smoking. Smoking is

C. A. Gurnett
St. Louis Children's Hospital, St. Louis, MO, USA
e-mail: gurnettc@neuro.wustl.edu

M. L. Williams
Podiatric Surgery/ Orthopedics, Kaiser Permanente Oakland Medical Center, Oakland, CA, USA

M. B. Dobbs (✉)
Paley Institute, St. Mary's Medical Center, West Palm Beach, FL, USA
e-mail: mdobbs@paleyinstitute.org



M. B. Dobbs et al. (eds.), *Clubfoot and Vertical Talus*,
https://doi.org/10.1007/978-3-031-34788-7_1

**Table 1.1** Environmental factors associated with clubfoot in some studies

- Maternal smoking
- Maternal exposure to selective serotonin uptake inhibitors
- Early amniocentesis
- Breech presentation
- Twin pregnancy
- First-born child
- Maternal obesity
- Low maternal socioeconomic status and educational attainment

well-known to be associated with small for gestational age births, and multiple studies have shown an association of smoking during pregnancy with an increased risk of clubfoot [4]. A small study of secondhand exposure to household smoke has also been associated with clubfoot [5]. Risk associated with smoking may also be accentuated by a concurrent family history of clubfoot [6]. Additionally, the presence of genetic variants in N-acetylation genes that result in slow metabolism of exogenous substances, including tobacco smoke, may also be weakly associated with clubfoot risk. Given the high incidence of maternal exposure to selective serotonin reuptake inhibitors (SSRIs) to treat depression and other psychiatric disorders in some countries, including the United States, there have been multiple studies of birth defects in infants whose mothers were exposed to these medications. Most of these studies have shown a small increase in incidence of clubfoot and an increased risk of other birth defects, including cleft lip and palate, in exposed fetuses [7]. However, other studies have shown conflicting data [4].

First-born children have a higher risk for clubfoot compared to their later born siblings. The underlying cause of this association is unknown but may reflect lower maternal age, which is associated with increased risk of clubfoot in some studies [5]. First-born children are also at increased risk of hip dysplasia, with some investigators hypothesizing that this may be due to intrinsic intrauterine factors such as crowding. Crowding due to oligohydramnios, as seen in the Potter sequence, can result in clubfoot, with the duration and temporal timing of oligohydramnios also influencing both the risk and the co-occurrence of hand contractures, which appears to only occur in later exposures [8]. Oligohydramnios is not typically seen in isolated clubfoot and therefore is not a common mechanistic cause of clubfoot. Breech presentation [9] and twinning [10] have also been associated with increased risk of clubfoot in some but not all studies.

Low socioeconomic status and less maternal education are also associated with a small increase in the risk of clubfoot [5], though the specific factors responsible have not been identified. Potential confounders exist for this association, however, including the fact that clubfoot is also associated with first-born status and smoking, which are both tied to lower socioeconomic status. Maternal obesity has also been implicated with slight elevated risk for clubfoot [11].

## Mechanistic Studies of Isolated Clubfoot

Detailed morphological evaluation of tissue from patients with isolated clubfoot, performed using a variety of modalities including immunohistochemistry and magnetic resonance imaging, suggests that isolated clubfoot is not a single entity with a single known cause. More likely, the diverse pathologies represent different underlying etiologies that all lead to a common phenotype. Graded differences in the severity of the underlying pathological abnormalities also greatly impact the phenotype, such that some individuals with clubfoot may have much more rigid deformities or newly described clinical exam findings, such as drop toe sign or the Samir-Adams sign that are highly suggestive of poor outcome. Nearly 40 years ago, Ippolito and Ponseti performed anatomic evaluations of clubfoot in the human fetus and proposed the term "retracting fibrosis" to describe their findings. Increased connective tissue and thickening of the tendo Achilles and posterior tibial tendons were noted. Shortening of the tibionavicular and plantar calcaneonavicular ligaments were noted in many of the feet they examined. Decreased muscle size was also often associated with the retracting fibrosis that they argued was the primary etiological factor for clubfoot deformity [12]. Others reported similar contracted fibrotic tissue, maximal in the talocalcaneal region that appeared "disc-like" due to its similarity to intervertebral disc tissue [13]. More recent studies using modern immunohistochemical analysis to evaluate the molecular composition of the fibrous tissue yielded results showing increased vimentin and myofibroblastic characteristics in the ligamentous cells of biopsied clubfoot patients [14]. Other studies focused on differences in the collagen composition of this fibrotic tissue [15]. Comprehensive studies using high-resolution mass spectrometry of the fibrotic tissue revealed an abundance of more than 20 different extracellular matrix proteins, which could all be potentially targeted for the development of novel therapeutics [16].

Because limbs were often noted to be small in clubfeet, muscle abnormalities have also been evaluated through a study of muscle biopsy of affected clubfoot limbs. Although individual muscle biopsies are occasionally abnormal suggesting an underlying myopathy, collectively these are rare in clubfoot, and muscle biopsies are typically normal [17]. Using both histological and electron microscopy, some investigators have found evidence for neurogenic abnormalities [18]. Overall, however, microscopic abnormalities are not common in clubfoot, and the role for muscle biopsy in the evaluation of clubfoot, particularly in the age of noninvasive imaging and comprehensive genetic testing, is questionable.

Anatomic abnormalities of muscle have also been occasionally described in clubfeet. A surgical series of more than 200 patients treated in Sudan revealed the presence of a flexor digitorum accessorius longus muscle in approximately 13% of all cases [19] (Fig. 1.1). The presence of this accessory muscle was also associated with clinical exam differences in the posture of the great toe in extension, which was referred to as the Samir-Adam sign. Since the flexor digitorum accessorius longus muscle can only be definitively identified during surgical treatment, its frequency has not been well described in nonsurgically treated cases. However, now that a

**Fig. 1.1** Flexor dig
access long

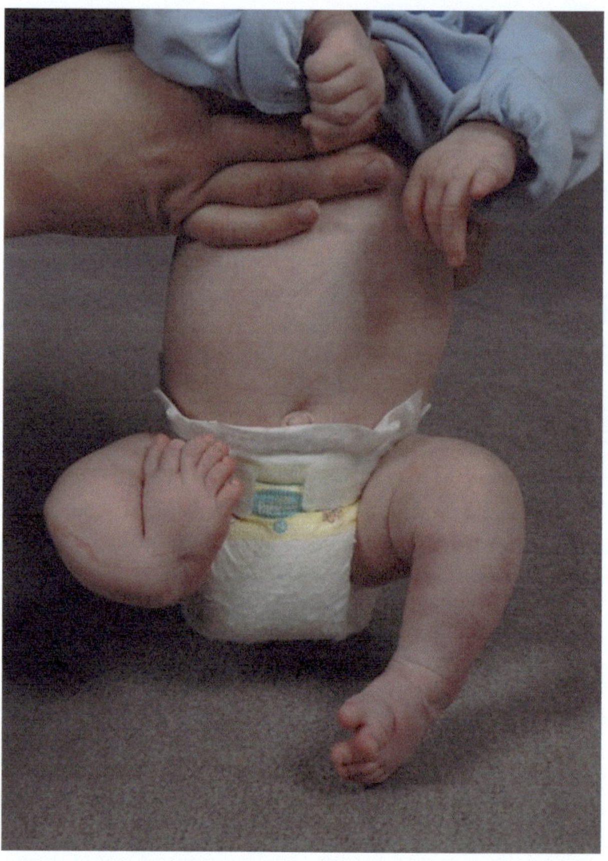

clinical sign has been reliably associated with its presence, its study in a larger cohort can be performed to determine the degree to which it is associated with higher rates of resistance to conservative treatments. The role of the flexor digitorum accessorius longus in the pathoetiology of clubfoot is unclear, although it is more common in familial clubfoot [20]. While no genetic abnormalities have been directly linked to the presence of this accessory muscle, it is notable that several genes recently implicated in clubfoot etiology are responsible for patterning defects in the limb, which may explain these large-scale anatomic abnormalities.

Careful observations of clubfeet with poor clinical outcome revealed the presence of a clinical examination finding called that drop toe sign that was present in a small number of infants with clubfoot [21] (Fig. 1.2). The drop toe sign is present when there is absence of active dorsiflexion of the toes after plantar stimulation of the foot. The resting posture of the toes is typically in plantarflexion. Exploration of the peroneal nerve revealed anatomic abnormalities that explained some of these cases. We evaluated 208 clubfeet and demonstrated absence of either dorsiflexion with stimulation of the dorsal or plantar aspect of the foot in 3% of all cases, though there was a slight reduction in movement in an additional 6% of cases [22]. The rate

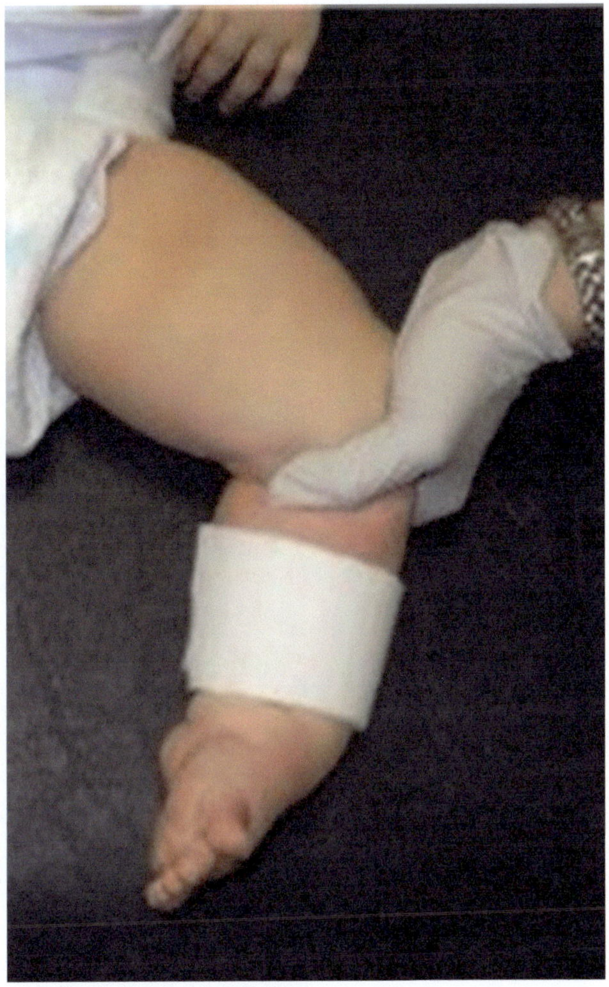

**Fig. 1.2** Drop toe sign photo

of motor deficits was slightly higher in unilateral cases, with nearly 6% of patients having unilateral deficits on systematic testing prior to brace initiation. In some patients described by Edmonds et al., the foot is also smaller, with reduced muscle mass and leg length discrepancy, and therefore, it is not entirely clear that the peroneal neuropathy is in isolation without other developmental abnormalities of the leg or whether the growth differences are a consequence of the primary nerve deficit. Familial unilateral peroneal nerve neuropathy has been reported at least once in a father and son pair [23]. Patients with peroneal nerve abnormalities typically have feet that are more difficult to correct, often require Achilles tendon lengthening, permanent bracing, and/or extensive surgery to maintain correction.

Vascular abnormalities have been described in both clubfoot and vertical talus and are important to recognize due to the risk of increased surgical complications

[24]. Doppler ultrasound and ankle brachial index were evaluated on 50 patients with clubfoot (74 ft) and showed abnormal flow in the anterior tibial artery and dorsalis pedis artery in 39% of cases and none of the controls. In severe clubfoot cases, the vascular flow abnormalities increased to 76% of cases [19], which was consistent with an earlier study [25]. Smaller studies revealed correlation between specific vascular anomalies and the presence of either clubfoot or vertical talus. Clubfoot appeared more commonly with absent anterior tibial artery while an absent posterior tibial artery was more common in vertical talus (Fig. 1.3) [26], although

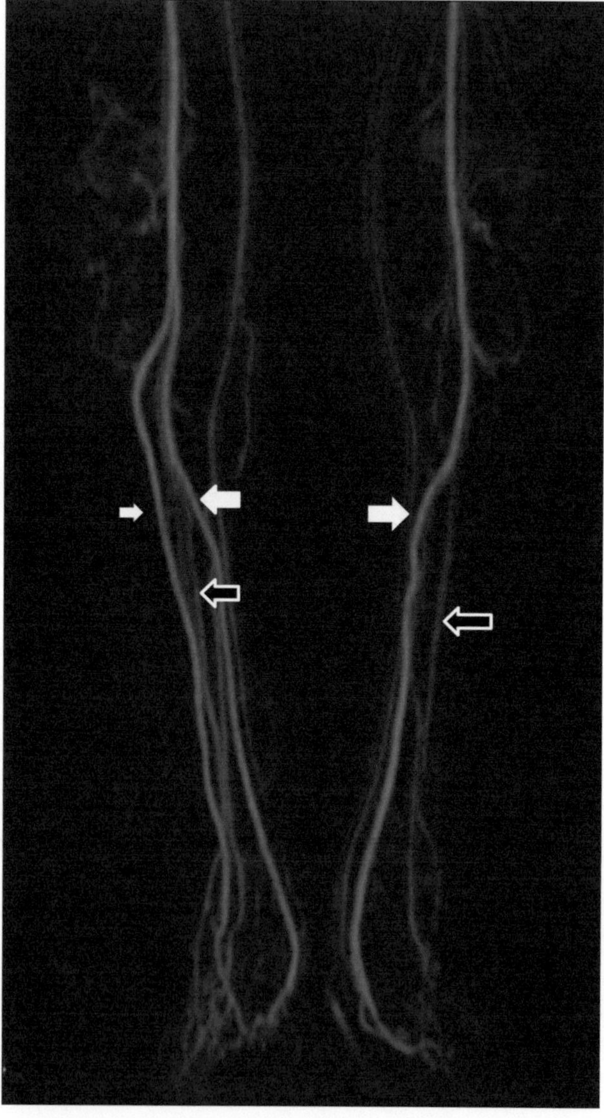

**Fig. 1.3** Absent anterior tibial artery in a child unilateral right-sided clubfoot with sacral agenesis as demonstrated by magnetic resonance angiography of the lower extremities. Large white arrow = posterior tibial artery, large black arrow = peroneal artery, small white arrow = anterior tibial artery. Left leg is on the left side of image

other cases have shown that these correlations are not absolute [27]. When evaluated with magnetic resonance angiography and magnetic resonance imaging, vascular abnormalities also correlated with reduced soft-tissue volumes [28].

For many years, it has been observed that unilateral clubfoot limbs are often smaller than unaffected limbs [29]. While size differences in the limb become much more obvious as a child grows, Ippolito found that these abnormalities were present very early in development, even prior to birth by studying fetuses with clubfoot [30]. Therefore, they argued that size difference was intrinsic to the underlying condition and could not be attributed to the possibility of iatrogenic effects of treatment [30]. By evaluating patients with both easily treated clubfoot and treatment resistant clubfoot, differences in soft-tissue volumes were found to correlate strongly with treatment response [31] (Fig. 1.4). Unilateral clubfeet with greater size discrepancy were found to have more difficulty achieving initial correction and sustaining correction over time. This effect is similar to past reported association of poor treatment response with greater reduction in calf size in children with unilateral clubfeet [29]. In addition to reduced muscle volumes, patients with treatment-resistant clubfoot also had greater increase in epimysial and intracompartment fat compared to patients with treatment-responsive clubfoot [31]. In most cases with treatment-responsive clubfeet, if reduced muscle volume was present, it was seen globally throughout all muscles in the calf. However, specific patterns of muscle-compartment aplasia/hypoplasia were highly correlated with treatment-resistant clubfoot (Fig. 1.5). Notably, clubfoot cases were identified in which the entire anterior,

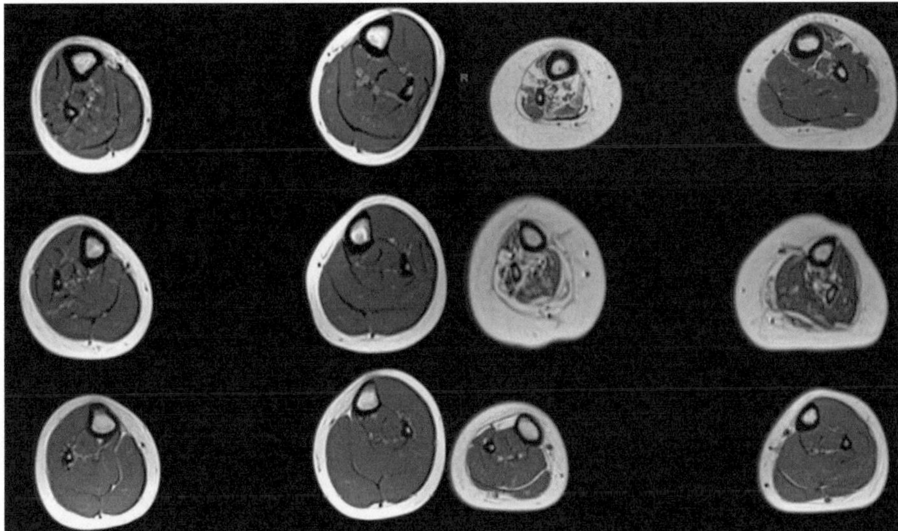

**Fig. 1.4** Clubfoot responsive clubfoot is associated with fewer soft-tissue abnormalities on magnetic resonance imaging compared to treatment resistant clubfoot. Cross-sectional images of the bilateral calves of three individuals with clubfoot that responded well to Ponseti method (left side) and three individuals with clubfoot whose feet responded poorly to clubfoot, with either poor initial correction or relapse or both (right side)

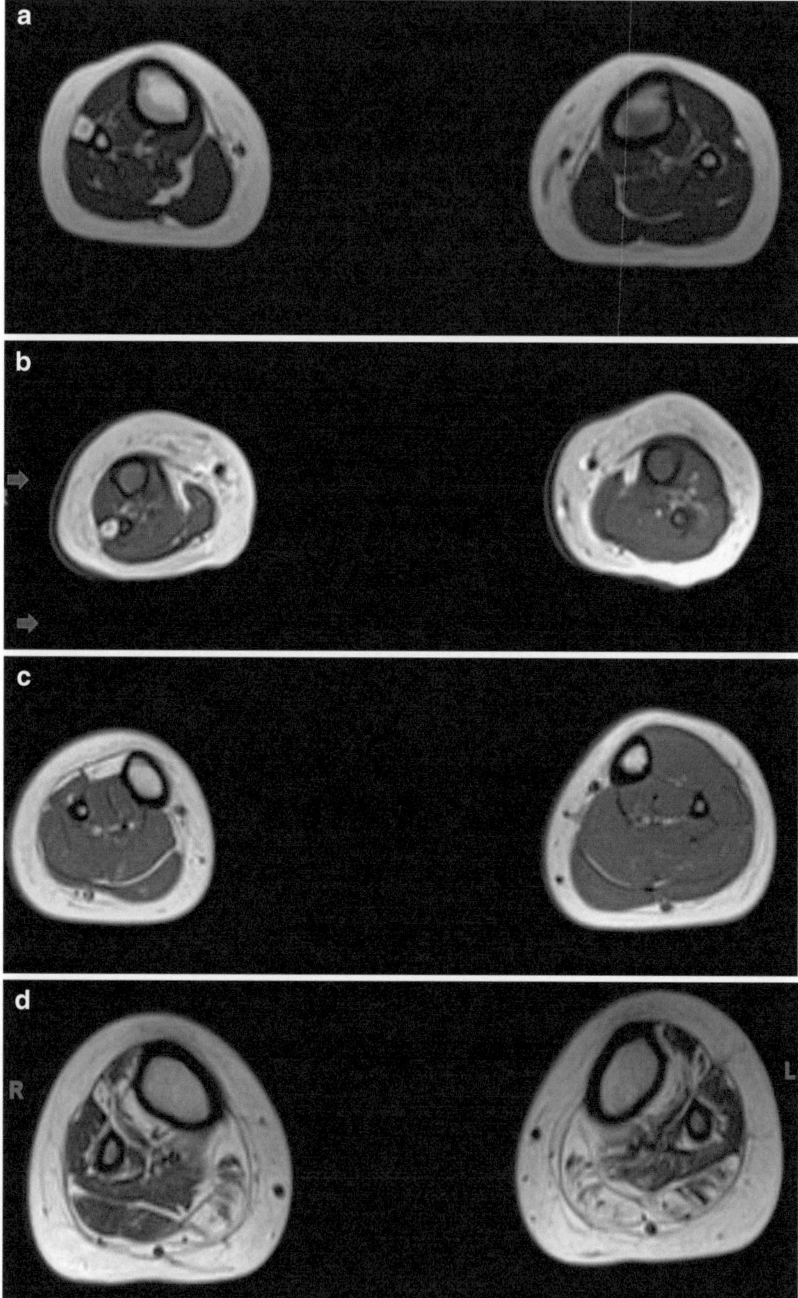

**Fig. 1.5** Specific muscle hypoplasia in four clubfoot cases as shown by magnetic resonance imaging. (**a**, **b**) Lateral muscle compartment replaced by fat (bright signal) on right leg (left image). (**c**) Anterior muscle compartment replaced by fat on the right leg (left image). (**d**) Posterior muscle compartment mostly replaced by fat bilaterally

lateral, or posterior muscle compartments were mostly or entirely replaced by fat. Individuals with specific muscle hypoplasia were also found to have clinical exam deficits, including drop toe sign and weak foot everter function. Some of these patients were later found to have genetic abnormalities in the PITX1-TBX4 pathway that will be described later in this chapter. Overall, soft-tissue abnormalities are common in clubfoot limbs, and the severity of these abnormalities correlates with both subtle clinical exam abnormalities and treatment response. Interestingly, soft-tissue abnormalities were remarkably conserved within families as demonstrated by the concordant magnetic resonance images (see Fig. 1.9 below).

## Familial Inheritance of Clubfoot

Strong evidence of a genetic predisposition for clubfoot is provided by twin and family studies. Monozygotic concordance for clubfoot is 33% compared to just 3% in dizygotic twins [32]. Approximately, 20% of all cases have a family history of clubfoot. Cardt et al. identified an affected first- or second-degree family history in 11% of all clubfoot cases [33], and we reported 14% incidence of having a first-degree relative with clubfoot [22]. In a study of 50 Maori kindreds all treated at the same hospital in New Zealand, the chance of subsequent children being affected was 4% when the index patient was a female compared to 9% if the index patient was a male and 30% when both a parent and a child were affected [3].

Mendelian forms of isolated clubfoot with multiple generations of affected individuals are rare, which suggests that most cases of clubfoot have complex inheritance or could be sporadic events reflecting environmental or somatic events. Segregation analysis of multiple clubfoot pedigrees supported a single dominant major gene model with low penetrance [34], particularly in Maori and Hawaiian populations [35], though recessive models have also been proposed [36]. Overall, a multifactorial or oligogenic model in which multiple genes are involved, with the added influence of environmental factors, appears likely to explain the majority of clubfoot cases. Multifactorial inheritance with a threshold effect is supported by identification of the Carter effect, in which females, who are less often affected with clubfoot, require a higher genetic load in order to be affected [37]. Studies supporting the Carter effect show that affected females are more likely to have an affected family member than males, which would be predicted to occur if females harbor a greater genetic load [33]. However, the Maori data from Beals do not show the Carter effect [3], suggesting the possibility of a different genetic landscape in this high-risk population.

## Syndromic Versus Isolated Clubfoot

The vast majority of clubfoot cases occur in isolation, meaning that the patient has no other structural abnormalities or malformations or known underlying disorder. However, nearly 25% of all clubfoot cases are associated with known syndromes, such as myelomeningocele and distal arthrogryposis (Table 1.2) [38]. Distal arthrogryposis is a relatively common condition in which clubfoot occurs along with distal hand contractures and can be subdivided into many different types with varying characteristics [39]. Clubfoot is also more common in connective tissue disorders, including Marfan syndrome, Ehlers-Danlos syndrome, and Loeys Dietz syndrome, but it is not an essential feature of these disorders [40] Other disorders in which an increased incidence rate of clubfoot has been reported include brain malformations (i.e., Dandy Walker malformation and perisylvian syndrome), Costello syndrome, and osteogenesis imperfecta. Chromosomal abnormalities, such as Klinefelter's syndrome (47, XXY) and trisomy 18, can be associated with clubfoot, although the latter is most classically associated with vertical talus [41]. While prenatal evaluations may identify some of these diagnoses prior to birth, some syndromes cannot be identified until birth or later in childhood [42].

**Table 1.2** Common syndromic causes of clubfoot

| |
|---|
| • Myelomeningocele |
| • Muscle abnormalities |
|   – Distal arthrogryposis |
|   – Myotonic dystrophy |
| • Larsen syndrome |
| • Arthrogryposis multiplex congenita |
| • Chromosomal abnormalities |
|   – Trisomy 18 |
|   – Trisomy 21 (Down syndrome) |
|   – DiGeorge Syndrome (Chromosome 22q11.2 deletion) |
|   – 47, XXY (Klinefelter syndrome) |
| • Connective tissue disorders |
|   – Ehlers-Danlos Syndrome |
|   – Marfan syndrome |
| • Brain malformations |
|   – Dandy Walker malformation |
|   – Perisylvian syndrome |

# Expansion of Syndromic Phenotypes to Include Isolated Clubfoot

As genetic testing becomes increasingly sophisticated and comprehensive, the identification of patients with known genetic diagnoses is likely to increase, particularly as patients with subtle or nonclassical clinical findings become diagnosed through genetic testing. It is becoming increasingly clear that the phenotypic spectrum resulting from mutations in Mendelian disease genes is broader than initially described. For example, we identified a mutation in MYH3, a gene responsible for distal arthrogryposis in a family with predominantly isolated clubfoot [43]. While some family members had mild hand contractures, which is typical of distal arthrogryposis, other family members had normal hands with no evidence for hand contractures, even upon careful examination. The absence of mutations in MYH3 and other contractile genes implicated in distal arthrogryposis in larger cohorts of clubfoot cases suggests that mutations in the coding regions of these genes are uncommon cause of isolated clubfoot [44]. Evaluation of common variants in the regulatory regions of 15 muscle contractile genes showed several positive associations with clubfoot [45], particularly around tropomyosin-1 (TPM1) and tropomyosin-2 (TPM2), including some variants having functional effects on promoter activity depending on allelic combination [46]. Overall, while genetic variation in the coding sequence of skeletal muscle contractile genes may on rare occasions be identified in individuals with isolated clubfoot, the vast majority of individuals with coding mutations in these genes also have hand, upper limb, or facial contractures or other features that are much more typical and consistent with a diagnosis of distal arthrogryposis.

A second example of expanding the phenotype of a known disease gene to include isolated clubfoot is provided by mutations in filamin B (FLNB). Yang et al., described a mutation in FLNB that segregated with isolated clubfoot in six affected members of an extended Chinese family [47]. Autosomal dominant FLNB mutations are responsible for Larsen syndrome, which is characterized by joint dislocations, cervical vertebral anomalies, spatulate fingers, and clubfoot, as well as atelosteogenesis type 1 and type 3 [48]. Additional investigations are needed to determine whether the lack of additional skeletal anomalies in clubfoot patients with these FLNB mutations is due to genotype–phenotype correlations with the exact mutation specifying the phenotype or whether the phenotypes are modified by the presence of additional protective or risk alleles in the same gene or at other loci. The presence of concordant mild phenotypes segregating throughout the entire family suggests a genotype–phenotype correlation for the FLNB mutation. Expanded phenotypes of Mendelian disorders are likely to become more common as patients with milder isolated birth defects are being sequenced, since the initial publications often describe the most severely affected individuals.

## PITX1

Several years ago, we identified a large family with multiple affected members with isolated clubfoot (Fig. 1.6) [38]. In addition, the proband's phenotype was much more severe, as he had tibial hemimelia and preaxial polydactyly, along with bilateral clubfoot. The family consisted of slightly more affected males than females, as is typical with clubfoot. In addition, there were several incidences of incomplete penetrance, with carrier females having normal feet, despite passing the genetic inheritance of clubfoot to their children. Inheritance was characterized as autosomal dominant with reduced penetrance. Clubfoot was occasionally unilateral, which demonstrates that even genetic cases can be influenced by environmental factors or other stochastic processes capable of modifying the phenotype. Interestingly, right-sided clubfoot was more common in the family with PITX1 mutation and was more often severely involved. Collection and analysis of DNA markers from all family members revealed linkage of clubfoot to a small region on chromosome 5 with a

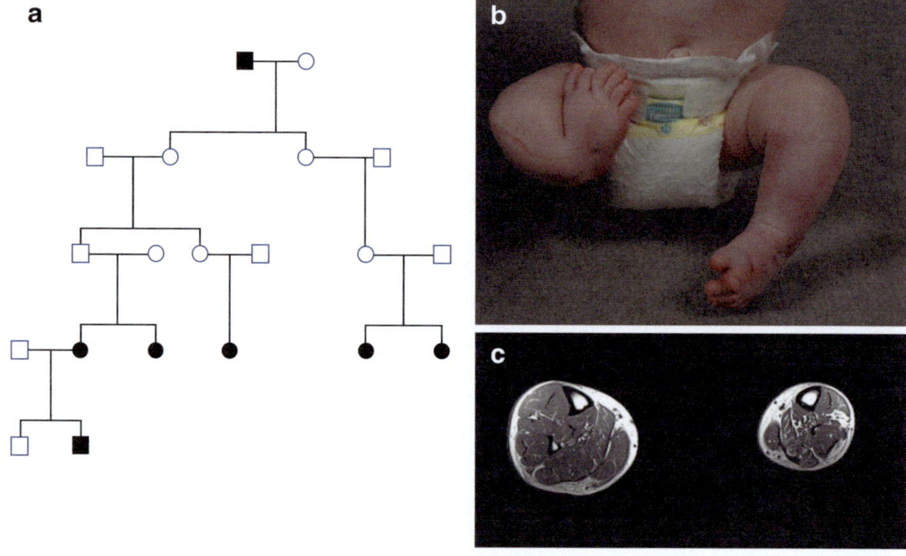

**Fig. 1.6** PITX1 missense mutation segregates in a large family with a spectrum of lower limb malformations, including predominantly isolated clubfoot, but also tibial hemimelia, preaxial polydactyly, hip dysplasia, and pes planus (flatfoot). (**a**) Pedigree showing eight individuals with lower limb malformations spanning five generations. Multiple carriers of the PITX1 mutation are unaffected. (**b**) Proband with PITX1 mutation is most severely affected family member and has bilateral preaxial polydactyly and right-sided tibial hemimelia along with bilateral clubfoot. (**c**) Magnetic resonance image of an affected member of this family with unilateral, left-sided clubfoot (right side of image) shows decreased muscle volume of the affected limb, along with a nearly absent peroneus muscle that has been replaced by fat on the affected left leg

high degree of statistical significance, which was due to the large number of family members showing inheritance of this region. Candidate gene sequencing of the more than 30 genes within the linkage region was undertaken, with the knowledge and recognition that PITX1 (paired-like homeodomain 1), a gene known to be critical for lower limb development, was located within the region. A missense mutation in a single copy of PITX1 was identified in the proband and every affected family member, and had never previously been seen in any healthy populations.

PITX1 is one of only a handful of genes that is expressed preferentially in the lower limb, with little or no expression in the upper limb [49]. High levels of expression of PITX1 are seen during early limb development. Studies in mice demonstrated that complete loss of PITX1 resulted in malformed hindlimbs [50], and PITX1 was also shown to determine the morphology of muscle, tendon, and bones in the hindlimb [51]. In contrast to mice which had loss of the first digit in the absence of PITX1, all but one individual in our family with the PITX1 had normal digit number. The proband in our family had additional digits as a form of preaxial polydactyly, which was nearly the opposite of the mouse oligodactyly phenotype and remains unexplained. Further evidence of a role for PITX1 in clubfoot etiology was shown by our identification of a microdeletion involving PITX1 that segregated with isolated clubfoot in a small family and identification of additional patients with clubfoot having either nonsense mutations in PITX1 or microdeletions involving this gene [41, 43]. Additional features common in patients with PITX1 variants include the presence of short stature, which is not surprising because common genetic variation around PITX1 has been independently associated with human height [52] and hip dysplasia. However, too few patients have been described to accurately predict the risk of additional features or the risk of clubfoot.

Pitx1 haploinsufficiency also results in a clubfoot or clubfoot-like phenotype in mice [43] (Fig. 1.7), although it only occurs in about 10% of mice missing one copy of the gene, which explains why the phenotype was not described in the initial publication describing Pitx1 knockout mice [50]. Interestingly, clubfoot was often unilateral in mice missing a copy of Pitx1, though it was equally likely to involve either the right or the left leg. Loss of both copies of Pitx1 results in early neonatal lethality and severe limb hypoplasia, which is much more severe on the right side [50]. Right-sided predominance of the limb defect in the Pitx1 haploinsufficient mice is likely explained by compensation by the closely related gene, Pitx2, which is asymmetrically expressed as it plays a major role in right–left asymmetry and heart development [53]. Micromagnetic resonance imaging was used to evaluate the morphological abnormalities associated with the clubfoot-like phenotype in the Pitx1 mice. Vascular anomalies, consisting of peroneal artery hypoplasia, were present in the affected clubfoot limb using magnetic resonance angiography [43]. MicroCT also showed reduced tibial and fibular bone volumes. However, there were no obvious patterning defects, as mice had the full complement of bones and polydactyly was not present. However, quantification of muscle and fat volumes revealed

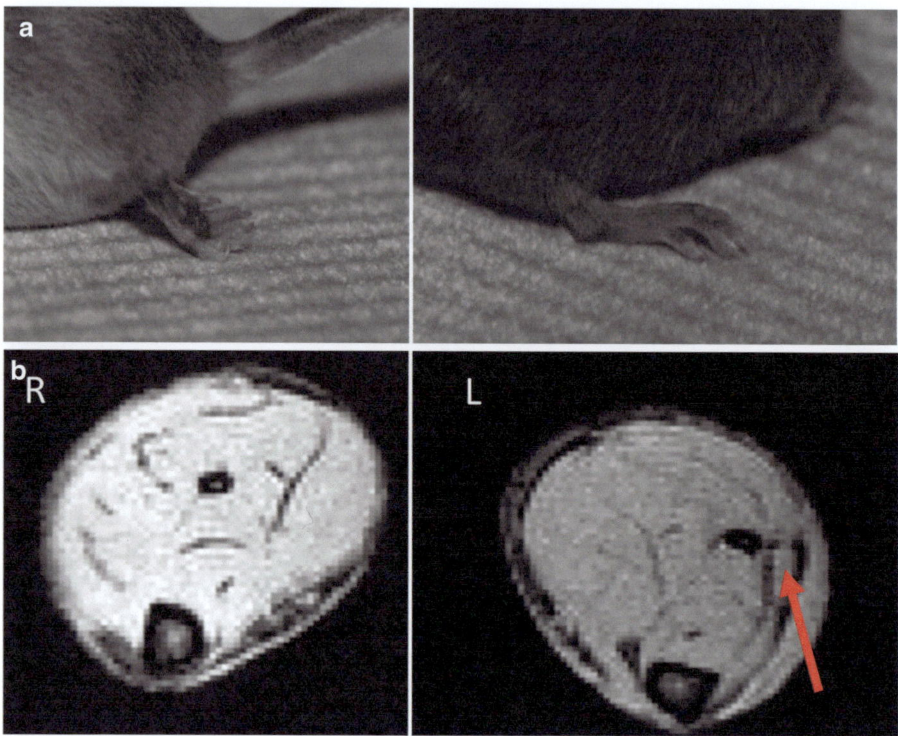

**Fig. 1.7** PITX1 haploinsufficient mice have clubfoot. (**a**) Left hindlimb from a Pitx1−/+ mouse demonstrating a unilateral clubfoot-like malformation (left image) and right hindlimb that is normal (right image). (**b**) Magnetic resonance image of the hindlimb of an affected Pitx1−/+ mouse showing hypoplastic peroneus muscle (arrow) present on affected left hindlimb but not on the unaffected right hindlimb

hypoplasia of the lateral muscle compartment containing the peroneus muscle. Compensatory increase in fat content in the lateral compartment was noted. Interestingly, unlike our human family with PITX1 mutation, mice with clubfoot were slightly more likely to be female. Overall, the morphological abnormalities were more obvious over the lateral aspect of the leg, consistent with what geneticists and developmental biologists describe as a developmental field defect [54]. In mice with Pitx1 haploinsufficiency, the developmental field defect resulted in hypoplastic peroneal artery, peroneus muscles, and small tibial volumes and is consistent with an abnormality occurring very early in development that affected nearly all tissues arising from a small number of precursor cells. Based on data from mouse studies showing that Pitx1 normally promotes cellular proliferation in the lateral limb bud [50], reduction in the number of cells likely resulted in defects in all of the tissues that subsequently arose from these lateral limb bud cells, including muscle, bone, and vasculature.

## Chromosome 17q23.1q23.2 Microdeletions and Microduplications

Further evidence of a role of transcriptional regulators of early limb development in clubfoot pathogenesis was provided by the identification of recurrent chromosome 17q23.1q23.2 microduplications and microdeletions (also called copy number variants) in families with isolated clubfoot (Fig. 1.8) [55]. Chromosome 17q23 copy number variants were identified in a research-based genome-wide chromosomal microarray analysis of 400 clubfoot cases [41, 55]. Overall, approximately 5% of all familial isolated clubfoot families were found to have copy number variants, mostly microduplications, of chromosome 17q23.1q23.2 [55]. Limb phenotypes of patients with chromosome 17q23.1q23.2 microduplications consist predominantly of clubfoot, although some females had hip dysplasia without clubfoot. Incomplete penetrance, particularly in females, is common. In contrast to patients with the chromosome 17q23.1q23.2 microdeletion who tend to have long narrow toes, patients with chromosome 17q23.1q23.2 microduplications

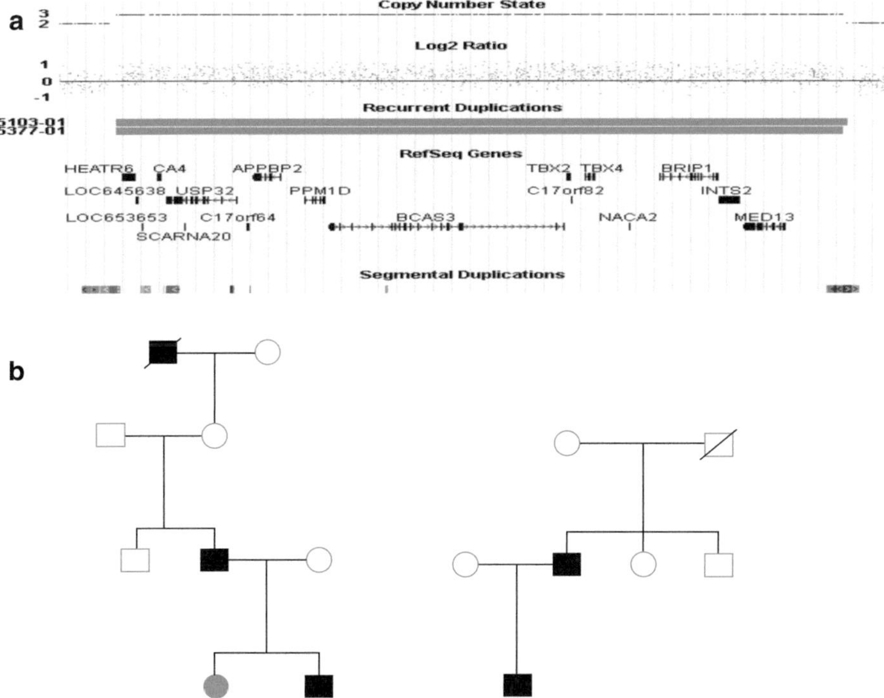

**Fig. 1.8** Recurrent chromosome 17q23.1q23.2 microduplication is associated with familial clubfoot. (**a**) Identical 2.2 Mb microdeletion in patients 5103-01 and 5377-01 who have isolated clubfoot. This microdeletion results in the duplication of 14 genes within the interval. (**b**) Two pedigrees showing segregation of the chromosome 17q23 microdeletion in individuals with clubfoot (black) and hip dysplasia (gray)

have short toes and wide feet. The chromosome 17q23.1q23.2 recurrent copy number variant contains 17 genes and is flanked by segmental repeats that likely mediate nonallelic homologous recombination that results in identically sized 2.2 megabase duplications and deletions. Although multiple genes are located within the chromosome 17q23.1q23.2 interval, including TBX4 (T-box transcription factor 4) and TBX2 (T-box transcription factor 2), TBX4 over- or under-expression is likely responsible for the limb phenotype. Evidence in support of TBX4 as the etiological gene within the interval includes multiple lines of data demonstrating that TBX4 is transcriptional target of PITX1 [56], and like PITX1, TBX4 is one of only a few genes that are preferentially expressed in the hindlimb and not in the forelimb [57], making it an ideal candidate gene for clubfoot. Chromosome 17q23.1q23.2 microdeletion was first described in a series of patients with developmental delay and a variety of limb anomalies and congenital heart defects and early onset pulmonary hypertension [58]. Point mutations and loss-of-function mutations in TBX4 were previously described in small patella syndrome [59]. There has not been any evidence demonstrating a role for noncoding regions near TBX4 in clubfoot pathogenesis [60].

## HOXC Microdeletions and Missense Mutations in Clubfoot

A single patient with a microdeletion involving the HOXC gene cluster was identified in the genome-wide research study of copy number variants of 400 patients with clubfoot in which the chromosome 17 recurrent copy number variants and PITX1 deletion were identified [41] (Fig. 1.9). Additional microdeletions of the HOXC gene cluster were identified in vertical talus families and a proband with fibular hemimelia, and a rare missense mutation in HOXC11 was found to segregate with clubfoot in a single large family [61]. HOXC10 and HOXC11 are developmentally expressed homeobox genes whose expression is altered by PITX1 expression [56] and are also, like PITX1 and TBX4, preferentially expressed in the hindlimb.

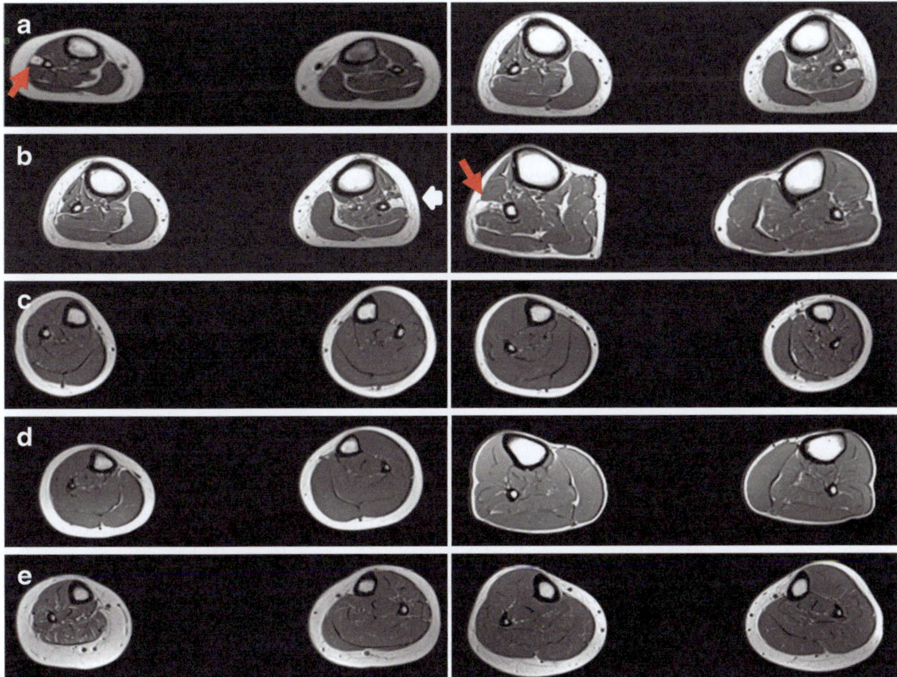

**Fig. 1.9** Soft-tissue abnormalities are strongly concordant between family members with familial clubfoot. (**a**) Two generations both with clubfoot and peroneus muscle replaced with fat (arrows) and increased epimysial fat. (**b**) Child and grandfather with clubfoot secondary to HOXC deletion with peroneus muscle replaced with fat (arrows) and increased epimysial fat. (**c**) Two siblings with unilateral clubfoot (right and left, respectively) and likely pathogenic HOXC missense mutation. (**d**) Child with unilateral clubfoot (right) and father with bilateral clubfoot. (**e**) Child with clubfoot (right) and mother with bilateral clubfoot

## Common Genetic Variants in Clubfoot

Prior to the use of large-scale genome-wide association studies of common variants for clubfoot, candidate studies of common variants were undertaken. Only one genome-wide association study of common variants for clubfoot has been published [62]. This was the result of a multicenter collaboration and consisted of approximately 400 clubfoot cases, all of whom were of European American descent because single ethnicities are required to avoid spurious results in genome-wide association studies. The genome-wide study of common variants in clubfoot pathogenesis did not reveal any genetic variants that reached genome-wide significance, although there were single nucleotide variants that replicated the association in a larger clubfoot cohort. These single nucleotide variants were in noncoding regions near the transcriptional regulators NCOR2 and ZNF664, as well as near FOXN3, SORCS1, and MMP7/TMEM123. None of these genes had previously been implicated in clubfoot etiology. Further studies are needed, particularly using much larger sample sizes, in order to confirm these associations and to identify additional common variants that may influence clubfoot susceptibility.

Association studies of clubfoot with selected candidate common variants have also been performed, though most are also with relatively small sample sizes. Studies of the regulatory regions of 15 muscle contractile genes showed several positive associations with clubfoot, particularly around tropomyosin-1 (TPM1) and tropomyosin-2 (TPM2) [45], including some variants that had functional effects on promoter activity depending on allelic combination.

## PITX1-TBX4-HOXC Mutations and Treatment Resistance

When PITX1 mutations were first identified in a large family with clubfoot, it was noted that the affected individuals often had stiff clubfeet that were difficult to treat [38]. Subsequently, treatment resistance, with high rates of recurrence after noninvasive treatment with the Ponseti method, was also noted in clubfoot patients with chromosome 17q23.1q23.2 microduplications [55] and both clubfoot and vertical talus patients with HOXC microdeletions (described below in vertical talus). Structural abnormalities, including tibial or fibular hemimelia, or hip dysplasia, were also found in a minority of affected family members with PITX1-TBX4-HOXC mutations, suggesting that the genetic abnormalities had effects on limb patterning that resulted in feet that were more difficult to treat.

As morphological abnormalities and patterning defects were noted in the limbs of mice with mutations in transcriptional regulators of early limb development (p. 180) [43, 51], we sought to obtain magnetic resonance images (MRI) of patients with these abnormalities to more clearly define the morphological abnormalities underlying the clubfoot or vertical talus phenotype. Morphological abnormalities in the feet of a patient with PITX1 mutations show abnormal muscle, bone, and vasculature that is more prominent over the lateral aspect of the leg, including the peroneus muscles that are similar to those that we described in mice that are missing a copy of Pitx1 [43]. These abnormalities correlate with exam findings that include weak foot everter function and are likely to contribute to the difficulty in attaining clubfoot correction after treatment with the Ponseti method.

Morphological abnormalities are often quite consistent within families, even though clinical phenotypes may vary slightly (Fig. 1.9). MRI scans were performed on two affected members of five families. MRI obtained from an affected grandfather and grandson showed both had increased intramysial fat and lateral muscle hypoplasia that was more marked over the lateral aspect of the leg, with increased fat near the peroneus muscle. Similar results were seen with two members of a family with suspected genetic clubfoot, although the genetic etiology has not been elucidated. Paired MRI samples from two affected individuals from three families showed no obvious morphological abnormalities, although the leg was often smaller on the affected limb in unilateral cases. These data show remarkable intrafamilial consistency in the morphological features of the lower leg in familial clubfoot.

## Vertical Talus

Vertical talus is nearly 20 times less common than clubfoot, and therefore, fewer studies have investigated its demographics and frequency. Merrill et al. published a series of >60 patients, in which two-thirds were male, which reflects a similar gender imbalance as clubfoot [28]. The cause of this gender imbalance is unknown. Vertical talus was bilateral in two-thirds of cases and was unilateral left-sided in 20% of cases and unilateral right-sided in 10% of cases.

Unlike clubfoot which occurs in isolation without other birth defects or known etiology in the vast majority of cases, vertical talus occurs in isolation only about 35–50% of the time [28]. The most common etiologies are cerebral palsy, myelomeningocele, caudal regression syndrome, distal arthrogryposis, and multiple pterygium syndrome. Polydactyly, syndactyly, or missing phalanges occur in rare cases. Chromosomal abnormalities, including trisomy 13, trisomy 18, and trisomy 21, are relatively common. In fact, in the pediatric literature, vertical talus is often referred to as "rocker-bottom" foot and is a classic sign of trisomy 18.

Environmental factors associated with vertical talus have been poorly studied due to the lower frequency of this birth defect and lack of sufficient number of patients for adequate study.

Evidence for shared etiology and pathogenesis of clubfoot and vertical talus is provided by the description of multiple patients who have been identified who have clubfoot on one limb and vertical talus on the other [28]. In addition, we identified several families who have affected members with either clubfoot or vertical talus. Clubfoot and vertical talus share in common a high rate of vascular abnormalities, which may point to a common etiology and support the recent implication of genes encoding closely related transcriptional regulators of early limb development in both disorders. Finally, the response of clubfeet and feet with vertical talus to similar, but opposite, conservative noninvasive manipulations and interventions suggests a conserved underlying biology.

Only a few studies have been undertaken to evaluate anatomic abnormalities in vertical talus. Similar to clubfoot, vascular anomalies are more common in vertical talus, but they are not necessary for its pathogenesis. Vascular abnormalities have been documented in vertical talus, just as they are in clubfoot, and may increase the risk of surgical complications [24]. Too few studies have been performed to determine the exact incidence. While absent posterior tibial artery has been described in vertical talus [26], congenital vertical talus secondary to a CDMP-1 mutation was not associated with any vascular anomalies, suggesting the that distinct etiologies directly influence the resulting anatomy [27]. Muscle biopsies from vertical talus cases frequently show nonspecific nondiagnostic abnormalities that are often seen in arthrogryposis or congenital myopathy [28].

## Implication of Transcriptional Regulators of Early Limb Development in Vertical Talus

Traditional positional cloning led to the identification of HOXD10 as a gene responsible for vertical talus in a large family of Italian descent in which vertical talus segregated along with a cavovarus foot deformity that resembled Charcot-Marie-Tooth disease segregated [63]. Candidate gene sequencing of the large region on chromosome 2q31 led to identification of a single missense mutation M319K in the HOXD10 gene. HOXD10 is a homeobox gene that is part of the hox developmental program that leads to highly coordinated expression and limb development. Other hox genes implicated in human disease include hand-foot-uterus syndrome (HOXA13) [64] and synpolydactyly and brachydactyly (HOXD13). A second identical HOXD10 M319K mutation was identified in a British family with isolated congenital vertical talus, although this family did not have any evidence for Charcot-Marie-Tooth disease [22]. Sequencing of HOXD10 in multiple additional vertical talus families did not identify additional mutations, suggesting that this was an uncommon cause of congenital vertical talus. HOXD10 was also sequenced in a clubfoot cohort without identification of any genetic mutations [22].

Screening a large number of clubfoot and vertical talus cases for copy number variants revealed a small deletion of the 5′ genes of the HOXC gene cluster, including HOXC13 [41]. Additional testing for small copy number variants using a novel BAC-based capture method revealed three additional overlapping microdeletions around the 5′ HOXC gene cluster [61]. These microdeletions were fully penetrant and segregated with clubfoot in two families and vertical talus in two families. They ranged in size from 13 to 175 kb, which is often smaller than those detected or reported by some clinical microarray diagnostic testing laboratories. While most individuals had isolated clubfoot or vertical talus, variable expressivity included mild 2–3 toe syndactyly and hammertoes in 2 individuals who carried the microdeletion but did not have clubfoot. In several cases, the toes were overlapping. Structural abnormalities, including fibular hemimelia, were seen in one patient. Fingernail hypoplasia, previously noted in patients with isolated HOXC13 mutations or deletions, was noted in one male patient. The occurrence of either vertical talus or clubfoot in each family is likely related to differences in size of the microdeletion and the involvement of different genes, including HOXC13, HOXC12, and the HOTAIR long noncoding RNA. In addition, the regulatory region surrounding HOX gene clusters and the distances between regulatory regions and coding regions have previously been shown to be important for normal embryonic development, such that even noncoding deletions that do not involve any gene coding sequence are likely to be important. In addition, copy number analysis of a large number of healthy controls revealed few deletions of the 5′ HOXC genes, suggesting its overall importance for normal human development. Similar to patients with PITX1 genetic abnormalities, individuals with HOXC deletions had lateral muscle hypoplasia and treatment-resistant vertical talus (Fig. 1.10).

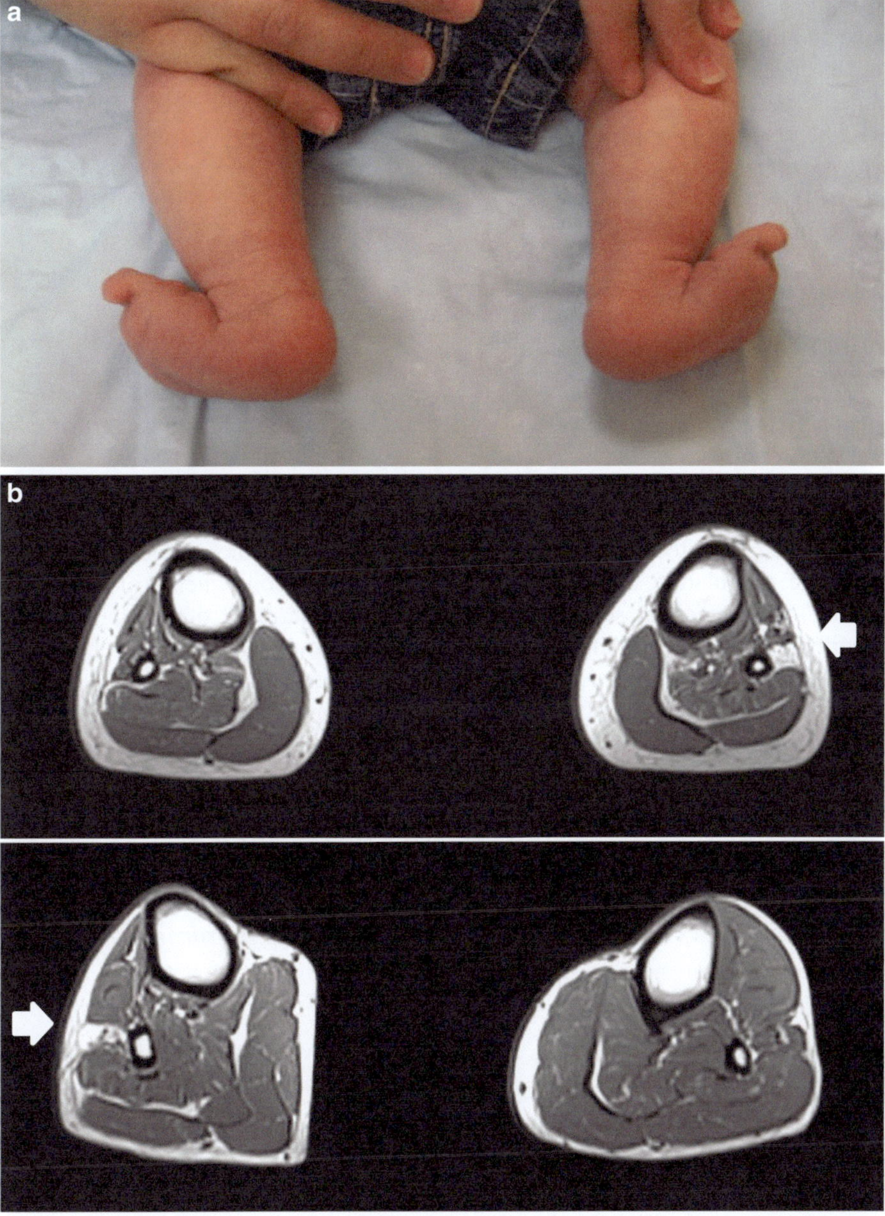

**Fig. 1.10** Vertical talus associated with HOXC deletion. (**a**) Infant with bilateral vertical talus and HOXC deletion. (**b**) Magnetic resonance images of two relatives with the same HOXC deletion and bilateral treatment resistant clubfoot. Lateral muscle compartment is replaced by fat, which is more prominent on the left leg of the child and the right leg of his grandfather (white arrows)

Other genes implicated in congenital vertical talus are found in patients who also have additional skeletal or non-orthopedic congenital anomalies. Deletions including the teashirt zinc finger homeobox 1 gene (TSHZ1) have been identified in patients with congenital vertical talus, though they appear to only occur in individuals who also have congenital aural atresia. Vertical talus has also been described with GDF5 mutations (also called cartilage-derived morphogenetic protein-1 or CDMP-1), though most also have mild hand anomalies, including brachydactyly type C or clinodactyly [20].

## Conclusions

The pathogenesis and etiology of clubfoot and vertical remains a mystery for most cases, despite decades of study using a variety of innovative approaches. Recent advances in genetics have improved recognition of the PITX1-TBX4-HOX pathway in rare cases of clubfoot and vertical talus (Fig. 1.11). Studies of these rare cases revealed insight as to how developmental field defects, in which defects of the muscle, nerve, vasculature, and bone, can all be present as a consequence of abnormalities in these genes in some clubfoot patients. Regardless of whether genetic abnormalities are identified in a patient, the presence of clinical exam abnormalities, including drop toe sign and weak abductor function signals the likelihood of a problematic foot that may be difficult to treat. Many of these treatment-resistant

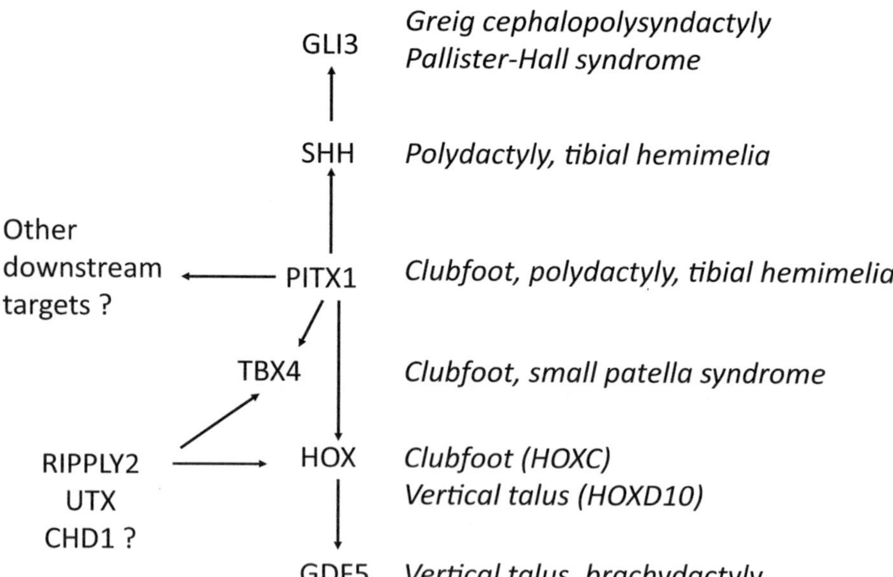


**Fig. 1.11** Genetic pathways leading to clubfoot and vertical talus

patients have corresponding morphological abnormalities, such as hypoplasia of specific muscle groups that likely explain the treatment difficulties. Additional investigations to explain the etiology and pathogenesis are needed to advance precision medicine for children with clubfoot and vertical talus.

# References


1. Smythe T, Kuper H, Macleod D, Foster A, Lavy C. Birth prevalence of congenital talipes equinovarus in low- and middle-income countries: a systematic review and meta-analysis. Trop Med Int Health. 2017;22(3):269–85. https://doi.org/10.1111/tmi.12833. Epub 2017 Jan 22. PMID: 28000394.
2. Carey M, Bower C, Mylvaganam A, Rouse I. Talipes equinovarus in Western Australia. Paediatr Perinat Epidemiol. 2003;17(2):187–94. https://doi.org/10.1046/j.1365-3016.2003.00477.x. PMID: 12675786.
3. Beals RK. Club foot in the Maori: a genetic study of 50 kindreds. N Z Med J. 1978;88(618):144–6. PMID: 280791.
4. Reefhuis J, Honein MA. Maternal age and non-chromosomal birth defects, Atlanta--1968-2000: teenager or thirty-something, who is at risk? Birth Defects Res A Clin Mol Teratol 2004 ;70(9):572–9. https://doi.org/10.1002/bdra.20065. PMID: 15368555..
5. Palma M, Cook T, Segura J, Pecho A, Morcuende JA. Descriptive epidemiology of clubfoot in Peru: a clinic-based study. Iowa Orthop J. 2013;33:167–71. PMID: 24027478; PMCID: PMC3748874.
6. Prakalapakorn SG, Rasmussen SA, Lambert SR, Honein MA, National Birth Defects Prevention Study. Assessment of risk factors for infantile cataracts using a case-control study: National Birth Defects Prevention Study, 2000-2004. Ophthalmology. 2010;117(8):1500–5. https://doi.org/10.1016/j.ophtha.2009.12.026. Epub 2010 Apr 3. PMID: 20363508; PMCID: PMC2994269.
7. Yazdy MM, Mitchell AA, Louik C, Werler MM. Use of selective serotonin-reuptake inhibitors during pregnancy and the risk of clubfoot. Epidemiology. 2014;25(6):859–65. https://doi.org/10.1097/EDE.0000000000000157. PMID: 25171134; PMCID: PMC4180776.
8. Slaney SF, Goodman FR, Eilers-Walsman BL, Hall BD, Williams DK, Young ID, Hayward RD, Jones BM, Christianson AL, Winter RM. Acromelic frontonasal dysostosis. Am J Med Genet. 1999;83(2):109–16. PMID: 10190481.
9. Nguyen MC, Nhi HM, Nam VQ, Thanh do V, Romitti P, Morcuende JA. Descriptive epidemiology of clubfoot in Vietnam: a clinic-based study. Iowa Orthop J. 2012;32:120–4. PMID: 23576932; PMCID: PMC3565392.
10. Lochmiller C, Johnston D, Scott A, Risman M, Hecht JT. Genetic epidemiology study of idiopathic talipes equinovarus. Am J Med Genet. 1998;79(2):90–6. PMID: 9741465.
11. Werler MM, Yazdy MM, Mitchell AA, Meyer RE, Druschel CM, Anderka M, Kasser JR, Mahan ST. Descriptive epidemiology of idiopathic clubfoot. Am J Med Genet A. 2013;161A(7):1569–78. https://doi.org/10.1002/ajmg.a.35955. Epub 2013 May 17. PMID: 23686911; PMCID: PMC3689855.
12. Ippolito E, Ponseti IV. Congenital club foot in the human fetus. A histological study. J Bone Joint Surg Am. 1980;62(1):8–22. PMID: 7351421
13. Hersh A. The role of surgery in the treatment of club feet. 1967. Foot Ankle Int. 1995;16(11):672–81. https://doi.org/10.1177/107110079501601103. PMID: 8589806.
14. Sano H, Uhthoff HK, Jarvis JG, Mansingh A, Wenckebach GF. Pathogenesis of soft-tissue contracture in club foot. J Bone Joint Surg Br. 1998;80(4):641–4. https://doi.org/10.1302/0301-620x.80b4.8526. PMID: 9699828.

15. Suzuki M, Miyazaki Y, Miyake T, Kido H, Yamaguchi K, Kagawa H, Yanabu M, Nomura S, Fukuhara S. Uptake of fibrinogen by circulating platelets. Vox Sang. 1994;67(2):243. https://doi.org/10.1111/j.1423-0410.1994.tb01673.x. PMID: 7801625.

16. Ošt'ádal M, Eckhardt A, Herget J, Mikšík I, Dungl P, Chomiak J, Frydrychová M, Burian M. Proteomic analysis of the extracellular matrix in idiopathic pes equinovarus. Mol Cell Biochem. 2015;401(1–2):133–9. https://doi.org/10.1007/s11010-014-2300-3. Epub 2014 Dec 4. PMID: 25472880.

17. Herceg MB, Weiner DS, Agamanolis DP, Hawk D. Histologic and histochemical analysis of muscle specimens in idiopathic talipes equinovarus. J Pediatr Orthop. 2006;26(1):91–3. https://doi.org/10.1097/01.bpo.0000188994.90931.e8. PMID: 16439910.

18. Isaacs H, Handelsman JE, Badenhorst M, Pickering A. The muscles in club foot--a histological histochemical and electron microscopic study. J Bone Joint Surg Br. 1977;59-B:465–72.

19. Shaheen S, Mursal H, Rabih M, Johari A. Flexor digitorum accessorius longus muscle in resistant clubfoot patients: introduction of a new sign predicting its presence. J Pediatr Orthop B. 2015;24(2):143–6. https://doi.org/10.1097/BPB.0000000000000129. PMID: 25493703.

20. Dobbs MB, Walton T, Gordon JE, Schoenecker PL, Gurnett CA. Flexor digitorum accessorius longus muscle is associated with familial idiopathic clubfoot. J Pediatr Orthop. 2005;25(3):357–9. https://doi.org/10.1097/01.bpo.0000152908.08422.95. PMID: 15832155.

21. Edmonds EW, Frick SL. The drop toe sign: an indicator of neurologic impairment in congenital clubfoot. Clin Orthop Relat Res. 2009;467(5):1238–42. https://doi.org/10.1007/s11999-008-0690-9. Epub 2009 Jan 7. PMID: 19130157; PMCID: PMC2664423.

22. Dobbs MB, Gurnett CA. The 2017 ABJS Nicolas Andry Award: advancing personalized medicine for clubfoot through translational research. Clin Orthop Relat Res. 2017;475(6):1716–25. https://doi.org/10.1007/s11999-017-5290-0. Epub 2017 Feb 24. PMID: 28236079; PMCID: PMC5406347.

23. Matar HE, Garg NK. Congenital talipes equinovarus associated with hereditary congenital common peroneal nerve neuropathy: a literature review. J Pediatr Orthop B. 2016;25(2):108–11. https://doi.org/10.1097/BPB.0000000000000250. PMID: 26588839.

24. Hootnick DR, Levinsohn EM, Crider RJ, Packard DS Jr. Congenital arterial malformations associated with clubfoot: a report of two cases. Clin Orthop Relat Res. 1982;167:160–3.

25. Munajat I, Yoysefi M, Nik Mahdi NM. Deficient dorsalis pedis flow in severe idiopathic clubfeet: does Ponseti casting affect the outcome? Foot (Edinb). 2017;32:30–4. https://doi.org/10.1016/j.foot.2017.05.003. Epub 2017 Jun 8. PMID: 28672132.

26. Dobbs MB, Gordon JE, Schoenecker PL. Absent posterior tibial artery associated with idiopathic clubfoot. A report of two cases. J Bone Joint Surg Am. 2004;86(3):599–602. https://doi.org/10.2106/00004623-200403000-00022. PMID: 14996890.

27. Kruse L, Gurnett CA, Hootnick D, Dobbs MB. Magnetic resonance angiography in clubfoot and vertical talus: a feasibility study. Clin Orthop Relat Res. 2009;467:1250–5. https://doi.org/10.1007/s11999-008-0673-x2664419.

28. Merrill LJ, Gurnett CA, Siegel M, Sonavane S, Dobbs MB. Vascular abnormalities correlate with decreased soft tissue volumes in idiopathic clubfoot. Clin Orthop Relat Res. 2011;469:1442–9. https://doi.org/10.1007/s11999-010-1657-1.

29. Porter RW. Congenital talipes equinovarus: I. Resolving and resistant deformities. J Bone Joint Surg Br. 1987;69(5):822–5. https://doi.org/10.1302/0301-620X.69B5.3680351. PMID: 3680351.

30. Ippolito E, Maio F, Mancini F, Bellini D, Orefice A. Leg muscle atrophy in idiopathic congenital clubfoot: is it primitive or acquired? J Child Orthop. 2009;3:171–8. https://doi.org/10.1007/s11832-009-0179-42686819.

31. Moon DK, Gurnett CA, Aferol H, Siegel MJ, Commean PK, Dobbs MB. Soft-tissue abnormalities associated with treatment-resistant and treatment-responsive clubfoot: findings of MRI analysis. J Bone Joint Surg Am. 2014;96:1249–56. https://doi.org/10.2106/JBJS.M.012574116564.

32. Wynne-Davies R. Genetic and environmental factors in the etiology of talipes equinovarus. Clin Orthop Relat Res. 1972;84:9–13. https://doi.org/10.1097/00003086-197205000-00003.
33. Cardy AH, Sharp L, Torrance N, Hennekam RC, Miedzybrodzka Z. Is there evidence for aetiologically distinct subgroups of idiopathic congenital talipes equinovarus? A case-only study and pedigree analysis. PLoS One. 2011;6(4):e17895. https://doi.org/10.1371/journal.pone.0017895. PMID: 21533128; PMCID: PMC3080359.
34. Wang JH, Palmer RM, Chung CS. The role of major gene in clubfoot. Am J Hum Genet. 1988;42(5):772–6. PMID: 3358425; PMCID: PMC1715171.
35. Yang HY, Chung CS, Nemechek RW. A genetic analysis of clubfoot in Hawaii. Genet Epidemiol. 1987;4(4):299–306. https://doi.org/10.1002/gepi.1370040408. PMID: 3666436.
36. Rebbeck TR, Dietz FR, Murray JC, Buetow KH. A single-gene explanation for the probability of having idiopathic talipes equinovarus. Am J Hum Genet. 1993;53(5):1051–63. PMID: 8213831; PMCID: PMC1682321.
37. Kruse LM, Dobbs MB, Gurnett CA. Polygenic threshold model with sex dimorphism in clubfoot inheritance: the Carter effect. J Bone Joint Surg Am. 2008;90(12):2688–94. https://doi.org/10.2106/JBJS.G.01346. PMID: 19047715; PMCID: PMC2663333.
38. Gurnett CA, Alaee F, Kruse LM, Desruisseau DM, Hecht JT, Wise CA, Bowcock AM, Dobbs MB. Asymmetric lower-limb malformations in individuals with homeobox PITX1 gene mutation. Am J Hum Genet. 2008;83:616–22. https://doi.org/10.1016/j.ajhg.2008.10.0042668044.
39. Bamshad M, Van Heest AE, Pleasure D. Arthrogryposis: a review and update. J Bone Joint Surg Am. 2009;91(Suppl 4):40–6. https://doi.org/10.2106/JBJS.I.00281. PMID: 19571066; PMCID: PMC2698792.
40. Janecke AR, Li B, Boehm M, Krabichler B, Rohrbach M, Müller T, Fuchs I, Golas G, Katagiri Y, Ziegler SG, Gahl WA, Wilnai Y, Zoppi N, Geller HM, Giunta C, Slavotinek A, Steinmann B. The phenotype of the musculocontractural type of Ehlers-Danlos syndrome due to CHST14 mutations. Am J Med Genet A. 2016;170A(1):103–15. https://doi.org/10.1002/ajmg.a.37383. Epub 2015 Sep 16. PMID: 26373698; PMCID: PMC5115638.
41. Alvarado DM, Buchan JG, Frick SL, Herzenberg JE, Dobbs MB, Gurnett CA. Copy number analysis of 413 isolated talipes equinovarus patients suggests role for transcriptional regulators of early limb development. Eur J Hum Genet. 2013;21:373–80. https://doi.org/10.1038/ejhg.2012.177.
42. Paton RW, Fox AE, Foster A, Fehily M. Incidence and aetiology of talipes equino-varus with recent population changes. Acta Orthop Belg. 2010;76(1):86–9. PMID: 20306970.
43. Alvarado DM, McCall K, Aferol H, Silva MJ, Garbow JR, Spees WM, Patel T, Siegel M, Dobbs MB, Gurnett CA. Pitx1 haploinsufficiency causes clubfoot in humans and a clubfoot-like phenotype in mice. Hum Mol Genet. 2011;20:3943–52. https://doi.org/10.1093/hmg/ddr3133177645.
44. Dobbs MB, Gurnett CA. Update on clubfoot: etiology and treatment. Clin Orthop Relat Res. 2009;467(5):1146–53. https://doi.org/10.1007/s11999-009-0734-9. Epub 2009 Feb 18. PMID: 19224303; PMCID: PMC2664438.
45. Weymouth KS, Blanton SH, Bamshad MJ, Beck AE, Alvarez C, Richards S, Gurnett CA, Dobbs MB, Barnes D, Mitchell LE, Hecht JT. Variants in genes that encode muscle contractile proteins influence risk for isolated clubfoot. Am J Med Genet A. 2011;155A(9):2170–9. https://doi.org/10.1002/ajmg.a.34167. Epub 2011 Aug 10. PMID: 21834041; PMCID: PMC3158831.
46. Weymouth KS, Blanton SH, Powell T, Patel CV, Savill SA, Hecht JT. Functional assessment of clubfoot associated HOXA9, TPM1, and TPM2 variants suggests a potential gene regulation mechanism. Clin Orthop Relat Res. 2016;474(7):1726–35. https://doi.org/10.1007/s11999-016-4788-1. Epub 2016 Mar 28. PMID: 27020427; PMCID. PMC4887369.
47. Liu YB, Zhao L, Ding J, Zhu J, Xie CL, Wu ZK, Yang X, Li H. Association between maternal age at conception and risk of idiopathic clubfoot. Acta Orthop. 2016;87(3):291–5. https://doi.org/10.3109/17453674.2016.1153359. Epub 2016 Feb 22. PMID: 26901038; PMCID: PMC4900088.

48. Lu J, Lian G, Lenkinski R, De Grand A, Vaid RR, Bryce T, Stasenko M, Boskey A, Walsh C, Sheen V. Filamin B mutations cause chondrocyte defects in skeletal development. Hum Mol Genet. 2007;16(14):1661–75. https://doi.org/10.1093/hmg/ddm114. Epub 2007 May 17. PMID: 17510210.

49. Lanctot C, Lamolet B, Drouin J. The bicoid-related homeoprotein Ptx1 defines the most anterior domain of the embryo and differentiates posterior from anterior lateral mesoderm. Development. 1997;124:2807–17.

50. Szeto DP, Ryan AK, O'Connell SM, Rosenfeld MG. P-OTX: a PIT-1-interacting homeodomain factor expressed during anterior pituitary gland development. Proc Natl Acad Sci U S A. 1996;93:7706–10. https://doi.org/10.1073/pnas.93.15.770638811.

51. DeLaurier A, Schweitzer R, Logan M. Pitx1 determines the morphology of muscle, tendon, and bones of the hindlimb. Dev Biol. 2006;299(1):22–34. https://doi.org/10.1016/j.ydbio.2006.06.055. Epub 2006 Jul 14. PMID: 16989801.

52. Lango Allen H, Estrada K, Lettre G, Berndt SI, Weedon MN, Rivadeneira F, Willer CJ, Jackson AU, Vedantam S, Raychaudhuri S, Ferreira T, Wood AR, Weyant RJ, Segrè AV, Speliotes EK, Wheeler E, Soranzo N, Park JH, Yang J, Gudbjartsson D, Heard-Costa NL, Randall JC, Qi L, Vernon Smith A, Mägi R, Pastinen T, Liang L, Heid IM, Luan J, Thorleifsson G, Winkler TW, Goddard ME, Sin Lo K, Palmer C, Workalemahu T, Aulchenko YS, Johansson A, Zillikens MC, Feitosa MF, Esko T, Johnson T, Ketkar S, Kraft P, Mangino M, Prokopenko I, Absher D, Albrecht E, Ernst F, Glazer NL, Hayward C, Hottenga JJ, Jacobs KB, Knowles JW, Kutalik Z, Monda KL, Polasek O, Preuss M, Rayner NW, Robertson NR, Steinthorsdottir V, Tyrer JP, Voight BF, Wiklund F, Xu J, Zhao JH, Nyholt DR, Pellikka N, Perola M, Perry JR, Surakka I, Tammesoo ML, Altmaier EL, Amin N, Aspelund T, Bhangale T, Boucher G, Chasman DI, Chen C, Coin L, Cooper MN, Dixon AL, Gibson Q, Grundberg E, Hao K, Juhani Junttila M, Kaplan LM, Kettunen J, König IR, Kwan T, Lawrence RW, Levinson DF, Lorentzon M, McKnight B, Morris AP, Müller M, Suh Ngwa J, Purcell S, Rafelt S, Salem RM, Salvi E, Sanna S, Shi J, Sovio U, Thompson JR, Turchin MC, Vandenput L, Verlaan DJ, Vitart V, White CC, Ziegler A, Almgren P, Balmforth AJ, Campbell H, Citterio L, De Grandi A, Dominiczak A, Duan J, Elliott P, Elosua R, Eriksson JG, Freimer NB, Geus EJ, Glorioso N, Haiqing S, Hartikainen AL, Havulinna AS, Hicks AA, Hui J, Igl W, Illig T, Jula A, Kajantie E, Kilpeläinen TO, Koiranen M, Kolcic I, Koskinen S, Kovacs P, Laitinen J, Liu J, Lokki ML, Marusic A, Maschio A, Meitinger T, Mulas A, Paré G, Parker AN, Peden JF, Petersmann A, Pichler I, Pietiläinen KH, Pouta A, Ridderstråle M, Rotter JI, Sambrook JG, Sanders AR, Schmidt CO, Sinisalo J, Smit JH, Stringham HM, Bragi Walters G, Widen E, Wild SH, Willemsen G, Zagato L, Zgaga L, Zitting P, Alavere H, Farrall M, McArdle WL, Nelis M, Peters MJ, Ripatti S, van Meurs JB, Aben KK, Ardlie KG, Beckmann JS, Beilby JP, Bergman RN, Bergmann S, Collins FS, Cusi D, den Heijer M, Eiriksdottir G, Gejman PV, Hall AS, Hamsten A, Huikuri HV, Iribarren C, Kähönen M, Kaprio J, Kathiresan S, Kiemeney L, Kocher T, Launer LJ, Lehtimäki T, Melander O, Mosley TH Jr, Musk AW, Nieminen MS, O'Donnell CJ, Ohlsson C, Oostra B, Palmer LJ, Raitakari O, Ridker PM, Rioux JD, Rissanen A, Rivolta C, Schunkert H, Shuldiner AR, Siscovick DS, Stumvoll M, Tönjes A, Tuomilehto J, van Ommen GJ, Viikari J, Heath AC, Martin NG, Montgomery GW, Province MA, Kayser M, Arnold AM, Atwood LD, Boerwinkle E, Chanock SJ, Deloukas P, Gieger C, Grönberg H, Hall P, Hattersley AT, Hengstenberg C, Hoffman W, Lathrop GM, Salomaa V, Schreiber S, Uda M, Waterworth D, Wright AF, Assimes TL, Barroso I, Hofman A, Mohlke KL, Boomsma DI, Caulfield MJ, Cupples LA, Erdmann J, Fox CS, Gudnason V, Gyllensten U, Harris TB, Hayes RB, Jarvelin MR, Mooser V, Munroe PB, Ouwehand WH, Penninx BW, Pramstaller PP, Quertermous T, Rudan I, Samani NJ, Spector TD, Völzke H, Watkins H, Wilson JF, Groop LC, Haritunians T, Hu FB, Kaplan RC, Metspalu A, North KE, Schlessinger D, Wareham NJ, Hunter DJ, O'Connell JR, Strachan DP, Wichmann HE, Borecki IB, van Duijn CM, Schadt EE, Thorsteinsdottir U, Peltonen L, Uitterlinden AG, Visscher PM, Chatterjee N, Loos RJ, Boehnke M, McCarthy MI, Ingelsson E, Lindgren CM, Abecasis GR, Stefansson K, Frayling TM, Hirschhorn JN. Hundreds of variants clustered in genomic loci and biological pathways

affect human height. Nature. 2010;467(7317):832–8. https://doi.org/10.1038/nature09410. Epub 2010 Sep 29. PMID: 20881960; PMCID: PMC2955183.

53. Marcil A, Dumontier E, Chamberland M, Camper SA, Drouin J. Pitx1 and Pitx2 are required for development of hindlimb buds. Development. 2003;130(1):45–55. https://doi.org/10.1242/dev.00192. PMID: 12441290.

54. Castori M, Rinaldi R, Cappellacci S, Grammatico P. Tibial developmental field defect is the most common lower limb malformation pattern in VACTERL association. Am J Med Genet A. 2008;146A(10):1259–66. https://doi.org/10.1002/ajmg.a.32288. PMID: 18386801.

55. Alvarado DM, Aferol H, McCall K, Huang JB, Techy M, Buchan J, Cady J, Gonzales PR, Dobbs MB, Gurnett CA. Familial isolated clubfoot is associated with recurrent chromosome 17q23.1q23.2 microduplications containing TBX4. Am J Hum Genet. 2010;87:154–60. https://doi.org/10.1016/j.ajhg.2010.06.0102896772.

56. Logan M, Tabin CJ. Role of Pitx1 upstream of Tbx4 in specification of hindlimb identity. Science. 1999;283:1736–9. https://doi.org/10.1126/science.283.5408.1736.

57. Margulies EH, Kardia SL, Innis JW. A comparative molecular analysis of developing mouse forelimbs and hindlimbs using serial analysis of gene expression (SAGE). Genome Res. 2001;11:1686–98. https://doi.org/10.1101/gr.192601311149.

58. Kerstjens-Frederikse WS, Bongers EM, Roofthooft MT, Leter EM, Douwes JM, Van Dijk A, Vonk-Noordegraaf A, Dijk-Bos KK, Hoefsloot LH, Hoendermis ES, Gille JJ, Sikkema-Raddatz B, Hofstra RM, Berger RM. TBX4 mutations (small patella syndrome) are associated with childhood-onset pulmonary arterial hypertension. J Med Genet. 2013;50(8):500–6. https://doi.org/10.1136/jmcdgcnet-2012-101152. Epub 2013 Apr 16. PMID: 23592887; PMCID: PMC3717587.

59. Bongers EM, Duijf PH, Beersum SE, Schoots J, Kampen A, Burckhardt A, Hamel BC, Losan F, Hoefsloot LH, Yntema HG, Knoers NV, Bokhoven H. Mutations in the human TBX4 gene cause small patella syndrome. Am J Hum Genet. 2004;74:1239–48. https://doi.org/10.1086/4213311182087.

60. Lu W, Bacino CA, Richards BS, Alvarez C, VanderMeer JE, Vella M, Ahituv N, Sikka N, Dietz FR, Blanton SH, Hecht JT. Studies of TBX4 and chromosome 17q23.1q23.2: an uncommon cause of nonsyndromic clubfoot. Am J Med Genet A. 2012;158A:1620–7. https://doi.org/10.1002/ajmg.a.354183381434.

61. Alvarado DM, McCall K, Hecht JT, Dobbs MB, Gurnett CA. Deletions of 5′ HOXC genes are associated with lower extremity malformations, including clubfoot and vertical talus. J Med Genet. 2016;53(4):250–5. https://doi.org/10.1136/jmedgenet-2015-103505. Epub 2016 Jan 4. PMID: 26729820; PMCID: PMC4955942.

62. Zhang TX, Haller G, Lin P, Alvarado DM, Hecht JT, Blanton SH, Stephens Richards B, Rice JP, Dobbs MB, Gurnett CA. Genome-wide association study identifies new disease loci for isolated clubfoot. J Med Genet. 2014;51:334–9. https://doi.org/10.1136/jmedgenet-2014-102303.

63. Shrimpton AE, Levinsohn EM, Yozawitz JM, Packard DS Jr, Cady RB, Middleton FA, Persico AM, Hootnick DR. A HOX gene mutation in a family with isolated congenital vertical talus and Charcot-Marie-tooth disease. Am J Hum Genet. 2004;75:92–6. https://doi.org/10.1086/4220151182012.

64. Mortlock DP, Innis JW. Mutation of HOXA13 in hand-foot-genital syndrome. Nat Genet. 1997;15(2):179–80. https://doi.org/10.1038/ng0297-179. PMID: 9020844.

# Chapter 2
# Classification of Clubfoot

Alain Dimeglio and Federico Canavese

## Introduction

At birth, only 35% of the foot is ossified, and bones are still cartilaginous, soft, and flexible, whereas fibrous structures are stiff and resistant. The condition is variable in its clinical course. Within the spectrum of all possible congenital clubfoot conditions, there are different degrees of involvement, ranging from the stiffest to the supplest foot [1–9]. Clubfeet classically have been divided into four categories: benign, moderate, severe, and very severe. However, the criteria defining them are generally inaccurate and do not change treatment. Therefore, a severity scale is very useful to differentiate feet accurately.

## Clinical Evaluation

### *Postural Clubfoot*

At birth, postural clubfoot should be differentiated from congenital clubfoot in which the deformity is usually rigid, with limited range of movement.

The so-called postural clubfoot shows inversion of the hind foot, it shows adduction and inversion of the forefoot, and the entire foot is plantar flexed at the level of the ankle. Usually, there are neither abnormal skin creases nor calf atrophy. On passive manipulations, the deformity is reducible.

A. Dimeglio (✉)
Faculty of Medicine, University of Montpellier, Montpellier, France

F. Canavese
Pediatric Orthopedic Surgery Department, University Hospital Jeanne de Flandre and Faculty of Medicine, Lille, France

© The Author(s), under exclusive license to Springer Nature Switzerland AG 2023
M. B. Dobbs et al. (eds.), *Clubfoot and Vertical Talus*,
https://doi.org/10.1007/978-3-031-34788-7_2

## *Congenital Clubfoot*

The so-called congenital clubfoot is a diagnosis by elimination in the same way as idiopathic scoliosis. Family history is positive in about 5% of cases, and the search for a cause is a pressing concern.

Palpation is the most important step since there is no substitute for the tactile feeling by an expert hand. Feet must be manipulated gently and gradually; during clinical examination, babies must be relaxed. It must be remembered that the difficulty with which a clubfoot corrects is not always directly dependent upon the degree of deformity. It is more related to the rigidity secondary to taut soft tissue structures. Assessing a clubfoot, especially in the neonatal period, requires an exhaustive checklist where **inspection**, **palpation**, and **reducibility** are the key points.

However, it must be kept in mind that clinical assessment should not be limited to a simple orthopedic evaluation of the foot deformity. It is a misnomer that clubfoot is a deformity limited to the foot. It is, therefore, necessary to assess the child as a whole.

A neonatal ultrasound assessment is strongly recommended to check the medullary axis, the state of the brain, and the state of the heart. Certain affections can be revealed secondarily. The stiffness of the hind foot could suggest a nonvisible neonatal synostosis [1–3].

When dealing with clubfoot deformity, the examiner should keep in mind the following basic steps:

(a) Palpate the heel to check out if calcaneus is present or not ("empty heel").
(b) Evaluate the external face of the talus on the anterior-external portion of the foot ("convex lateral border").
(c) Assess the reducibility of the foot on the horizontal plane (rotation of the calcaneotarsal complex and adduction), on the sagittal plane (equinus), and on the frontal plane (varus).
(d) Test the tonicity of the muscles.

## *Clubfoot Assessment*

Clubfoot examination can be easily performed with the baby prone. In order to assess clubfoot deformity, the examination should start with the tibia, noting the position of the tibial tubercule, medial, and lateral malleolus. Having oriented the tibia, the deformities in the hind foot can be established by noting the position of the head of the talus and the alignment of the calcaneus and its orientation. The position of the forefoot in relationship to the hind foot can now be assessed and the deformity noted. It should be remembered that recurvatum of the knee and external rotation of the leg can mask equinus and forefoot deformity, respectively.

The forefoot and midfoot are inverted and adducted. The big toe appears to be relatively shortened. The lateral border of the foot is convex, and the medial one is concave. The forefoot is in equinus. The heel is drawn up and inverted, and a deep crease is usually present on the posterior aspect of the ankle joint. The calf is atrophic.

Posterior and medial plantar ankle creases are usually present. The heel is high, drawn up by a retracted Achilles tendon (equinus deformity). The hind foot is in varus; the forefoot is adducted and inverted with the navicular bone abutting the medial malleolus (varus deformity). The normal space between the medial malleolus and the navicular bone is absent as the navicular is displaced medially and plantarward, and it is tethered to the medial malleolus. The lateral malleolus and the calcaneus are tethered as well, and the hallux appears shortened because of the proximal displacement (adduction and inversion deformity) of the medial column of the foot. The skin on the lateral aspect of the foot in front of the lateral malleolus is thin, with a prominent body of the talus under it. Moderate to severe calf atrophy is present. Calf atrophy when significant is a pejorative criterion.

Dorsalis pedis and tibial artery pulses are usually present but vascular dysgenesis is possible, so it is important to assess circulation of the foot and ankle.

Muscle testing for motor strength is difficult to perform in a newborn infant. However, because ruling out neuromuscular nonidiopathic clubfoot is important, a muscle test should be performed even though it is difficult to carry out. Some feet have hardly any reactive muscles, fibrotic. The quality and the activity of the muscles are decisive factors for deformity progression.

Other joints (hips, knees, elbows, shoulders) should be examined to rule out subluxation or dislocation.

At the end of this complete evaluation, the examiner should be able to identify the following clinical figures:

– Short, fat feet versus long, thin feet
– Severity of the equinus (over 20%)
– Reducibility of the foot less than 50% versus more than 50%
– Severity of the atrophy of calf muscles and degree of reactivity of the peroneal muscles
– Absence versus presence of creases (posterior, medial, and/or plantar)


## Clubfoot Classification

Within the spectrum of all possible talipes equinovarus conditions, there are different degrees of involvement, from the stiffest to the softest foot. Classification is, therefore, essential to both score clubfoot at birth and to assess the impact of treatment.

A classification is required, but all classifications are necessarily arbitrary. To place discussions in a context, to assess results objectively, clubfeet have been nowadays codified in ascending order of severity, from the mildest to the most severe, to quickly identify feet to be treated [4]. It must be remembered that the difficulty with which a clubfoot corrects is not always directly dependent upon the degree of deformity. It is more related to rigidity.

Prerequisites of a system for evaluating clubfoot are: (a) it must be simple; (b) it must be easy to teach; (c) observation must be repeatable by various observers.

## *Ponseti and Smoley Classification System (1963)*

Ponseti and Smoley reported the results of treatment of congenital talipes equinovarus. Their classification system is based on ankle dorsiflexion (>10°, 0–10°, or 0°), heel varus (0°, 0°–10°, or >10°), forefoot adduction (0–10°, 10–20°, or >20°), and tibial torsion (neutral, moderate, or severe). Feet are classified on the basis of these measurements as good, acceptable, or poor [6].

## *Manes, Costa, and Innao Classification System (1975)*

Manes, Costa, and Innao introduced their classification system in 1975 [7]. The severity of the clubfoot is assessed on the sagittal plane only, and three degrees of severity can be identified, from the mildest to the most severe. The deformity can be rated as mild, completely reducible (Grade I); moderate, partially reducible (Grade II); or severe, not reducible (Grade 3).

## *Harrold and Walker Classification System (1983)*

Harrold and Walker system is based on the reducibility of the equinovarus deformity by manipulations. Patients with a foot that is reducible to or beyond neutral is described as grade I (mild); those with a varus or equinus deformity correctable to within 20° of neutral is described as grade II (moderate patients whose deformity (either varus or equinus) could not be manipulated to within 20° of neutral is described as grade III (severe) [8].

## *Catterall Rading System (1991)*

Catterall described four patterns of congenital clubfoot depending on the evolution of the deformity: resolving pattern, tendon contracture, joint contracture, and false correction [9]. To classify the foot in each category, the hind foot and the forefoot need to be assessed as follows:

(a) Hindfoot: lateral malleolus (mobile or posterior); equinus (yes or no); posterior, medial, and plantar creases (yes or no);
(b) Forefoot: lateral border (straight or curved); mobility (present or absent); cavus (yes or no); supination (yes or no).

## *Goldner and Fitch System (1994)*

Goldner and Fitch method of classification and evaluation of congenital clubfoot provides an index of severity that can be used as a guide to treatment. The system includes eight clinical and two radiographic parameters. Each parameter is rated as absent (0 points), mild (1, 2, or 3 points according to the severity), moderate (2, 4, or 6 points), or severe (3, 6 or 9 points), and the total score gives the severity of the deformity.

Clinical items are: (1) skin, ligaments, creases, elasticity; (2) calf size, ease of cast application; (3) muscles activity; (4) position of the head of the talus; (5) tibial-navicular interval; (6) foot alignment with ankle joint; (7) equinus; (8) cavus.

Radiographic items are: (1) evaluation of hindfoot (position of the talus, the calcaneus and their relationship; (2) abduction and adduction, spurious correction of forefoot.

## *Dimeglio's et al. grading System (1995)*

At birth, clubfeet are classified in ascending order of severity, from the mildest to the more severe, with a score on a scale from 0 to 20 as described by Dimeglio et al [4] (Fig. 2.1).

In order to establish a final score, each of the following parameters receives a score from 1 (completely reducible) to 4 (nonreducible):

(a) *Adduction of the forefoot compared with the hindfoot.* One point is given if the forefoot reaches 20° of abduction, two if it reaches 0° (neutral position), three points if it stops at −20°, and four points if hindfoot forefoot adduction does not exceed −45° (Fig. 2.2).
(b) *Varus of the hindfoot.* One point is given if hindfoot reaches 20° of valgus, two if it reaches 0° (neutral position), three points if it stops at −20°, and four points if hindfoot varus does not go above −45° (Fig. 2.3).
(c) *Internal rotation of the calcaneotarsal complex.* One point is given if calcaneotarsal complex reaches 20° of external rotation, two if it reaches 0° (neutral position), three points if it stops at −20°, and four points if internal rotation does not go above −45° (Fig. 2.4).
(d) *Equinus.* One point is given if dorsiflexion reaches 20°, two if it reaches 0° (neutral position), three points if it stops at −20°, and four points if dorsiflexion does not go above −45° (Fig. 2.5).

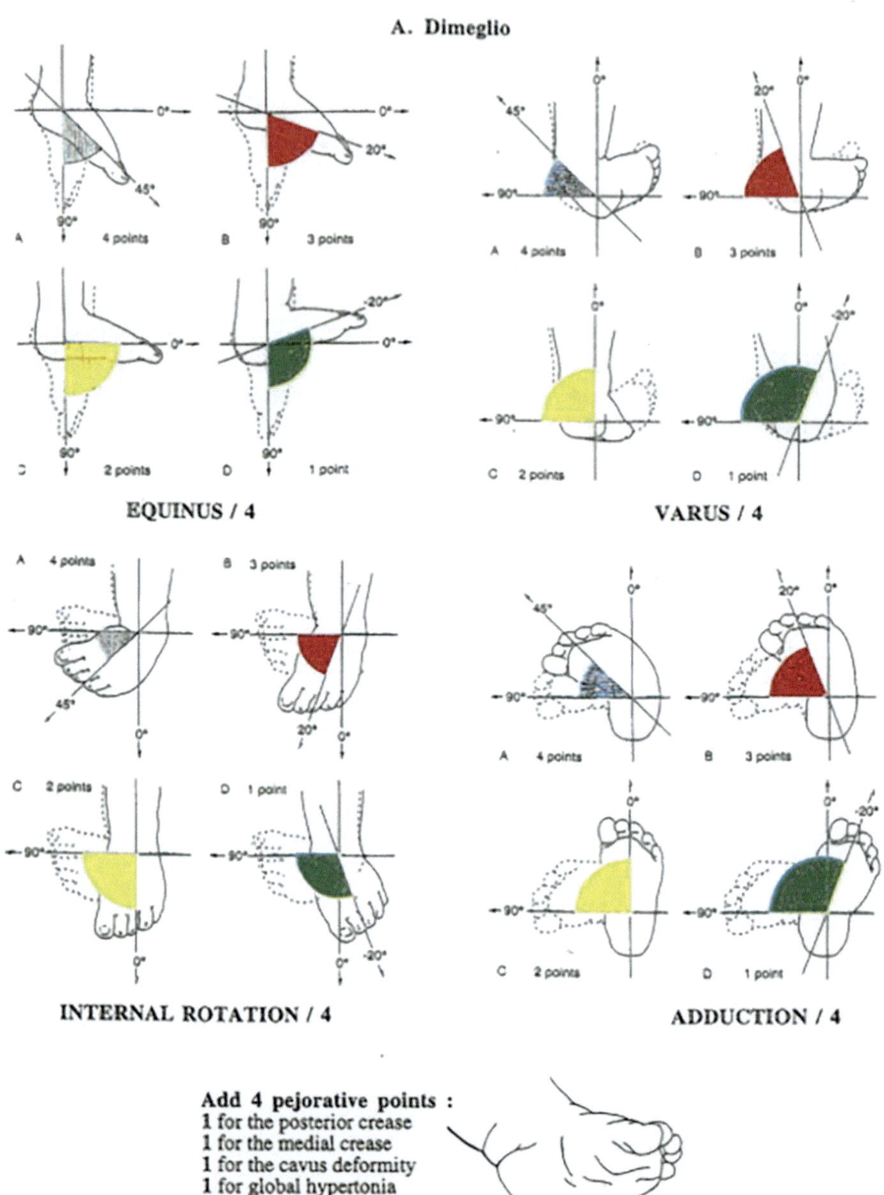


Fig. 2.1 Dimeglio classification system

**Fig. 2.2** Rating of forefoot adduction according to Dimeglio et al.

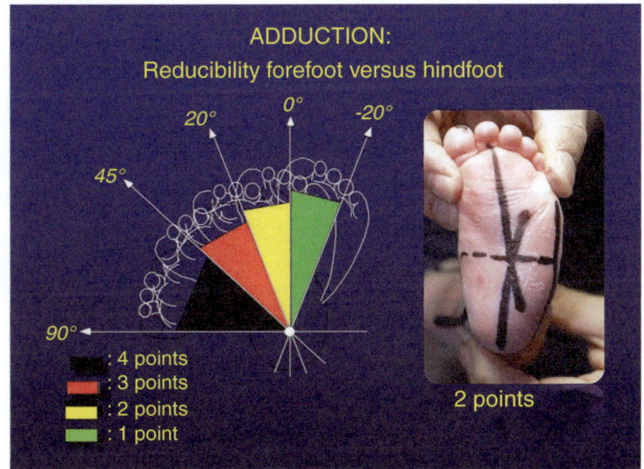


**Fig. 2.3** Rating of hindfoot varus according to Dimeglio et al.

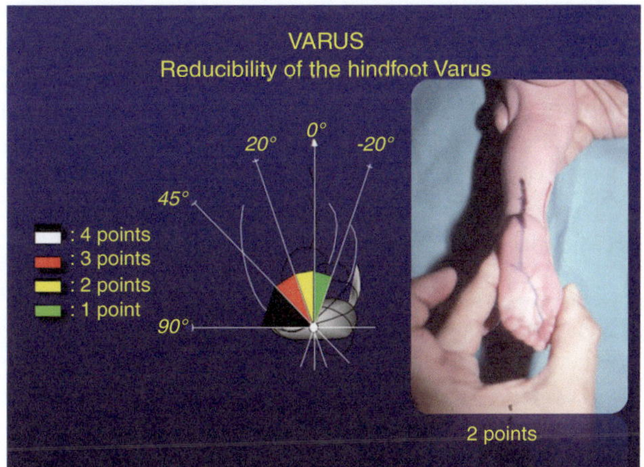


**Fig. 2.4** Rating of internal rotation according to Dimeglio et al.

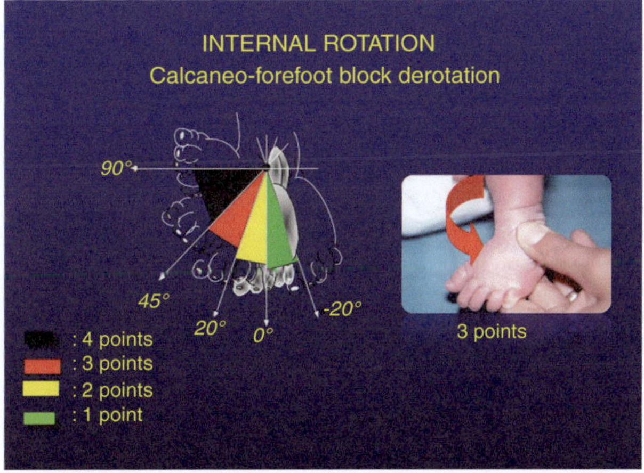

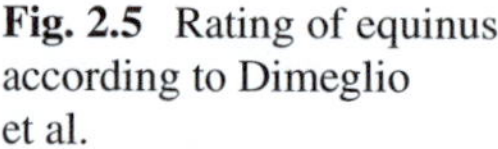

**Fig. 2.5** Rating of equinus according to Dimeglio et al.

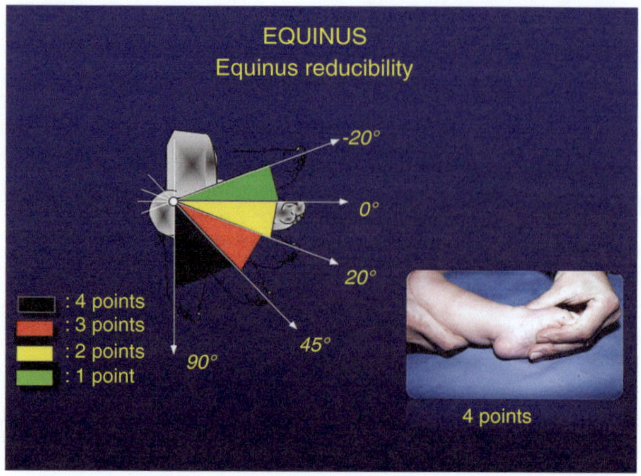


These parameters must be assessed in terms of reducibility, without forcing the foot. A small goniometer allows one to measure angulation precisely before and after the reducibility test. To these four parameters, four pejorative points are added to obtain a score out of 20: (1) one for the medial (or plantar) crease; (2) one for the posterior crease; (3) one for the cavus; (4) one for the infant's global hypertonia or muscle weakness or short, fat foot.

This classification allows surgeons to distinguish and to predict outcomes between four categories of feet [4]:

1. *Postural feet* (also called soft-soft feet). The score is between 1 and 5. These feet can be completely reduced. Any treatment can correct the deformity, and it is exceptional that these feet are neglected and become stiff.
2. *Moderate feet* (also called soft-stiff feet). The score is between 6 and 10. These feet can be reduced but are partially resistant (more than 50% of reduction possible). Orthopedic treatment is effective and makes it possible to avoid surgery in about nine cases out of ten;
3. *Severe feet* (also called stiff-soft feet). The score is between 11 and 15. These feet are resistant and can be only partially reduced (less than 50% reduction possible). Orthopedic treatment is effective in half of the cases. Cases nonresponding to conservative treatment require surgery.
4. *Very severe feet* (also called stiff-stiff feet). The score is between 16 and 20. These are feet that virtually cannot be reduced. Only three cases out of ten avoid extensive surgery. In this group, about 30% of clubfeet are nonidiopathic.

This classification system is simple, reproducible, and reliable. It permits to assess the effectiveness of the orthopadic treatment day by day during the first 6 months of life, and it allows for reliable comparisons between study populations that use various treatment techniques. Wainwright et al. studied the reliability of four most commonly used clinical classification systems—those described by

Catterall [9], Dimeglio et al. [4], Harrold and Walker [8], and Ponseti and Smoley [6], and found the system of Dimeglio et al., the most reliable of the above four [10].

Flynn et al. [11] and Celebi et al. [12] have shown that after an initial learning curve Dimeglio et al.'s grading system, Pirani's score and International Clubfoot Study Group classification system have good interobserver and intraobserver reliability.

## *Pirani's Score (1995)*

The Pirani's clubfoot score rates the severity of the congenital clubfoot by assessing three components of the hind foot and three components of the midfoot [13].

The three parameters that need to be assessed at the level of the hind foot are:

- Severity of posterior crease
- Emptiness of the heel
- Rigidity of the equinus

The three parameters that need to be assessed at the level of the midfoot include:

- Curvature of the lateral border of the foot
- Severity of the medial crease
- Position of the lateral part of the head of the talus

These parameters must be assessed in terms of reducibility, without forcing the foot. In order to establish a final score, each of the following parameters receives a score of 0 (absent or no abnormality), 0.5 (moderate abnormality), or 1 (present or severe abnormality).

This classification system is simple, and it has shown good inter- and intraobserver reliability.

## Clubfoot Evaluation During Growth

A realistic approach is crucial. The family should understand that congenital clubfoot is an in uterodeformation of the foot and that it can never be completely normal. Some residual atrophy of the calf remains. The foot will be smaller than an unaffected limb. Normal range of motion will be somewhat restricted. Even corrected, a congenital clubfoot remains a clubfoot throughout life.

An objective evaluation is necessary, but such an objective evaluation is difficult to appreciate when there is an interval of 1 or 2 years. Regular clinical assessment is, therefore, mandatory.

The functional assessment should consider any deformities of the hindfoot and the mobility of the subtalar joint.

The functional assessment involves an appreciation of toe walking, heel walking, walking down the stairs, standing on one leg, ability or inability to jump a rope, walking on uneven terrain, the wear of the shoes, the gait, and atrophy of the calf.

It is evidently necessary to check for a recurvatum of the knee that can conceal an equinus foot, a weakness of the triceps that is always detrimental, and a weakness of the flexors of the toes.

The radiographic assessment plays an essential role in the evaluation; the divergence between talus and calcaneus on anteroposterior and lateral view should be appreciated as well as the morphology of the bones, particularly a crushing of the talus, or a subluxation of the navicular bone, which is always a pejorative factor.

Around the age of 5 years, the ossification of the navicular bone permits a more precise radiographic evaluation of the foot. This evaluation should be repeated at the age of 10 years. This often comprehensive assessment carried out at the age of 5 years and repeated at the age of 10 years may lead to a worse judgment on some good results; in fact, the limited mobility of these feet can be striking.

While congenital idiopathic clubfoot is usually described as a defect in the foot, the musculature between the knee and the ankle is affected to some degree, and most importantly, the size difference in the affected leg persists for the life of the patient.

## *Carroll's System for Evaluating Clubfoot Results*

The system developed by Norris Carroll is based on a 20-point grading scale. The system takes into account 20 parameters, ranging from calf circumference to ability of the patients to walk on heels or toes. The ability to do a given activity (i.e., walk on toes) or anatomical parameters close to normal (i.e., less than 0.5 cm leg length discrepancy between clubfoot and contralateral side) are rated 1 point while abnormal parameters/inability to perform adequately an activity scores 0 point. A perfectly normal foot would score 20 points. A foot that scores 5 points or less may require further treatment, including surgery [14–16].

## Conclusion

- A meticulous and repetitive clinical examination is essential before classifying clubfoot.
- Whatever classification system you choose, it is essential to differentiate results of treatment according to the clinical severity of the foot: mild, moderate, severe, or very severe.
- From a practical point of view, a checklist with drawings is helpful to point out all the clinical parameters. Classification allows one to predict the impact of the conservative treatment, to follow the progress of treatment, and to estimate the **surgical risk**. The higher the score, the more severe the clubfoot, and the less

effective is the conservative treatment. It has been shown that the initial severity score is predictive of the clinical outcome in patients treated by the Ponseti method. When the Dimeglio's score is between 6 and 8 and between 9 and 13, 100% and 90% of clubfeet, respectively, can be corrected by the Ponseti method. However, when the score is 14–15 or more than 16, only 68% and 60% of clubfeet, respectively, can be successfully corrected by the Ponseti technique. The surgical risk is important information to give to the family in order to avoid any deception.

# References


1. Dimeglio A. Le pied bot. Montpellier: Sauramps Médical diffusion Vigot; 1985.
2. Charles YP, Canavese F, Dimeglio A. Frühfunktionnelle Behandlung beim angeborenen Klumpfuß. Orthopade. 2006;35:665–74.
3. Dimeglio A, Canavese F. Pie zambo: revision de los tratamientos actuals. Rev Ortop Traumatol. 2006;50:156–63.
4. Dimeglio A, Canavese F. The French functional physical therapy method for the treatment of congenital clubfoot. J Pediatr Orthop B. 2012;21:28–39.
5. Dimeglio A, Bensahel H, Souchet P, et al. Classification of clubfoot. J Pediatr Orthop B. 1995;4:129–36.
6. Ponseti IV, Smoley EN. Congenital club foot: the results of treatment. J Bone Joint Surg Am. 1963;45:261–344.
7. Manes E, Costa CM, Innao V. Treatment of congenital clubfoot during the first year of life. Chir Organi Mov. 1975;62(3):301–14.
8. Harrold AJ, Walker CJ. Treatment and prognosis in congenital club foot. J Bone Joint Surg Br. 1983;65-B:8–11.
9. Catterall A. A method of assessment of the clubfoot deformity. Clin Orthop. 1991;264:48–53.
10. Wainwright AM, Auld T, Benson MK, Theologis TN. The classification of congenital talipes equinovarus. J Bone Joint Surg Br. 2002;84:1020–4.
11. Flynn JM, Donohoe M, Mackenzie WG. An independent assessment of two clubfoot classification systems. J Pediatr Orthop B. 1998;18:323–7.
12. Celebi L, Muratli HH, Aksahin E, Yagmurlu MF, Bicimoglu A. Evaluation of treated clubfoot: assessment of interobserver and intraobserver reliability. J Pediatr Orthop B. 2006;15:34–6.
13. Pirani S, Outerbridge H, Moran M, Sawatsky B. A method of evaluating virgin clubfoot with substantial interobserver reliability. In: POSNA (Abstract); 1995
14. Tarraf Y, Carroll N. Analysis of the components of residual deformity in clubfeet presenting for reoperation. J Pediatr Orthop. 1992;12(2):207–16.
15. Dimeglio A. Le pied bot varus equin : regard sur le monde actuel. Acta Orthop Belg. 1998;64:80–2.
16. Goldner JL, Fitch RD. Classification and evaluation of congenital talipes equinovarus. In: Simons GW, editor. The clubfoot. The present and View of the future. Berlin: Springer; 1994. p. 120–9.

# Chapter 3
# From the Ponseti Method to the French Method: Research of a Consensus

Alain Dimeglio and Federico Canavese

## Introduction

Clubfoot has multiple clinical facets. Conservative treatment of clubfoot has established itself as the primary treatment of choice, that is, the treatment by plasters, the method of Ponseti or by manipulations, the French functional physical therapy (FFPT) method.

These two protocols revolve around different philosophies of treatment, and both have shown pros and cons. However, despite their differences, both protocols share the same basic goals and aim to achieve a pain-free supple plantigrade foot with as little surgery as practicably possible. Surgical treatment is only needed when the orthopedic treatment is no longer effective and/or when the foot shows no further improvement [1, 2]. Long-term studies have highlighted that clubfeet patients treated with an extensive soft-tissue release have poorer long-term foot function compared to patients undergoing conservative treatment [3, 4]. However, both FFPT and Ponseti treatment protocols do not completely eliminate the need for posterior and/or posteromedial releases. It has been shown that after the Ponseti method, 21% of children will require a conventional surgery, Achilles tenotomy excluded. In particular, 10% of severe clubfeet (11–15 points as per Dimeglio's grading scale) will need a posterior release and 10% a posteromedical release (20% rate of extensive surgery, overall). In addition, 23% of very severe clubfeet (16–20 points) will need a posterior release and a 15% posteromedial release (38% rate of extensive surgery, overall). *The challenge, today, is how can we improve these figures?*

A. Dimeglio (✉)
Faculty of Medicine, University of Montpellier, Montpellier, France

F. Canavese
Pediatric Orthopedic Surgery Department, University Hospital Jeanne de Flandre and Faculty of Medicine, Lille, France



M. B. Dobbs et al. (eds.), *Clubfoot and Vertical Talus*,
https://doi.org/10.1007/978-3-031-34788-7_3

## Can We Reconcile the French Functional Physical Therapy Method and the Ponseti Method?

The Ponseti method and the FFPT method have proven their efficacy. Both protocols have shown good efficacy, reliability, and lasting outcomes and are reported to perform comparably with initial correction rates of up to 90%. Rather than comparing the method of Ponseti and the FFPT method, the time has come to reconcile the differences between the two methods in order to merge the advantages of both and apply them in the same strategy. There are much more convergences than divergences between the two methods.

Richards et al. and Steinman et al. compared the Ponseti and FFPT method for idiopathic clubfeet. The study showed that no significant difference was found between the two techniques. Initial correction rates were 94.4% for the Ponseti method and 95% for the FFPT method. Relapses occurred in 37% and 29% of feet treated with the Ponseti technique and the FFPT method, respectively. At the latest follow-up, outcomes with the Ponseti method were good in 72% of cases, fair in 12%, and poor in 16%. For the FFPT method, outcomes were good in 67%, fair in 17%, and poor in 16% [5–8]. They concluded that crossover treatment between FFPT and Ponseti method has proven beneficial and that early triceps surae lengthening may decrease the need for future posterior release [5, 6, 8].

There is no scientific reason to limit the place of physiotherapy in the Ponseti method. The fundamental concept of Dr. Robert Salter that "motion is life" must be kept in mind as **it is easier to get the reduction although much more difficult is to maintain it.** A delicate, active, precise physiotherapy can be helpful and alter this very last statement in a positive light.

- During the reduction stage, before performing the plaster, the session of physiotherapy should not last 2 or 3 min only; a careful manipulation by a skilled physical therapy for 30 min before the application of a plaster is likely to improve results and to speed up the reduction of the foot. In the Ponseti protocol, physiotherapy has a very limited place. Physiotherapy before cast application increases the reducibility of the foot, the skin becomes more elastic, and the overall number of casts will possibly be reduced.
- After reduction has been achieved and Denis Brown shoes are being worn, physiotherapy plays an active role and reduces the risk of relapses. During manipulation, the foot should be mobilized on all planes, and lateral peroneal muscles should be stimulated regularly to prevent internal rotation.

At this stage, manipulations are not dangerous; manipulations can be taught to families by the physiotherapist, with the help of the skeleton specimens designed by Dr. Ignacio Ponseti. In our institution, a video highlighting manipulations and complementary exercises is given to each family, and the progress of treatment is assessed at each follow-up visit. With this strategy, relapses can be substantially reduced, as the primary reason for a relapse is the inability of families to maintain the correction originally obtained.

Lassitude is a risk and responsible of noncompliance. In some specific cases, when the family has a tendency to give up the Ponseti protocol, the FFPT method can be a valid option, and the reverse is also true.

By taking advantage of the bridges and overlapping between the two methods, it is possible to get out from a strategic deadlock. If the child refuses to wear the Denis Brown shoes, an ankle foot orthosis, designed with the hindfoot platform in external rotation and a hinge to stimulate the foot dorsiflexion, can be successfully used instead. Strategic flexibility is the key to success in the management of congenital clubfoot.

## Can the "Hybrid Method" Improve the Outcome of Conservative Treatment?

Canavese and Dimeglio, using the "hybrid protocol," that is, combining the advantages of both Ponseti method and FFPT method, found that fewer patients needed surgery than previously reported and that those who did required less extensive releases. Compared to Ponseti's method, the *hybrid method* adds regular manipulations and radiographs. The frequent manipulations overcome the periods of cast immobilization, which are similar to those reported for the Ponseti's technique alone. Compared to the FFPT method, the *hybrid method* borrows the advantages of serial casting and ankle foot orthosis during follow-up. According to Canavese and Dimeglio, the *hybrid method* (92 treated feet) was able to correct all clubfoot deformities rated 12/20 and less. Eight cases of posterior releases were needed in feet rated 13/20 and above (24.2%), but the overall rate of posterior release in this cohort of patients (8.7%) was lower than previously published rates. None of the hybrid-method patients needed a posteromedial release. They concluded that the *hybrid method* can improve the morphology and suppleness of the foot and, by doing so, minimizes both the extent of surgery and the risk of relapse [9].

Canavese and Dimeglio believe manipulations can help improve results for feet treated with the Ponseti method. Manipulations stimulate muscles that are otherwise immobilized by serial casting and several months of foot abduction orthosis treatment. Careful manipulation by a physiotherapist before cast application is likely to improve results and speed up the reduction of the foot. Given this evidence, centers should be creating clubfoot units to coordinate all treatments and follow-up visits. A clubfoot unit serves to centralize all patients, help inform and motivate the relatives, and play an education role for physiotherapists and an outreach role for the families who can, to a certain extent, also be enrolled in clubfoot treatment [7, 9].

The *hybrid method* is comparable to the Ponseti technique and the FFPT method in its aim to avoid surgery and the associated fibrosis. The conservative treatment of tomorrow is probably midway between the Ponseti method and the FFPT method and can therefore be expected to improve outcomes. These preliminary results are encouraging, but larger cohorts of patients with longer follow-up are now needed to confirm this early promise [7, 9].

## Surgery "à La Carte"

The use of surgery for primary clubfoot correction should be limited to an "à la carte" approach. The term "surgery à la carte" was introduced by Bensahel et al. in 1987, and it belongs to the French method and philosophy of clubfoot treatment. Surgery is considered as a complementary procedure to nonoperative treatment, which aims to reduce the extent of surgery in case it is requested [10]. "Surgery à la carte" differs from the surgery proposed by Simons [11] and McKay [12], and those surgical strategies should not be mixed together. Dobbs et al. have shown that many patients with clubfoot treated with an extensive soft-tissue release have poor long-term foot function due to foot stiffness and osteoarthritis (moderate to severe in 56% of cases) [13]. With the "à la carte" approach, structures are released as needed to obtain correction as an adjunct to a more conservative treatment approach.

Six different principles must be remembered when surgery is planned [1, 2, 9, 14]:

(a) To avoid extensive surgical dissection. Clubfoot surgery should be assimilated to plastic surgery.
(b) To avoid long skin incision. Clubfoot surgery should be done by multiple skin mini-incisions.
(c) "Be gentle with the tendons!" (A. Dimeglio). Ligaments, tendons, and sheaths must be protected to avoid fibrosis. The surgeon should treat the delicate anatomical structures of the child's foot with plastic surgical respect, in the same spirit as the hand surgeon would treat the structures in "no man's land"; after surgery, physical therapy and splinting have to be maintained.
(d) In congenital clubfoot, equinus is the most difficult deformity to treat. Delpech first reported that all clubfoot deformities are interrelated and pointed out that the calcaneus is involved in the equinus, varus, and adduction of the deformed foot. In particular, varus is linked to the amount of residual equinus, and, if varus persists, forefoot supination and adduction will still be present [15].

Surgeons must remember the golden chance to correct a clubfoot deformity is the first surgery, and nothing can be permanently achieved before skeletal maturity.

Surgery should not be considered as a defeat of the conservative treatment but more like a complementary procedure to conservative treatment. The conservative treatment has positively modified the morphology of the foot and the skin and has prepared the ground for a possibly easier surgery.

At 1 year of age, three situations can be encountered:

1. The foot is completely corrected: splinting and regular follow-up visits have to be continued.
2. The foot has minimal residual imperfections: limited or absent dorsiflexion, tendency to internal rotation and/or lack of divergence between talus and calcaneus on plain radiographs. Manipulations and splinting must be continued. It is a wait-and-see situation.
3. The foot is resistant, and correction could not be achieved. In this worst-case scenario, it is possible to repeat the Ponseti method or to perform "surgery à la carte."

1. Residual Equinus: Achilles Tendon Lengthening

    Achilles tendon lengthening can be performed using different techniques: the percutaneous technique (Hooke), the Vulpius triceps lengthening, or the mini-open tenotomy at the distal part. In some complex cases, rated 15/20 or more, Achilles tendon can be combined with a fractional lengthening of the posterior tibialis tendon through a limited incision on the medial part of the leg.
2. Residual Equinus: Posterior Release

    Posterior release is indicated when hindfoot retraction is severe, when the lateral foot radiograph in maximum dorsiflexion shows a lack of talocalcaneal divergence, and when calcaneum is still elevated. It consists of lengthening of the Achilles tendon in association with a limited posterior capsular release of the subtalar joint, including both the posteromedial (up to the flexor hallucis longus tendon) and the posterolateral (up to peroneal tendons) corners. The tibialis posterior tendon, the flexor digitorum longus tendon, and the flexor hallucis longus tendon can be lengthened. A Kirschner wire is inserted through the posterior part of the talus to reduce the talonavicular joint (*Carroll maneuver*) [14]. A second Kirschner wire is inserted plantarly through the calcaneus and the talus to maintain the reduction. Immobilization is required for about 4–6 weeks [1, 2, 14].
3. Persistent Equinus and Adduction: Posteromedial Release

    Posteromedial release is indicated when the foot is not corrected and has equinus and adduction. Surgery should be performed through two different limited incisions, starting with the posterior release as described above and followed by a medial incision. It is important that the surgery is kept to a minimum. The medial incision is used to release the tibialis posterior tendon at its insertion and to reduce the talonavicular joint. The medial internal ligament or spring ligament and the interosseous ligament between the talus and the calcaneum should never be sacrificed. Tendon sheaths should remain intact. It is important to remove the plantar ramifications of the tibialis posterior tendon before reducing the talonavicular joint. Once the talonavicular joint is reduced, the tibialis posterior tendon can be reinserted at the level of the navicular bone (*lengthening effect*). A Kirschener wire maintains the reduction, and postoperative immobilization is required for 4–6 weeks. The cast and the Kirschener wire are removed under general anesthesia after 4–6 weeks. This allows the surgeon to check the skin incisions and the foot shape [14]. At this stage, it is essential to restore foot mobility.

4. Release of the Abductor Hallucis Longus

   Release of the abductor hallucis longus can be carried out by a supplementary mini-medial incision.
5. Residual Supination: Tibialis Anterior Tendon Transfer

   Patients with isolated residual adduction and dynamic supination benefit from transfer of the anterior tibialis tendon laterally to the lateral cuneiform due to its over activity associated to the under activity of the peroneal muscles. Anterior tibialis tendon transfer is indicated for dynamic supination. When a medial release is performed, the tendon transfer can be completed through the same incision. This procedure is usually performed around age 5 years, if supination persists [1, 2, 10, 14, 16–18].
6. Plantar Fascia Release

   Plantar fascia release can be performed through a mini-incision on the proximal medial part of the sole of the foot.
7. Bean-Shaped Foot: Cuboid Decancellation

   A long and convex lateral border and a short and concave medial side characterize the "bean-shaped foot." The long lateral column can be shortened by a variety of operations including Evans [19], Lichtblau [20], Simon, or cuboid decancellation [21]. Our favorite technique is to perform a closing wedge osteotomy of the cuboid. Alternatively, the medial column can be lengthened by an opening wedge osteotomy of the medial cuneiform as proposed by McHale [22].
8. Postoperative Immobilization

   Immobilization in plaster must be short and should not exceed 4–6 weeks.

   After surgery, splinting with hinged ankle foot orthosis and regular physiotherapy should be continued for 1 year, at least.

## Conclusions

A significant follow up is necessary to evaluate the effect of conservative treatment as deteriorations can occur. Despite some differences, all conservative treatment methods share the same basic principles:

1. The FFPT method is a combination of manipulations, splinting, and "surgery à la carte."
2. Not all clubfeet can be corrected by conservative treatment alone, that is, Ponseti technique, FFPT method, or *hybrid method*. Surgical treatment, that is, "surgery à la carte," is only needed when the orthopedic treatment is no longer effective and/or when the foot shows no more improvement.
3. The creation of a unit through which all treatment and follow-up for a patient with congenital clubfoot are coordinated shall be given priority. This centralizes all patients with clubfeet in the region, helps to inform and motivate the relatives, and is of vital importance in the education of physiotherapists.
4. Continuity of treatment is mandatory. Any slackening of treatment may be harmful.

5. Families, physiotherapists, and splints have the same impact on the treatment protocol. The primary reason for relapses is the inability of families to maintain the correction initially achieved.
6. After surgery, demobilization is disastrous; postoperative physiotherapy is essential.
7. The assessment at the third month is important, since a choice must be made between continuing the orthopedic treatment because it is effective and surgery can be avoided and keeping the orthopedic treatment going in order to preserve what has been achieved, while knowing that surgery is likely to be necessary.
8. Early triceps surae lengthening improves the outcome and decreases the rate of extensive surgery. Very severe feet (score, 16–20) are still a challenge. Daily manipulations and splinting contribute to make surgery less extensive.
9. A significant follow-up is necessary to evaluate the effect of treatment as deteriorations can be observed around and after 2 years of age. Nothing is permanently achieved before skeletal maturity.
10. Our experience has proven that these methods feed to each other. Casting to control reduction is now recommended every week while initially they were changed every 3 weeks. In the FFPT method, short-term cast immobilization and lengthening of the Achilles tendon (Vulpius technique) has been incorporated into the protocol, instigated by the Montpellier school. Following reduction by plaster, regular physical therapy can reduce the duration in splint and the risk of relapse in the Ponseti method. Physiotherapy optimizes by 30% the Ponseti method (efficiency coefficient). And by introducing changes in the original method, without denaturing the philosophy, the need of surgery can be reduced further.
11. The conservative treatment of tomorrow is probably halfway between the method of Ponseti and the FFPT method (*hybrid method*), and from this point, one can expect to improve results. There is no reason to stick in a sterile opposition between the Ponseti method and the FFPT method. Over time, both methods have evolved. A rigid position is a dramatic error. Strategic flexibility is the key to efficiency. Continuity is essential. To achieve a long-term correction with a foot that is fully functional and pain free, a combination of approaches that applies the strengths of Ponseti and FFPT method is needed.

# References


1. Charles YP, Canavese F, Dimeglio A. Frühfunktionnelle Behandlung beim angeborenen Klumpfuß. Orthopade. 2006;35:665–74.
2. Dimeglio A, Canavese F. Pie zambo: revision de los tratamientos actuals. Rev Ortop Traumatol. 2006;50:156–63.
3. Cooper DM, Dietz FR. Treatment of congenital idiopathic clubfoot. A thirty-year follow-up note. J Bone Joint Surg Am. 1995;77:1477–89.
4. Morcuende JA, Dolan LA, Dietz FR, Ponseti IV. Radical reduction in the rate of extensive corrective surgery for clubfoot using the Ponseti method. Pediatrics. 2004;113:376–80.

5. Richards S, Faulks S, Rathjen K, Karol LA, Johnston CE, Jones SA. A comparison of two nonoperative methods of idiopathic clubfoot correction: the Ponseti method and the French functional (physiotherapy) method. J Bone Joint Surg Am. 2008;90:2313–21.
6. Steinman S, Richards BS, Faulks S, Kaipus K. A comparison of two nonoperative methods of idiopathic clubfoot correction: the Ponseti method and the French functional (physiotherapy) method. Surgical technique. J Bone Joint Surg Am. 2009;91(Suppl 2):299–312.
7. Dimeglio A, Bonnet F, Mazeau P, de Rosa V. Orthopaedic treatment and passive motion machine: consequences for the surgical treatment of clubfoot. J Pediatr Orthop B. 1996;5:173–80.
8. Richards BS, Johnston CE, Wilson H. Nonoperative clubfoot treatment using the French physical therapy method. J Pediatr Orthop. 2005;25:98–102.
9. Canavese F, Mansour M, Moreau-Pernet G, Gorce Y, Dimeglio A. The hybrid method for the treatment of congenital talipes equinovarus: preliminary results on 92 consecutive feet. J Pediatr Orthop B. 2017;26(3):197–203.
10. Bensahel H, Csukonyi Z, Desgrippes Y, Chaumien JP. Surgery in residual clubfoot: one-stage medioposterior release 'à la carte'. J Pediatr Orthop. 1987;7:145–82.
11. Simons GW. The clubfoot. The present and view of the future. Berlin: Springer; 1994.
12. McKay DW. New concepts of and approach to clubfoot treatment: section II-correction of the clubfoot. J Pediatr Orthop. 1983;3:10–21.
13. Dobbs MB, Nunley R, Schoenecker PL. Long-term follow-up of patients with clubfeet treated with extensive soft-tissue release. J Bone Joint Surg Am. 2006;88(5):986–96.
14. Dimeglio A, Canavese F. The French functional physical therapy method for the treatment of congenital clubfoot. J Pediatr Orthop B. 2012;21:28–39.
15. Delpech JM. De l'orthomorphie par rapport à l'espèce humaine ou recherches anatomico-pathologiques sur les causes, les moyens de prévenir, ceux de guérir les principales difformités et sur les véritables fondements de l'art appelé: Orthopédie. Paris: Gabon; 1828.
16. Carroll NC. Pathoanatomy and surgical treatment of resistant clubfoot. AAOS Instr Course Lect. 1988;37:43–117.
17. Ponseti IV. Treatment of congenital club foot. J Bone Joint Surg Am. 1992;74:448–54.
18. Bensahel H, Guillaume A, Csukonyi Z, Thémar-Noel C. The intimacy ofclubfoot: the ways of functional treatment. J Pediatr Orthop B. 1994;3:155–60.
19. Evans D. Relapsed clubfoot. J Bone Joint Surg Br. 1961;43:722–33.
20. Lichtblau S. A medial and lateral release operation for clubfoot. J Bone Joint Surg Am. 1973;55:1377–84.
21. Hudson I, Catterall A. Posterolateral release for resistant clubfoot. J Bone Joint Surg Br. 1994;76:281–4.
22. Mubarak SJ, Dimeglio A. Navicular excision and cuboid closing wedge for severe cavovarus foot deformities: a salvage procedure. J Pediatr Orthop. 2011;31:551–6.

# Chapter 4
# Treatment of Clubfoot After Walking Age


Monica Paschoal Nogueira


## Delayed Treatment

In many countries, children with clubfeet are not always treated as newborns [1–4]. The term neglected for any condition carries a sense of poor care and or a patient's failure to present for treatment. Reasons for lack of treatment vary from lack of resources. One also must note that medical professionals are sparse in various locations [5–7]. As a child ages the deformity can become more rigid. Likewise, casting a toddler or ambulatory child poses increased challenges. As the child ages with such deformity uncorrected, they can become physically limited and socially ostracized. The term "neglected" carries a negative meaning that these children were intentionally not treated. There are many reasons in which children may not seek treatment until later in life.

The Ponseti method has become the standard of care in treating not only infants at birth with clubfoot but also children with secondary diagnoses [8, 9]. Ongoing research supports the utility of this method in treating older children with clubfeet and children with recurrences.

## Children Undergoing the Ponseti Method

Most surgeons from developing countries learned about the Ponseti method in newborns and found themselves in the situation of trying to apply those principles in older children. Many countries embarked on casting ambulatory children with more rigid and complex deformities. Important work from India, China, Brazil, Nepal, Turkey, Ethiopia, Egypt, Iran, and Malawi was published [1–3, 7, 10–19]. Further


M. P. Nogueira (✉)
Departament of Pediatric Orthopaedic and Limb Reconstruction, Instituto de Assistência
Médica ao Servidor Público Estadual (IAMSPE), São Paulo, SP, Brazil



M. B. Dobbs et al. (eds.), *Clubfoot and Vertical Talus*,
https://doi.org/10.1007/978-3-031-34788-7_4

cases from the Philippines, Colombia, Mexico, Guatemala, Nicaragua, Bolivia, Argentina, and Paraguay were presented at international meetings. Most of the studies came from national programs [20] or collaboration studies [21–23]. Surgeons shared the common goal of deformity correction via the Ponseti method (Fig. 4.1).

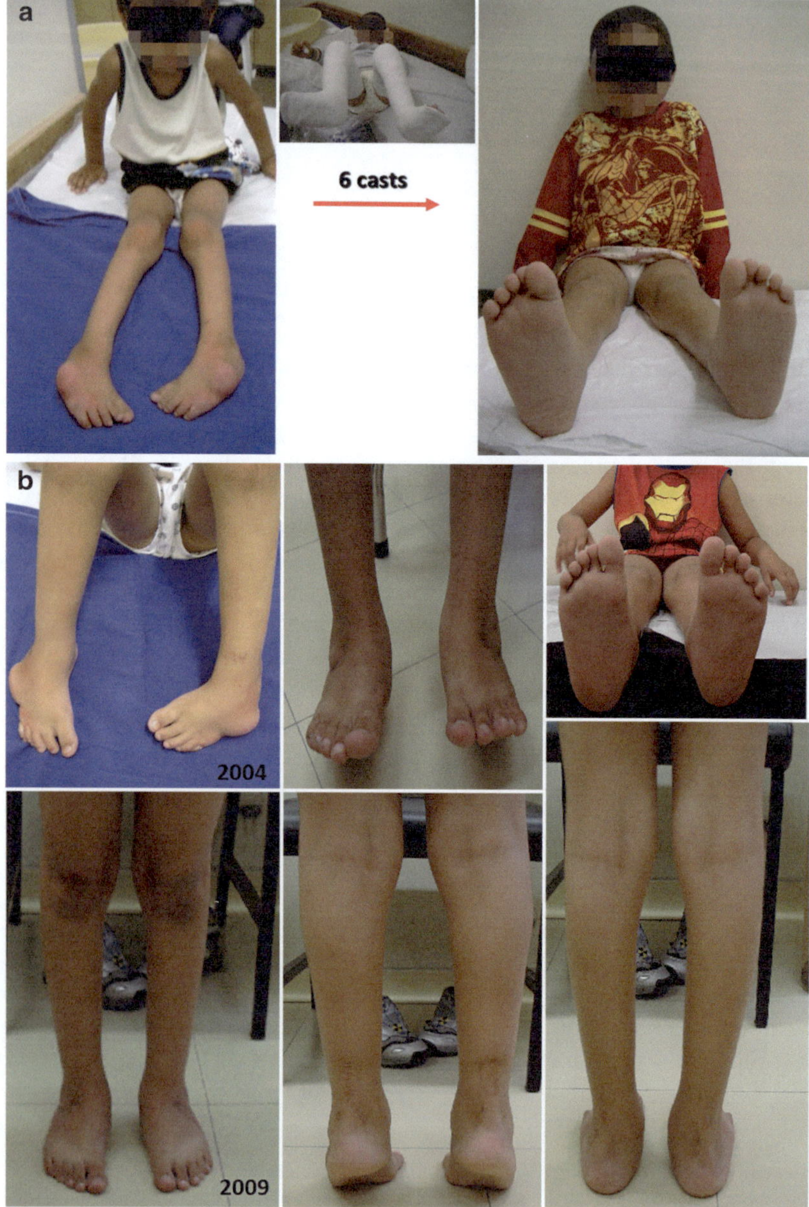


**Fig. 4.1** Clinical pictures of a 6-year-old boy pre- and posttreatment with six casts and percutaneous tenotomy. (**a**) Pictures pre- and posttreatment and long leg casts. (**b**) At 5 years of follow-up. (**c**) At 8 years of follow-up. (**d**) Radiographs pre- and posttreatment

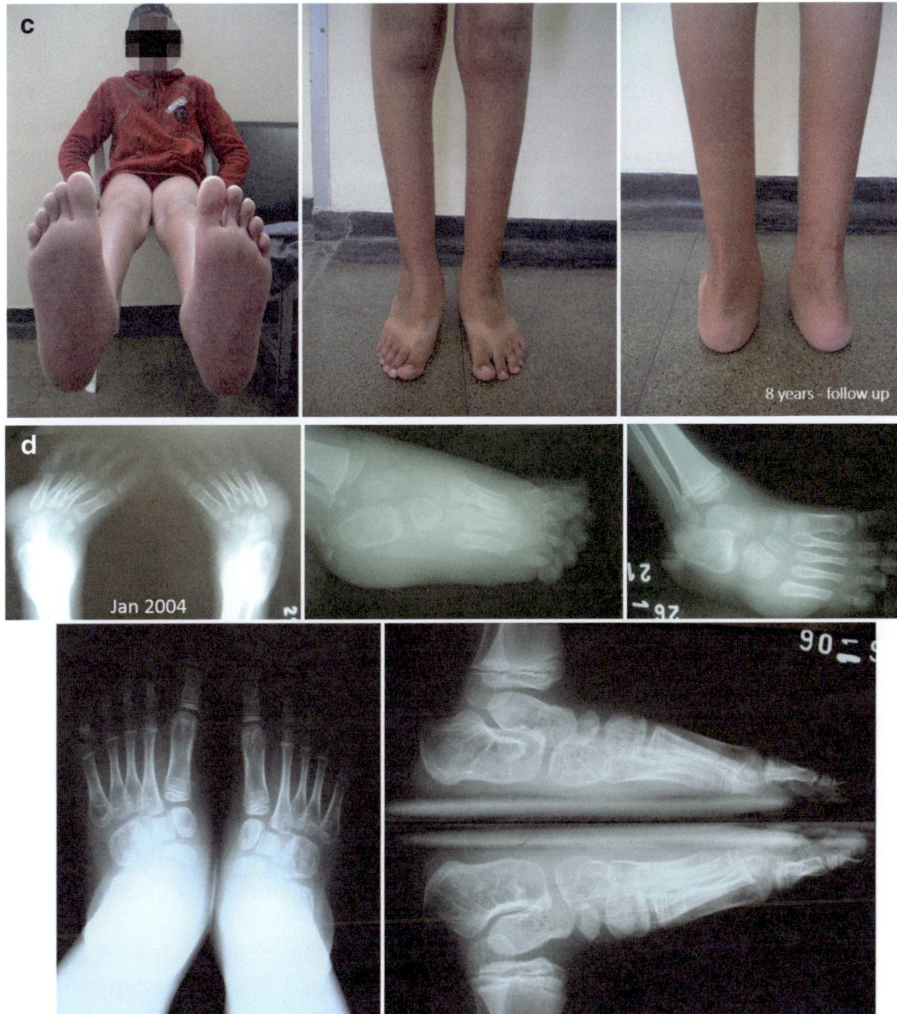


**Fig. 4.1** (continued)

## Scoring Systems for the Older Child with Clubfoot

Due to adaptation of joints and enhanced soft-tissue tightening with growth, the hindfoot is different as compared to a clubfoot in a newborn. The hindfoot features of Pirani's score remain misleading [24–26]. Rigidity and motor function are prognostic toward recurrence risks [24–26]. More rigidity often equates to more casts to achieve deformity correction; however, remodeling is possible and has been shown in older children with nontreated clubfeet [26]. Maintenance of deformity correction at a time of growth is assisted by bracing. Hygromas reflect soft tissues adaptation to the ground and are not considered in the scoring systems. Partial reducibility, motion, and function can be considered more important and are not evaluated in the scoring systems.

## Treatment Challenges

Patients may have economic constraints. Others relay transportation constraints and incredible geographic distances from treatment facilities. In many countries, patients are void of resources and lack medical education. Families may assume there is no available treatment for clubfoot or coexisting deformities [3].

The Ponseti method can successfully be executed in infants. Many practitioners start treatment the first several weeks of an infant's life to take advantage of diminished kicking strength and flexibility. As the child becomes stronger, the casting process can become more challenging, and techniques in soothing a child become quite essential. With growth, tightness can develop. Full correction of the deformity is key as with undercorrection the deformity can worsen with growth. This holds true when recurrences are examined beyond the current bracing recommendations.

Challenges exist with clinical visits and follow-up. Many patients have economic challenges, transportation constraints, and often could "use" the deformity to receive benefits from the health or social security, perpetuating the disease cycle of lack of resources and lack of health and education caused by a congenital deformity that can be treated effectively in the first months of life [3].

On the other hand, there is already evidence showing that some weeks or even months of delay in treatment do not interfere with good results in clubfoot treatment [27]. However, the recommendation is to start treatment in infancy, so providers can take advantage of the flexibility of soft tissues structures. Treatment in neonatal intensive care units requires evaluation of not only birth weight but also concomitant pathology that may require sooner care. Due to the myofibroblast-like cells described by [8, 28, 29], clubfeet would have the stubborn tendency to contract in the medial and posterior aspects of the foot and leg generating the growth of feet in the deformed position. Correction and maintenance strategies for any age remains key.

## Ponseti Method Pearls

The Ponseti method has proven to be effective in treating infants with clubfoot. Surgeons continue to explore its utility and benefits in the older population. Published literature in Latin America, the Middle East, and Asian countries report adult patients being corrected with long series of serial casts [22, 23, 30]. The potential for a mature foot to be corrected with casting can exist for the same reasons this foot may improve by progressive correction via external fixators. One may expect a more rigid foot with expected complications from extended casting. This will be further discussed.

Treatment continues to be very effective and requires attention to detail. As the foot is elongated, attention must be directed to the pressure on the head of the talus and plantar head of first metatarsal. Pressure must be gentle and well distributed, and the cast is well molded, to avoid irritation. The two-hand maneuver used for the treatment of complex feet could be indicated in those elongated feet. The molding of the plantar surface in a manner of "milking" the plantar fascia produces good correction of the cavus deformity.

The number of casts needed to achieve correction can be higher; it will vary depending on the foot flexibility and the provider's experience. Studies describe that the initial score or condition does not always relate to the power of correction after manipulations and casting.

Short leg casts are not as effective as long leg casts in correction of clubfeet. Capturing the appropriate rotation cannot take place in short leg casts. When the child internally rotates a leg with a well-molded short leg cast, the tissues in the medial and posterior compartments of the leg are relaxed. For the same reason, a less-flexed knee does not produce the highest tension on the posteromedial structures, and the correction is less effective.

The manipulation is skillful and gentle throughout the process. A well-molded cast will minimize creep. One should avoid excess pressure on and osseous structure. Because of that, manipulations and casting under anesthesia as defended by some authors [24] can be worrisome, for not allowing control of tension. Efficient molding is the secret to allow for balance in good tissue tensioning and good distribution of pressure.

The goal remains a plantigrade foot. Talar coverage is key despite age. The lateral border should not only be straight but also should not demonstrate any overload. Heel purchase should be present. Correction of equinus is possible biomechanically only if the anterior tuberosity of calcaneus is already lateral from the talus. Attempts to dorsiflex before the anterior tuberosity of calcaneus is lateral from the talus will result in flattening of talus and will not provide adequate equinus correction. Important consideration must be given to avoid overcorrection.

It is important to recommend skin care and hygiene and motion of the knee and ankle for several minutes between the cast changes. Removal of casts are removed just prior to a subsequent cast being applied [31]. The casting environment should be calm and soothing. This environment may look different based on the age of the child being casted. Infants can be soothed with containment techniques, bottle feeding, pacifiers, Sweet-Ease, and sound machines. In toddlers, one may need various toys or screens to assist. An electronic tablet or phone can be helpful for the older patient. Parents and caregivers can assist with these soothing tactics.

Older children need to demonstrate rectus to valgus alignment of the hindfoot. Varus should not persist. The foot should be plantigrade. The lateral border should be straight. Equinus should be resolved. Much like the infant, equinus is addressed last.

Some authors advocate changing the cast every 2 weeks, based on the premise that collagen takes a while to respond to stretch [3, 31], but the progression of correction can be achieved weekly. This protocol is performed by the majority of authors [14]. Complications associated with extended casting will be described. This protocol seems to be more indicated in the treatment of older children with clubfeet (Fig. 4.2).

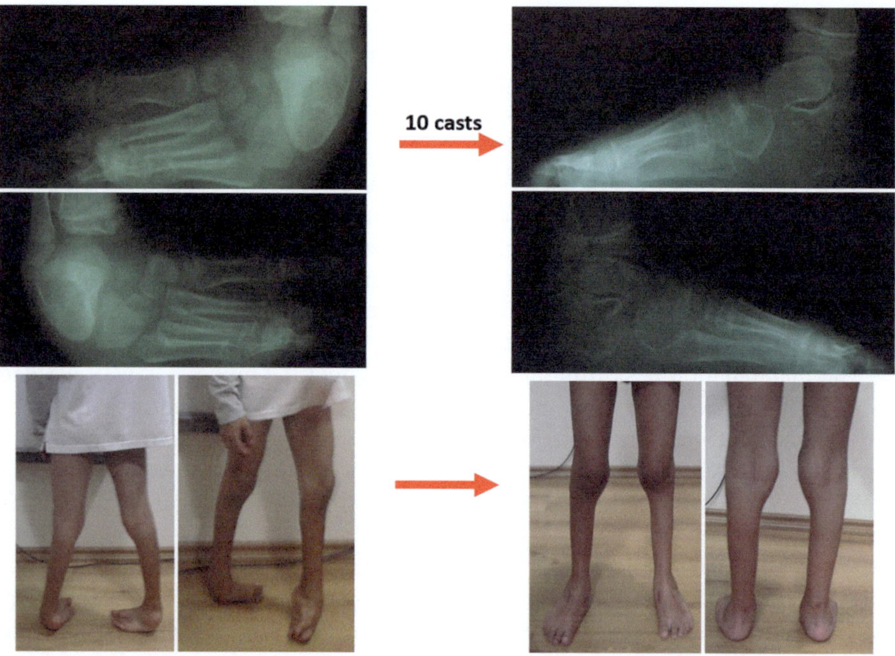



**Fig. 4.2** Pictures and radiographies of a 7-year-old boy with bilateral clubfoot before and after ten casts, complete Achilles percutaneous tenotomy, and anterior tibial tendon transfer

## Documentation Is Essential

Documentation of the progression of correction at every cast change is very important to determine progress and success. Failure of reduction may warrant other more invasive techniques to obtain a plantigrade foot. Every week, comparative photographs of the foot (plantar with the knee included to measure abduction, lateral from the medial side in maximal dorsiflexion, and axial view of the calcaneous) will show the progression of deformity correction (Fig. 4.3). As the feet could assume variable positions (depending on flexibility), pictures of the new casts and foot position will help.

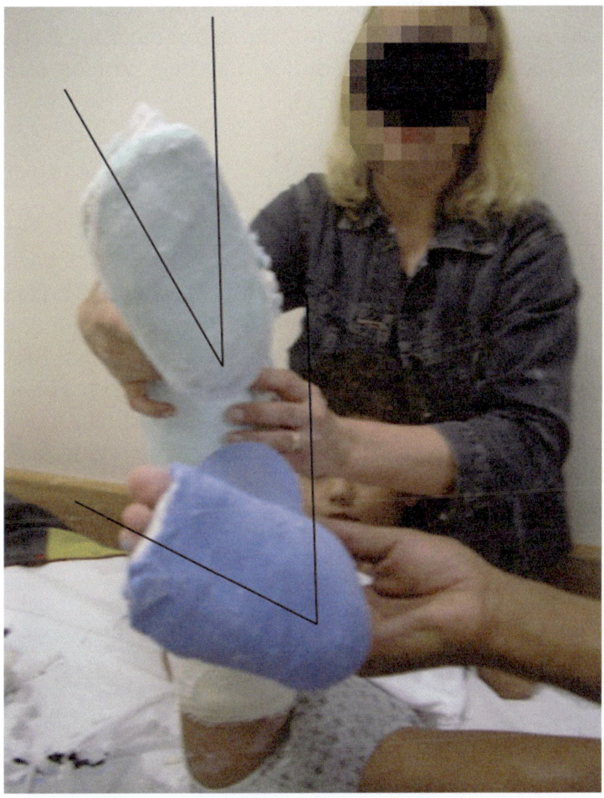

**Fig. 4.3** Carefully measuring the abduction and equinus/dorsiflexion is essential to document progression of deformity correction

## Complications with Extended Casting

Long leg casting for several weeks could lead to osteoporosis, proximal joint contractures, and more time to return to ambulation [3]. The loss of bony architecture will lead to increased risk of stress fractures when recovering to walk. Activities in the swimming pool are well recommended after taking out casts, to improve flexibility and strength, with less risk of fractures.

Stress fractures could be a cause of pain when children return to ambulation. Hip contractures can result from sitting and a sedentary lifestyle in wheelchairs. To minimize these contractures, patients may lie prone as much as possible and stretch hip flexors even with casts on, in a "parachuting" position to rest or watch television.

Knee contractures can be addressed only after cast removal. The child can lie prone and straighten the knees to activate quadriceps. Temporary weakness occurs, and the thigh can lose up to 2 cm in circumference after 4–6 weeks in cast. That is recovered continuously during the first months after treatment. Rehabilitation should focus on the whole child.

## Bracing Protocol

Brace protocol is challenging at this age, but it is crucial to maintain the correction. Bracing does not provide correction. Bracing simply attempts to maintain correction achieved from the casting or surgical process. Bracing immediately after casts is utilized for 23 h per day for 3 months [21]. This is recommended despite the patient's age of treatment [32]. This should be followed by a period of nighttime bracing for at least 12 months following treatment [33] (Fig. 4.4).

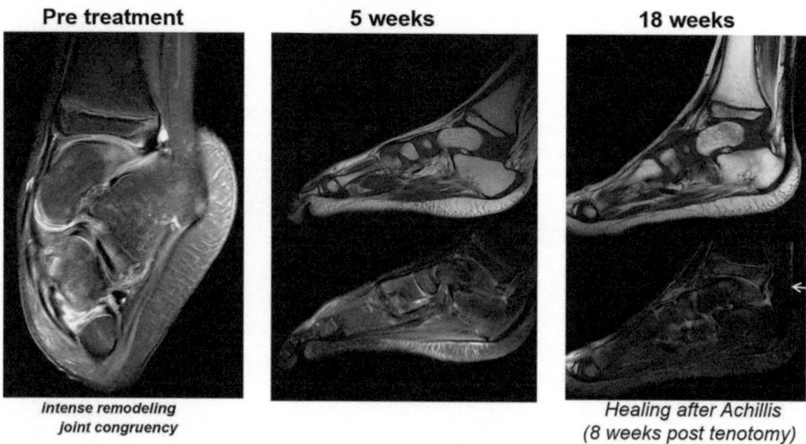


**Fig. 4.4** Magnetic resonance imaging of a clubfoot before, after 5 casts and 18 weeks (8 weeks after tenotomy) showing intense cartilage remodeling

Some studies propose the use of an ankle foot orthosis, including the foot, ankle, and the lower leg (AFO) can maintain correction [2, 3, 7] while we need a prospective study focused on such. The author questions the utility of an AFO and the stretch it provides on the medial column. This is also the reason we recommend long leg cast instead of short leg casts. Some studies support the use of short leg casts justifying that it is the only way those children can come walking to the clinic. The bracing phase can be challenging for families [33, 34]. Caregivers need guidance and reassurance in the process.

## Achilles Tendon Tenotomy

A complete percutaneous tenotomy of the Achilles tendon is performed to correct residual equinus after abduction of about 60–70° in the vast majority of children with clubfoot [1, 2, 10, 11, 13–16, 35–37]. The age limit for adequate healing and remodeling is not well defined. Complete percutaneous tenotomy of Achilles tendon in children with idiopathic clubfeet is a safe procedure with no subsequent planovalgus deformity, as reported by many authors [1, 2, 10, 11, 13–16, 35–37]. The Achilles tendon is not the only structure responsible for retraction. Capsular contractures of the ankle and foot can contribute to equinus deformity. Complete tenotomy should be reconsidered in children with cerebral palsy, who do not have capsular contractures. Some authors support that open lengthening of the Achilles would provide more controlled dorsiflexion [24].

## Anterior Tibial Tendon Transfer

Anterior tibial tendon transfer was described by **Garceau in 1967** [38] and described to be indicated for treatment of the second relapse in children with clubfeet [8]. This imbalance results in inversion of the foot, especially after the period the child is protected with the abduction brace.

A tendon transfer can function as an internal brace or a means at reducing a deforming force. This works best in a flexible foot where the architecture is plantigrade. The Tibialis Anterior tendon transfer is performed after adequate serial casting [39].

Transfer of the Tibialis Anetrior tendon must not be done to the cuboid bone to avoid overcorrection into eversion and valgus. Also, hemitendon transfers (like those described to treat equinovarus feet in children with cerebral palsy) are not recommended, because the main goal is to take out the deforming force from the medial part of the dorsum of the foot to a more lateral (more central) position in the foot.

Performing the Tibialis Anterior tendon transfer does not prevent all relapses. However, some surgeons elect to transfer the tendon at the end of casting especially in the older patient. One reason is the Achilles tenotomy is performed under general anesthesia, because of the age, and then performing the transfer would be under the same anesthetic episode. The benefits of the Tibialis Anterior tendon transfer in the protocol is also discussed for children with relapses after posteromedial releases [40].

## Psychological Aspects

Casting in the ambulatory child poses different obstacles as compared to infants. Casting leads to restriction of activities and impairment of mobility, which in return can produce frustration among all involved. Gentle manipulation and casting methods are utilized. Documentation should reflect one's progressive correction. Digital photos can also be utilized to uplift the patient and reiterate the progress. Educating children that they will need to reposition themselves for sleep will be helpful. Assistive devices can be used for children to attend school and not feel isolated.

By 5–7 years of age, many children have feelings toward medical treatments, as reported in the external fixation literature, referring to limb lengthening in children [41, 42]. Reasons for that could be related to previous experiences. Realistic expectations of all individuals involved will be important in developing a treatment pathway. The dynamics of the family will too be improved with clear dialogue.

## Surgical Correction

Some children require more invasive approaches to rebalance and restore more normal function in shoe gear [39, 40, 43–47]. Casting can be utilized to reduce various aspects of clubfoot and in return allow for smaller incisions to complete correction. Lateral column shortening, decortication of the cuboid bone, or calcaneocuboid fusions can help. A closing cuboid and opening medial cuneiform osteotomy can improve upon the adductus [44]. Calcaneal lateral closing wedge osteotomy [45] can be used to correct hindfoot varus.

External fixation offers progressive correction or also can provide stability following osseous procedures. External fixation has been used to correct clubfoot and studies in subtalar joint biomechanics assisted with understanding progressive correction. As the indications for the Ponseti method broadened, surgical procedures decreased.

In experienced centers for external fixation, the application of external fixators has been utilized with this strategy [41]. The hexapodal frames that use external rotation in the correction of clubfoot, with a hold on the talar head, mimic Ponseti casting and are becoming more popular among external fixation experts. The use of multiple osteotomies controlled by different hexapodal systems is versatile but still bulky for the patient.

## Future Directions

Certainly, as one of the most common orthopedic congenital deformities, clubfoot is a public-health problem. Health managers and stakeholders should include this deformity in the health agenda in every country. Clubfoot treatment via the Ponseti method is not expensive in comparison to other treatment modalities. Education remains important to continue advances in care.

**Acknowledgments** I would like to thank Dr. Davi Haje and Dr. Gabriel Ferraz for their dedication in this field of medicine.

## References


1. Khan SA, Kumar A. Ponseti's manipulation in neglected clubfoot in children more than 7 years of age: a prospective evaluation of 25 feet with long-term follow-up. J Pediatr Orthop B. 2010;19(5):385–9.
2. Bashi RH, Baghdadi T, Shirazi MR, Abdi R, Aslani H. Modified Ponseti method of treatment for correction of neglected clubfoot in older children and adolescents--a preliminary report. J Pediatr Orthop B. 2016;25(2):99–103.
3. Lourenço AF, Morcuende JA. Correction of neglected idiopathic club foot by the Ponseti method. J Bone Joint Surg Br. 2007;89(3):378–81.
4. Tindall AJ, Steinlechner CW, Lavy CB, Mannion S, Mkandawire N. Results of manipulation of idiopathic clubfoot deformity in Malawi by orthopedic clinical officers using Ponseti method: a realistic alternative for the developing world? J Pediatr Orthop. 2005;25(5):627–9.
5. Penny JN. The neglected clubfoot. Tech Orthop. 2005;20(2):153–66.
6. Adegbehingbe OO, Oginni LM, Ogundele OJ, Ariyibi AL, Abiola PO, Ojo OD. Ponseti clubfoot management: changing surgical trends in Nigeria. Iowa Orthop J. 2010;30:7–14.
7. Ayana B, Klungsoyr PJ. Good results after Ponseti treatment for neglected congenital clubfoot in Ethiopia. A prospective study of 22 children (32 feet) from 2 to 10 years of age. Acta Orthop. 2014;85(6):641–5.
8. Ponseti IV. Congenital clubfoot. Fundamentals of treatment. Oxford: Oxford University Press; 1996.
9. Morcuende JA, Dolan LA, Dietz FR, Ponseti IV. Radical reduction in the rate of extensive corrective surgery for clubfoot using Ponseti method. Pediatrics. 2004;113(2):376–80.
10. Verma A, Mehtani A, Sural S, Maini L, Gautam VK, Basran SS, et al. Management of idiopathic clubfoot in toddlers by Ponseti's method. J Pediatr Orthop B. 2012;21(1):79–84.
11. Sinha A, Mehtani A, Sud A, Vijay V, Kumar N, Prakash J. Evaluation of Ponseti method in neglected clubfoot. Indian J Orthop. 2016;50(5):529–35.
12. Faizan M, Jilani LZ, Abbas M, Zahid M, Asif N. Management of idiopathic clubfoot by Ponseti technique in children presenting after one year of age. J Foot Ankle Surg. 2015;54(5):967–72.
13. Wang YZ, Wang XW, Zhang P, Wang XS. Application of Ponseti method in patients older than 6 months with congenital talipes equinovarus. Beijing Da Xue Xue Bao. 2009;41(4):452–5.
14. Spiegel DA, Shrestha OP, Sitoula P, Rajbhandary T, Bijukachhe B, Banskota AK. Ponseti method for untreated idiopathic clubfeet in Nepalese patients from 1 to 6 years of age. Clin Orthop Relat Res. 2009;467(5):1164–70.
15. Yagmurlu MF, Ermis MN, Akdeniz HE, Kesin E, Karakas ES. Ponseti management of clubfoot after walking age. Pediatr Int. 2011;53(1):85–9.

16. Hassan MK, Ibrahim AH, Mostafa MM, Bakr HA. Ponseti method for management of neglected idiopathic clubfoot. Curr Orthop Pract. 2013;24(3):295–7.
17. Hegazy M, Nasef NM, Abdel-Ghani H. Results of treatment of idiopathic clubfoot in older infants using the Ponseti method: a preliminary report. J Pediatr Orthop B. 2009;18(2):76–8.
18. Gul A, Sambandam S. Results of manipulation of idiopathic clubfoot deformity in Malawi by orthopedic clinical officers using the Ponseti method: a realistic alternative for the developing world? J Pediatr Orthop. 2007;27(8):971; author reply 971–2.
19. Alves C, Battle AE, Rodriguez MV. Neglected clubfoot treated by serial casting: a narrative review on how possibility takes over disability. Ann Transl Med. 2021;9(13):1103.
20. Nogueira MP, Duarte PS, Lourenço AF, Tedesco AP, Ferreira LA, Forlin E, et al. Ponseti Brasil: a national program to eradicate neglected clubfoot – preliminary results. Iowa Orthop J. 2011;31:43–8.
21. Banskota B, Banskota AK, Regmi R, Rajbhandary T, Shrestha OP, Spiegel DA. The Ponseti method in the treatment of children with idiopathic clubfoot presenting between five and ten years of age. Bone Joint J. 2013;95-B(12):1721–5.
22. Ferreira GF, Stéfani KC, Haje DP, Nogueira MP. The Ponseti method in children with clubfoot after walking age - systematic review and metanalysis of observational studies. PLoS One. 2018;13(11):e0207153.
23. Haje DP, Maranho DA, Ferreira GF, Rocha Geded AC, Aroojis A, Queiroz AC, et al. Ponseti method after walking age - a multi-centric study of 429 feet: results, possible treatment modifications and outcomes according to age groups. Iowa Orthop J. 2020;40(2):1–12.
24. Agarwal A. Ponseti method for late presentation of clubfoot. Int Orthop. 2014;38(1):207–9.
25. Pirani S, Zeznik L, Hodges D. Magnetic resonance imaging study of congenital clubfoot treated by Ponseti method. J Pediatr Orthop. 2001;21(6):719–26.
26. Dimeglio A, Bensahel H, Souchet P, Mazeau P, Bonnet F. Classification of clubfoot. J Pediatr Orthop B. 1995;4(2):129–36.
27. Alves C, Escalda C, Fernandes P, Tavares D, Neves MC. Ponseti method: does age at the treatment make a difference? Clin Orthop Relat Res. 2009;467(5):1271–7.
28. Zymny ML, Willig SJ, Roberts JM, D'Ambrosia RD. An eletron microscopic study of the fascia from the medial and lateral side of clubfoot. Pediatr Orthop. 1985;5:577.
29. Fukuhara K, Schollmeier G, Uhthoff H. The pathogenesis of clubfoot. A histomorphometric and immunobiochemical study of fetus. J Bone Joint Surg. 1994;76B:450.
30. Haje DP. Neglected idiopathic clubfoot successfully treated by Ponseti method: a case report of an adult patient who started treatment at 26 years of age. J Orthop Case Rep. 2020;10(4):74–7.
31. Dragoni M, Farsetti P, Vena G, Bellini D, Maglione P, Ippolito E. Ponseti treatment of rigid residual deformity in congenital clubfoot after walking age. J Bone Joint Surg Am. 2016;98(20):1706–12.
32. Terrazas-Lafargue G, Morcuende JÁ. Effect of cast removal timing in the correction of idiopathic clubfoot by the Ponseti method. Iowa Orthop J. 2007;27:24–7.
33. Nogueira MP, Amaral DT. How much remodeling is possible in a clubfoot treatment? Magnetic resonance imaging study in a 7-year-old child. J Limb Lengthening Reconstr. 2018;4(1):49–54.
34. Ponseti International Association. Clinical practice guidelines for the management of clubfoot deformity using the Ponseti method. Iowa: Ponseti International Association; 2015. http://www.ponseti.info/publications---resources.html.
35. Nogueira MP, Farcetta M, Fox MH, Miller KK, Pereira TS, Morcuende JA. Treatment of congenital clubfoot with the Ponseti method: the parents' perspective. J Pediatr Orthop B. 2013;22(6):583–8.
36. Nogueira MP, Fox MH, Miller KK, Morcuende JA. The Ponseti method in Brazil: barriers to bracing compliance. Iowa Orthop J. 2013;33:161–6.
37. Faldini C, Traina F, Nanni M, Sanzarello I, Borghi R, Perna F. Congenital idiopathic talipes equinovarus before and after walking age: observations and strategy of treatment from a series of 88 cases. J Orthop Traumatol. 2016;17(1):81–7.

38. Qureshi AR, Warriach SB. Evaluation of Ponseti method for management of idiopathic clubfoot in toddlers. Pak J Med Health Sci. 2013;7(3):730–2.
39. Garceau GJ, Palmer RM. Transfer of the anterior tibial tendon for recurrent clubfoot. A long-term follow-up. J Bone Joint Surg Am. 1967;49(2):207–31.
40. van Bosse HJ. Treatment of the neglected and relapsed clubfoot. Clin Podiatr Med Surg. 2013;30(4):513–30.
41. Dwyer FC. Osteotomy of the calcaneum for pes cavus. J Bone Joint Surg Br. 1959;41(1):80–6.
42. Ganger R, Radler C, Handbauer A, Grill F. External fixation in clubfoot treatment: a review of the literature. J Pediatr Orthop B. 2012;21(1):52–8.
43. Nogueira MP, Ey AB, Alves C. Is it possible to treat recurrent clubfoot with the Ponseti technique after posteromedial release? - a preliminary study. Clin Orthop Relat Res. 2009;467(5):1298–305.
44. Morton AA. Psychological considerations in the planning of staged reconstruction in limb deficiencies. In: Herring JA, Birch JB, editors. The child with a limb deficiency. 1st ed. Rosemont, IL: American Academy of Orthopaedic Surgeons; 1998. p. 195–205.
45. Richard HM, Nguyen DC, Birch JG, Roland SD, Samchukov MK, Cherkashin AM. Clinical implications of psychosocial factors on pediatric external fixation treatment and recommendations. Clin Orthop Relat Res. 2015;473(10):3154–62.
46. Köse N, Günal GE, Seber S. Treatment of severe residual clubfoot deformity by trans midtarsal osteotomy. J Pediatr Orthop B. 1999;8(4):251–6.
47. Mc Hale KA, Lenhart MK. Treatment of residual clubfoot deformity—the "bean-shaped" foot by opening wedge medial cuneiform osteotomy and closing wedge cuboid osteotomy. Clinical review and cadaver correlations. J Pediatr Orthop. 1991;11(3):374–81.

# Chapter 5
# Management of Atypical Clubfoot: Challenges and Solutions

Nitza N. Rodriguez, Robert J. Spencer, and Matthew B. Dobbs

## Introduction

Congenital talipes equinovarus (CTEV), also known as clubfoot, is one of the most common serious orthopedic birth defects. The standard treatment for clubfoot is manipulation with serial casting as outlined by Ponseti [1, 2]. The Ponseti method has gained popularity for its simple and inexpensive but effective treatment [3–7]. This method is considered the gold standard for treating all clubfeet regardless of the type and etiology [1, 3, 7–11].

Although CTEV is recognizable at birth, the severity may differ widely from mild to extremely rigid and resistant to manipulation and treatment. Most CTEV (~80%) occur as an individual birth defect and are referred to as **isolated clubfoot** (commonly known as idiopathic) [12, 13]. The remaining are **atypical clubfeet** and have been described in the literature as syndromic, neurogenic, non-idiopathic, and treatment-resistant clubfoot [14–18]. Atypical CTEV includes patients with related malformations, chromosomal abnormalities, and known genetic syndromes [14, 19, 20]. There is a small subset of atypical clubfeet referred to as treatment-resistant with soft-tissue abnormalities that display weakness with minor neurological manifestations without associated or identifiable conditions or syndromes [16, 17, 21]. The atypical clubfoot is intrinsically distinct in muscle length, function, and pathoanatomy, often resulting in rigidity of the deformity.

Historically, atypical clubfoot has been described in the literature as difficult to treat and too rigid to correct with the traditional Ponseti method resulting in extensive surgical interventions including radical bony procedures such as arthrodesis or

N. N. Rodriguez (✉) · R. J. Spencer
Southern California Foot and Ankle Specialists, Ladera Ranch, CA, USA

M. B. Dobbs
Paley Institute, St. Mary's Medical Center, West Palm Beach, FL, USA
e-mail: mdobbs@paleyinstitute.org



M. B. Dobbs et al. (eds.), *Clubfoot and Vertical Talus*,
https://doi.org/10.1007/978-3-031-34788-7_5

talectomy [22–26]. Despite the immediate resolve of the deformity, these patients had high recurrence rates and stiff painful feet long term [27–32]. More recent studies have shown promising results with short-term outcomes of treating atypical clubfeet with a modified Ponseti method [14, 20, 33, 34]. The goal for treating atypical clubfoot is to provide a braceable, plantigrade foot with the least amount of invasive surgery and complications. Ideally, correction should be accomplished before walking age to impede the adaptive bone changes. Certain modifications to the treatment are recommended as these clubfeet are more challenging to treat, may require more casts, and require closer monitoring due to higher recurrence rates and potential complications [14, 16, 20, 35, 36]. The heterogeneous nature and characteristics of atypical clubfeet and the challenges and solutions for treatment are discussed in this chapter.

## Atypical Clubfoot

There is a vast range of conditions associated with atypical clubfoot, which include, but are not limited to, arthrogryposis, spina bifida, myelomeningocele, sacral agenesis, amniotic band syndrome, diastrophic dysplasia, congenital myotonic dystrophy, fibular hemimelia, and other neurological disorders [12, 13, 37, 38]. However, arthrogryposis and myelomeningocele are the predominant associations seen [37]. Of the known etiologies of atypical clubfoot, disorders involving the nervous system are the majority [37]. The development of a clubfoot has been postulated to be the final result of a disruption or hit along a common pathway at any point in the neuromuscular unit including the brain, spinal cord, nerve, or muscle [12].

**Arthrogryposis multiplex congenita (AMC)** represents a large group of heterogeneous disorders with multiple non-progressive congenital joint contractures of two or more separate areas of the body. The word "arthrogryposis" is derived from the Greek language for the words joint (arthro-) and crooked or hooked (gryposis). Arthrogryposis is not a specific diagnosis, rather a clinical finding of rigid deformities present at birth and can be characteristic of a group of more than 400 different disorders with a variety of etiologies [39–42]. However, the commonality of all these disorders is fetal akinesia (reduction of spontaneous intrauterine movement) [42, 43]. This lack of movement in the developing fetus causes scarring to occur intra-articularly. More than 320 genes have been linked proving the genetic heterogeneity of the condition [44]. The overall prevalence of arthrogryposis is around 1 in 3000 live births with a high percentage of these being nonprogressive and responsive to physical therapy [45, 46]. The etiology of arthrogryposis is thought to be most likely multifactorial and includes extrinsic and intrinsic factors. The cause can also be associated with pathology in the muscles, connective tissue, and central or peripheral nervous system. Defects in neuromuscular transmission, compromised space in utero or fetal vascular supply, maternal disease, and external factors such as medications and drugs have also been reported [42, 47]. The inheritance and outcomes of arthrogryposis vary among these disorders, so it is crucial to make a specific diagnosis to aid in treatment [40].

Multiple congenital joint contractures are often separated into three different groups: Amyoplasia, Distal Arthrogryposis, and Syndromic (central nervous system and progressive neurological etiology). *Amyoplasia* is the most common form of arthrogryposis multiplex congenita with distinct clinical features comprising about one third of all cases [41, 42]. Amyoplasia occurs sporadically without a pattern of inheritance and is specifically defined as the lack of muscle formation [41, 46]. There is a replacement of skeletal muscle with fibrous tissue and fat. The clinical picture usually presents as affecting all four limbs with the shoulders being internally rotated and adducted, elbows extended, forearms pronated with the wrists ulnarly deviated, and fingers fixed, with the thumbs located in the palm. In the lower extremities, the hips and knees can be dislocated. The knees tend to be extended, and the feet are frequently in a severe equinovarus deformity [41]. The limbs usually have symmetric positioning and a decreased overall muscle mass with a fusiform appearance. These patients lack joint creases and have skin dimpling over joints (Fig. 5.1). Sensation is normal, and most patients have normal mental development [41].

*Distal Arthrogryposis (DA)* is a group of autosomal dominant disorders that are characterized by predominantly distal congenital joint contractures in the hands and feet without a primary neurological and/or muscle disease [40, 41]. DA affects the fast twitch muscle proteins. DA was initially described by Hall et al. in 1982 as arthrogryposis with congenital hand and foot involvement and subdivided them into two categories [45]. They further classified DA into five subgroups (Type IIA–IIE) with distal limb contractures and additional characteristic manifestations [47]. Bamshad et al. further revised and expanded this classification in 1996 to differentiate DA disorders from other conditions with distal extremity contractures [40]. The most commonly described forms of DA are DA1 and DA2B (Sheldon–Hall syndrome). However, Freeman–Sheldon syndrome (DA2A) is deemed as the most severe type of DA [48].

All of the other genetic or nongenetic disorders of arthrogryposis are grouped into the *syndromic arthrogryposis* and can be divided into two categories: central nervous system etiology and progressive neurological etiology.

Though arthrogryposis affects multiple joints, the foot and ankle are the most commonly involved [39]. Clubfoot is the most frequent foot deformity in arthrogryposis and is usually stiffer and more severe when compared to isolated clubfoot [39, 49–53]. The presence of multiple deformities requiring treatment makes the management of these atypical clubfeet more difficult [54]. Clubfeet associated with arthrogryposis have been commonly treated with either a radical soft-tissue release or talectomy resulting in varying outcomes [50, 51, 55]. Radical soft-tissue releases are associated with higher rates of relapse, which lead to repeat soft-tissue releases or salvage procedures [23, 25, 39, 54, 56, 57]. Due to poor outcomes, there has been a gradual shift to conservative treatment with manipulation and serial casting before an extensive surgical procedure is considered [25, 39, 46, 50, 51, 53, 54, 56–62].

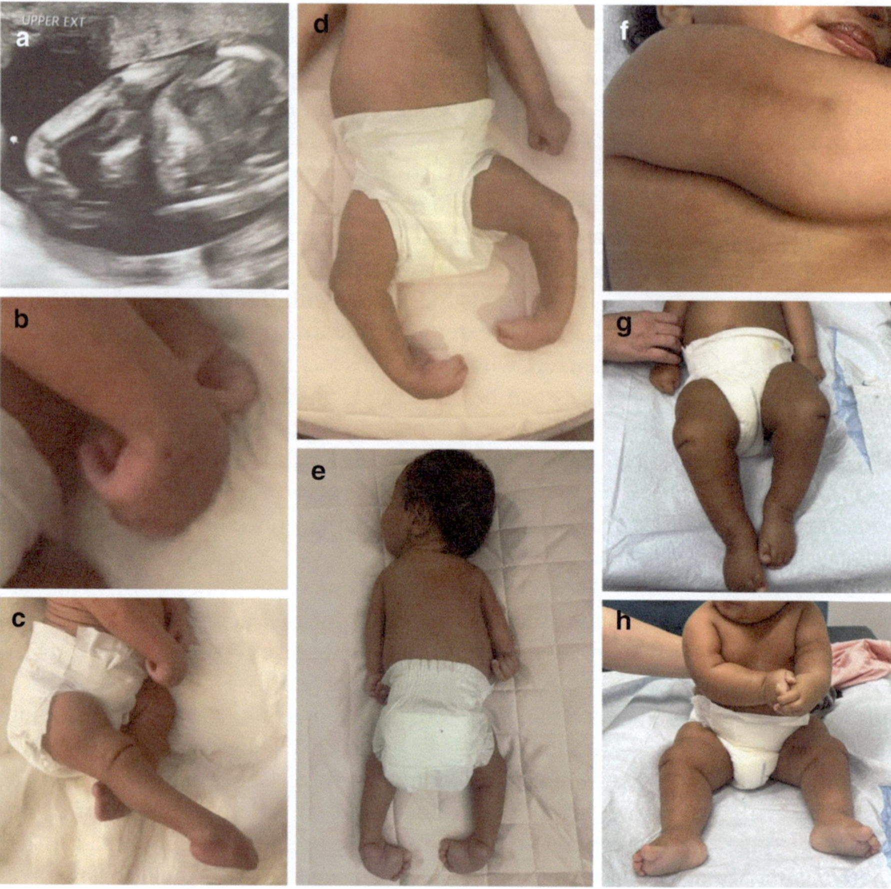

**Fig. 5.1** This is an infant with bilateral atypical clubfoot and arthrogryposis. (**a**) Ultrasound demonstrating the elbow extension and wrist involvement. (**b**) Newborn with wrist involvement. (**c**) Knee extended with severe equinovarus deformity. Note the dimple in the Right knee. (**d**, **e**) Showing the shoulders internally rotated and adducted, elbows extended, forearms pronated with the wrists ulnarly deviated and fingers fixed, with the thumbs located in the palm, and severe clubfoot bilateral. (**f**) Note a lack of joint crease at the elbow and prominent line along the arm. (**g**, **h**) At 2 months, after clubfoot correction and therapies initiated

Boehm et al. reported good outcomes in 92% of the children with distal arthrogryposis treated using the Ponseti method [14]. Van Bosse et al. also demonstrated promising results in all 19 clubfeet with arthrogryposis treated with a modified Ponseti method where they performed an initial percutaneous Achilles tenotomy before initiating the weekly Ponseti casting [63]. Church et al. compared 5-year outcomes between isolated clubfoot and clubfoot with arthrogryposis. They demonstrated successful treatment with the Ponseti method in creating a braceable foot that can delay the need for invasive surgical interventions [34].

There is a spectrum of severity and presentation in patients with arthrogryposis. The ultimate purpose of the treatment is to make a braceable foot with a plantigrade platform. This is done with the least amount of surgery and minimizes the chances of recurrence. Early treatment in these patients is recommended so that more fluid range of motion can be initiated sooner preventing adaptive changes [36]. Although it is best to make an accurate diagnosis to ensure understanding of all the components involved, this is not always possible. Patients with arthrogryposis are sensate and have an average or above intellect. Care is taken to evaluate all other joints involved and address any needed treatment accordingly. Managing expectations is imperative as it is impossible to restore an abnormally developed joint. Proper education helps families understand that relapses occur regardless of treatment.

**Spina Bifida** is another common condition associated with atypical clubfoot. Spina bifida is a congenital neural tube defect, which results in the vertebral column being open with possible spinal cord involvement. *Myelomeningocele,,* the most common and severe form, is a failure of the spinal neural tube closure leaving exposed neural tissue. This results in motor and sensory deficits below the level of the lesion affecting the motor function and ambulatory aptitude. Spina bifida is often associated with other spinal cord lesions or structural abnormalities of the brain (hydrocephalus) [64]. Hydrocephalus is present to some extent in up to 85% of these patients [65]. In the past, the combination of hydrocephalus and incomplete closure of the spinal column led to low survival rates or full-time use of a wheelchair. Presently, most children have the potential to be ambulatory with early surgical intervention allowing closure of the spinal defect and successful treatment to control the hydrocephalus [66].

The incidence of myelomeningocele varies geographically but has been decreasing overall and is around 1.9/10,000 births in the United States [64, 65]. Although the incidence is decreasing, it is still considered a significant chronic condition causing disability affecting between 70,000 and 100,000 people in the United States [64]. The largest known risk factors are genetics and dietary deficiencies [65]. Folic acid supplementation has been shown to significantly reduce the incidence of myelomeningocele [64, 67, 68]. The actual etiology of spina bifida is unknown; however, it is thought to be multifactorial with folate deficiency playing a key contributor along with both genetics and various environmental factors [64, 69, 70].

Most patients with myelomeningocele are born with various foot deformities including vertical talus and clubfoot [71, 72]. However, clubfoot is the most common foot deformity in myelomeningocele [22, 66]. The clubfoot deformity incidence is dependent on the neurological level of involvement [72]. Clubfoot develops in ~90% of thoracic or lumbar levels (L3 and L4 being the most common) and ~50% of patients with sacral level of involvement [72].

The combination of motor paralysis/spasticity, sensory loss, muscle imbalance and deformity in patients with myelomeningocele make their clubfoot treatment challenging. These feet are known to be severely rigid and resistant to treatment, comparable to the arthrogrypotic clubfoot [20, 72]. Due to the rigidity and severity of this deformity, historically clubfoot associated with myelomeningocele has also been treated with extensive surgical interventions [22, 24, 66, 73–75]. Starting in

2008, reports discussing the treatment of clubfoot associated with myelomeningocele with the Ponseti technique and minimal amount of extensive surgery have emerged [12, 15, 20].

Gerlach et al. reported on 16 patients with 28 clubfeet associated with myelomeningocele and compared the outcomes to 20 patients with 35 isolated clubfeet (control group), prospectively. Initial correction was obtained in 96% of the myelomeningocele. The mean number of casts for correction were similar for the two groups. The correction was maintained with either a standard or a dynamic foot abduction brace. The rate of relapse was found to be significantly higher (68%) in the myelomeningocele group compared with 26% in the isolated group. After final follow-up at an average of 34 months, successful treatment without the need for extensive soft-tissue release or tendon transfer was accomplished in 86% of the myelomeningocele group and 97% of the isolated clubfeet [20]. Other studies have also reported promising results in this patient population using the Ponseti technique [12, 15, 76–80].

The goal of treatment is a plantigrade, supple foot that is braceable with the greatest amount of range of motion. These insensate patients are at higher risk for complications and deformities during casting including tibial bowing, skin complications, and iatrogenic fractures [20]. The absence of nerve innervation affects the vascularity and thus the bone health resulting in fragile bones. This decrease or lack of sensation can also make it easy to be overly aggressive with manipulation during casting since the child does not resist or cry. The congenital impairment causing decreased sensation and muscular activity results in less axial load to their lower extremities predisposing them to low bone mineral density and possible fractures [81]. It is important to consider these characteristics to avoid possible complications in this population.

**Tethered Cord Syndrome (TCS)** occurs when the caudal section of the spinal cord attaches to the meninges resulting in a tethering effect, which limits its movement. This attachment leads to increased pressure and progressive stretching of the spinal cord with growth of the child resulting in varying neurological symptoms [82]. There has been evidence that clubfoot may be associated with TCS [83–86]. Jackson et al. demonstrated acceptable outcomes with using the Ponseti treatment for clubfoot associated with TCS compared with isolated clubfoot, however, they required an increased number of casts [87]. It is important to rule out space-occupying lesions that can be causing the tethered cord (Fig. 5.2). Clubfeet associated with tethered cord should be closely followed by a neurologist and/or neurosurgeon that can determine the proper treatment necessary as surgical intervention of the spine may be required to prevent or reverse progressive neurological symptoms helping to decrease clubfoot relapse.

**Sacral agenesis** is a rare birth defect resulting in absence of the sacrum or lower spine with varying degrees of severity. The incidence varies between 0.01 and 0.05 per 1000 live births and is highly associated with maternal diabetes [88]. Clinical manifestations are based on the severity of disease and may be associated with limb and joint contractures including clubfoot and less commonly vertical talus [89].

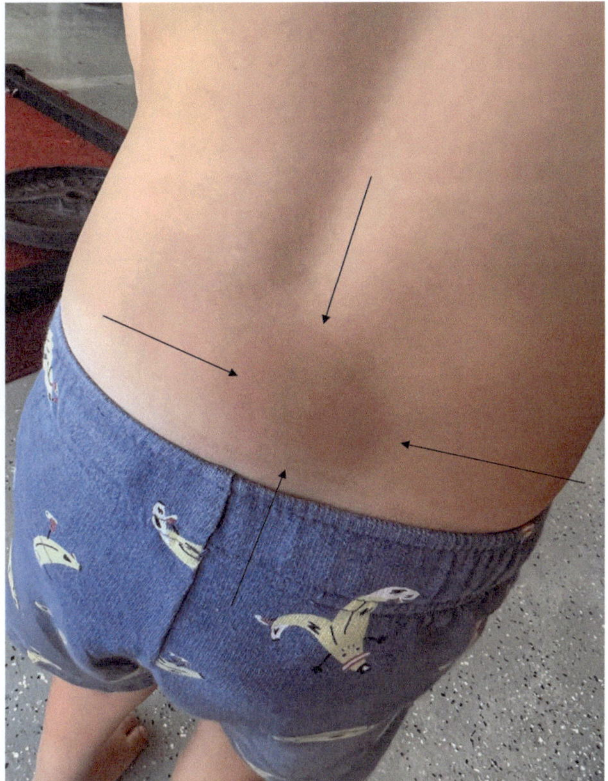

**Fig. 5.2** A 4-year-old boy with a lipoma at the L4–L5 vertebrae and tethered cord with atypical left clubfoot

Sacral agenesis is divided into four types with Type I characterized as partial or complete unilateral sacral agenesis. Type II involves partial bilateral symmetric agenesis of the sacrum. In Type III, there is total sacral agenesis and variable lumbar involvement with the ilia articulating with the lowest sides of the vertebra that is present. Type IV is similar to Type III except the caudal endplate of the vertebra rests above a fused ilia or an iliac amphiarthrosis [90]. With sacral agenesis, the neurological involvement is correlated with the corresponding level of involvement [90]. Patients with sacral agenesis usually have their protective sensation intact, which is a way to differentiate from myelomeningocele.

**Amniotic band syndrome (ABS)** is a congenital disorder thought to be a result of separation of the amnion from the chorion leading to the development of fibrous bands that are tied around the limbs or digits [91–93] (Fig. 5.3). The resultant oligo-hydramnios from the disruption of the fetal membrane is considered to be linked to a high incidence of clubfoot. Clubfoot deformity has been documented to be present with ABS in a range between 12% and 56% [23, 91, 94–98]. More current literature has supported the treatment of clubfoot associated with ABS using the standard Ponseti method [15, 92, 93, 99]. Physicians treating clubfoot associated with ABS should proceed with correcting the clubfoot using the modified Ponseti technique

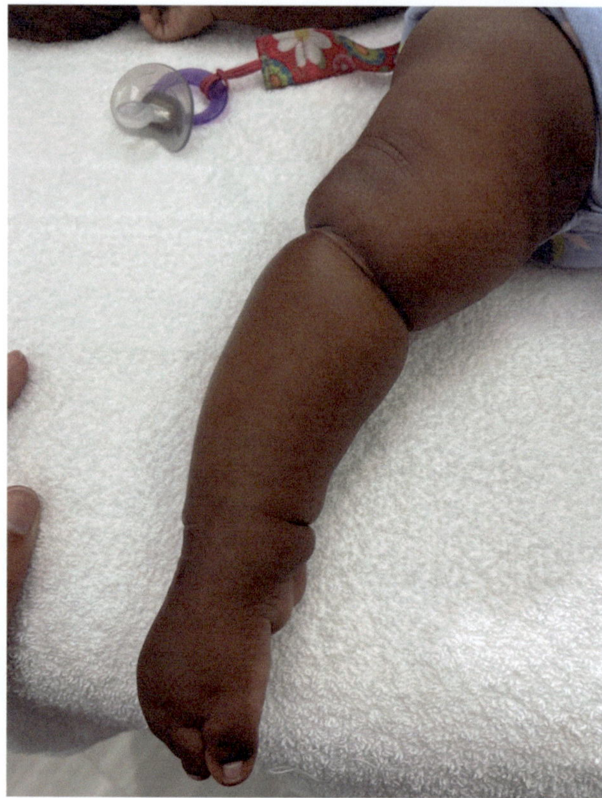

**Fig. 5.3** Infant with atypical clubfoot associated with amniotic band syndrome

and address the amniotic bands at the same time if possible. Depending on the location and severity of the bands, these can cause severe lymphedema, vascular compromise, and neurological symptoms, which may require immediate intervention.

**Diastrophic dysplasia** is an autosomal recessive disorder, which affects the development of cartilage and bone. The diagnosis relies on a combination of clinical, radiographic, and histopathologic features [100, 101]. This disorder is recognizable at birth with specific characteristics including an abducted, hypermobile, and proximally placed thumb. Other notable deformities include the absence of flexion creases and shortness of stature with micromelia, short broad hands with ankylosis of the proximal interphalangeal joints, and severe bilateral clubfoot deformity [101].

**Myotonic muscular dystrophy** is an autosomal dominant disorder of muscle that affects multiple systems in the body. The muscular dystrophies are characterized by muscle weakness and myotonia, cardiac abnormalities, cataracts, and other abnormalities. This disorder is divided into two forms: Myotonic muscular dystrophy Type 1 (DM1) and Myotonic muscular dystrophy Type 2 (DM2). Both forms are caused by different gene mutations resulting in varying clinical presentations. DM1 is generally more severe and associated with congenital disorders such as clubfoot, and DM2 is usually less common and with milder symptoms that appear later in adolescents or adulthood [102–104].

**Fibular hemimelia** is the most common congenital deficiency of long bones and may be associated with clubfoot. The primary characteristic of the condition ranges from mild shortening to complete absence of the fibula. Fibular hemimelia syndrome can be associated with varying degrees of fibular hypoplasia, shortening of the tibia and femur, genu valgum, lateral femoral condyle hypoplasia, ligament laxity of the knee, tibial bowing, a ball and socket ankle joint, tarsal coalitions, and missing lateral rays [105]. Children with fibular hemimelia always have a limb length inequality but ranges in severity from mild to severe. Mild limb length inequalities should be addressed with a full-length lift insert inside the shoe, and more severe limb length discrepancies greater than one-half inch should be treated with an additional modification to the sole of the shoe. If the physician fails to address the limb inequality, the shorter limb could lead to increased equinus, which would likely cause a recurrence of the clubfoot deformity. Once the child reaches an older age, a proximal tibial epiphysiodesis closure is considered for correction of the limb length discrepancy that are in general less than 3–4 cm. Predicted discrepancies greater than this can be addressed with limb lengthening surgery. When treating children with fibular hemimelia, it is important to rule out tarsal coalitions. Tarsal coalitions make corrections more challenging and bracing more difficult.

**Treatment-resistant atypical clubfoot with soft-tissue abnormalities** have been described as a subset of atypical clubfeet with minor neurological manifestations without associated conditions or syndromes [16, 17, 21]. Song et al. reported on a small group of patients having a "peroneal nerve palsy" with the loss of active dorsiflexion of the toes and ankle despite stimulation of the foot without a related syndrome or neuromuscular disorder. All of the patients had an abnormal electromyography (EMG) and nerve conduction velocity (NCV) tests and were difficult to treat with the traditional Ponseti method leading to surgical interventions [21]. Edmonds and Frick similarly described a small number of patients with a "drop toe sign" who lacked the ability to actively dorsiflex their toes and ankle with plantar stimulation and were unresponsive to the original Ponseti method. They performed magnetic resonance imaging (MRIs) of the cervical, thoracic, and lumbar spine in some of their patients, which all resulted in normal findings. They recommended using the modified Ponseti technique to correct these clubfeet [16]. More recent studies evaluated magnetic resonance (MR) Angiography (MRA) and MRIs of clubfeet, which demonstrated significant differences in soft-tissue anatomy in the treatment-responsive versus treatment-resistant clubfeet [17, 106]. In 2011, Merrill et al. evaluated MRAs of a small group of clubfeet and concluded that vascular anomalies correlated with decreased fat and muscle volumes and reduced tibial length. They postulated that these findings might be associated with recurrent clubfeet [106]. In another study, clubfeet with soft-tissue anomalies have been described as treatment-resistant with varying degrees of increased epimysial fat deposition, intramuscular fat deposition, or specific muscle compartment hypoplasia or any combination as seen on MRI of the lower extremity [17]. All of these studies reported a higher risk of treatment resistance and greater recurrence rate in this patient population [16, 17, 21, 106]. Patients that do not dorsiflex their toes or evert their foot are considered atypical even without a known underlying neurologic condition or syndrome. This is postulated to be a result of an altered transcription factor expression in early limb bud formation leading to varying clinical outcomes [106–108].

When comparing atypical to isolated clubfeet, they have been reportedly treated with extensive soft-tissue releases or even talectomy due to the rigid nature of the foot and resistance to casting [22–25]. However, research also shows that children respond better long term by avoiding the need for extensive surgery. Aggressive soft-tissue release and talectomy are associated with inconsistency and a high rate of short-term and long-term complications [27–29, 109]. These complications can lead to tibiocalcaneal arthritis, painful ambulation, spontaneous tibiocalcaneal fusion, and relapse of the deformity of the hindfoot requiring further surgery [50, 55, 110]. Treatment of clubfoot specifically in association with Arthrogryposis multiplex congenita is difficult. This is due to the foot and ankle rigidity and severity of deformity, resistance to correction, high rate of recurrence, and the combination of hip and knee contractures [36, 111].

In recent years, there have been more reports confirming that atypical clubfoot can be successfully treated with the Ponseti method [12, 14, 15, 20, 36, 77, 111, 112]. These studies have found that treating atypical clubfoot with the Ponseti method have short-term good results; however, they may require more casts and have a higher rate of recurrence when compared to isolated clubfoot [14]. Gurnett et al. found that there was no significant difference in the need for extensive surgery between atypical and isolated clubfoot [12]. Using the modified Ponseti casting method in atypical clubfoot will allow the greatest reduction of the severity of the deformity and thus reducing the magnitude of surgeries required. The goals for atypical clubfoot should be different than for isolated clubfoot. The goal of treatment is to have a neutral plantigrade braceable foot. In many of these atypical clubfeet, neutral or 5 degrees of dorsiflexion is acceptable as correction in the sagittal plane since many do not have active dorsiflexion ability.

## Treatment of Atypical Clubfoot

The management of all types of atypical clubfoot is challenging. Early recognition is paramount in achieving good outcomes in these patients. Some atypical clubfeet may not be recognized initially and start to develop complications when attempting the traditional Ponseti method. The modified Ponseti technique is recommended when treating atypical clubfoot.

A thorough history and physical exam is an integral component of treatment. Obtaining a family history and inquiring about prenatal testing, pregnancy and delivery complications, prior treatment history, and any known congenital defects or neuromuscular disorders are essential. A comprehensive physical exam is performed. The patient is completely undressed and examined from head to toe including the spine. The head, neck, and face are assessed for signs of torticollis or other indications of a syndrome. The spine is inspected from top to bottom for any masses,

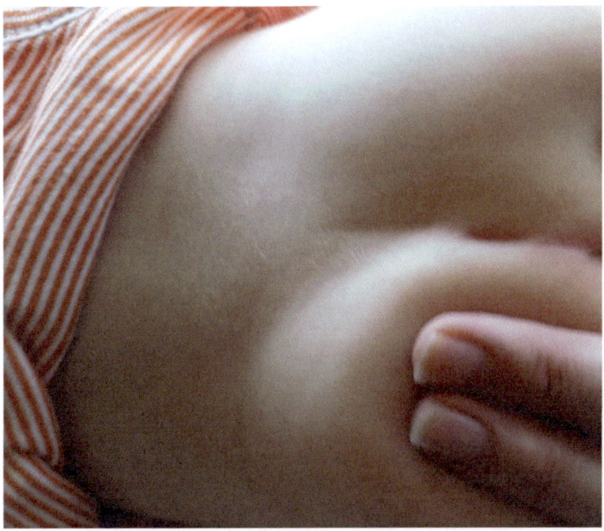

**Fig. 5.4** The photograph shows an infant with a sacral dimple

birthmarks, skin tags, tuft of hair, or sacral dimples (Fig. 5.4). It is important to rule out spinal cord abnormalities including tethered cord or sacral agenesis. The upper and lower limbs are examined for range of motion, tone, and deformity (Fig. 5.5a). A hip examination is performed to rule out hip dysplasia. Observations of the length of the legs and girth of the thighs and calves are documented. A comprehensive lower-extremity examination is performed to rule out any other pathology (Fig. 5.6).

These feet, especially with arthrogryposis, are generally more stiff and severe in appearance. Plantar stimulation is performed on all clubfeet to ensure the child dorsiflexes their ankles and splays their toes. A "drop toe" sign is observed in many atypical clubfeet resulting in the toes resting in a plantarflexed position (Fig. 5.7). Special attention is focused on assessing for "dimpling" of joints in particular the dorsal aspect of the metatarsophalangeal joints (Fig. 5.8). These findings are due to the lack of movement in utero, which may also be associated with glossy appearance of the skin devoid of wrinkles (Fig. 5.9). Evaluation of evertor muscle function is assessed and repeated at all subsequent office visits. The foot is examined for any plantar and posterior creases (Fig. 5.10). Identifying associated conditions is crucial in developing the proper treatment plan and predicting these patient's prognosis.

The materials used for treating atypical clubfoot are important. It is recommended to use plaster of paris, a material that allows shaping and molding, which is fundamental in identification of anatomic landmarks crucial for atypical clubfoot correction. Soft rolls and fiberglass casts do not allow the precise molding that is accomplished with plaster. This is especially important when treating atypical clubfoot since these are known to be more complicated and rigid. Soft rolls can be too soft allowing bending of the knee and movement increasing the chance of complications. Plaster cast application allows the provider to contour the entire leg preventing movement or slippage and capturing the desired corrected position. If plaster casts are used but not molded correctly, the efforts are futile and no different than

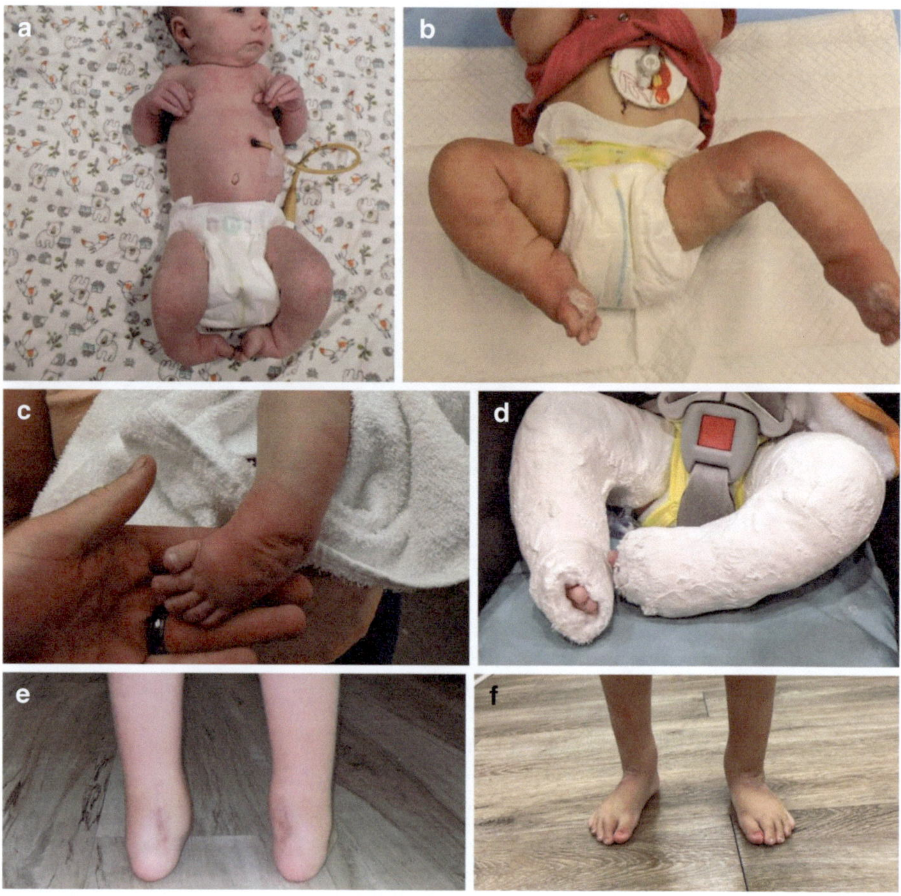

**Fig. 5.5** Patient with bilateral clubfoot associated with arthrogryposis. (**a**) Infant before treatment. Notice the hand involvement and severe clubfoot. (**b–d**) Patient started treatment at another institute. Notice excessive plaster used and the swelling after cast removal. (**e, f**) After transfer of care, the patient was corrected with the modified Ponseti technique. Patient suffered a relapse at 2 years old and was treated with the modified Ponseti technique and open tenotomies with posterior releases. Patient is 4 years old showing maintenance of correction

using the other materials, which may lead to complications (Fig. 5.5) and possible wounds especially in the insensate atypical clubfoot.

It is essential to use above-the-knee casts when treating atypical clubfoot. Casts are applied from toe to groin to prevent the ankle and talus from rotating. Above the knee casts allow for the best correction since the gastrocnemius muscle originates above the knee allowing for better immobilization and control of the deforming forces. If application is far below the groin or below the knee, treatment can also be compromised due to slipping causing various degrees of deformity. Another cause for slipping in patients who have full range of motion in their lower extremities is not achieving enough bend in the knee leading to motion and possible further

**Fig. 5.6** A 6-month-old male with atypical clubfoot and medial dislocation of the patella with noted dimpling and inability to fully extend his left leg

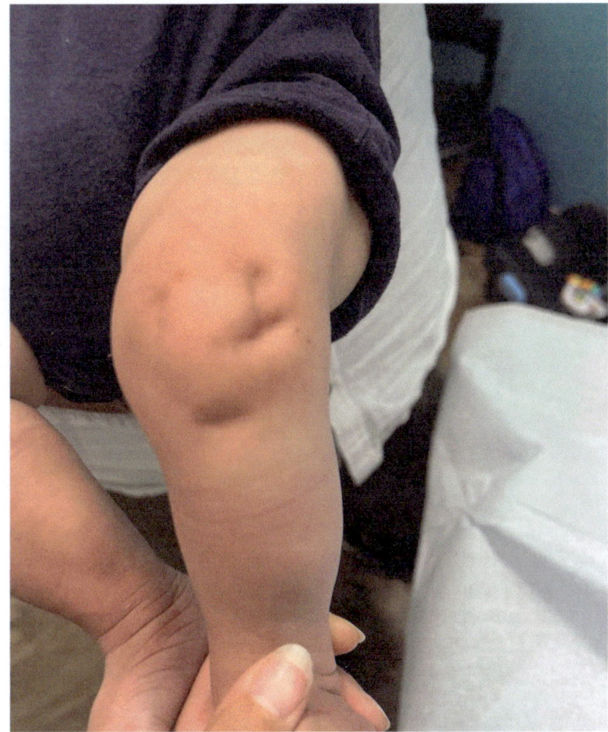

**Fig. 5.7** This photograph depicts a left atypical neurogenic clubfoot with a diagnosis of a tethered cord and a lipoma in the spine at the level of L4–5, the same patient from Fig. 5.2. The left foot is in a severe equinus position with a noted "drop toe" sign

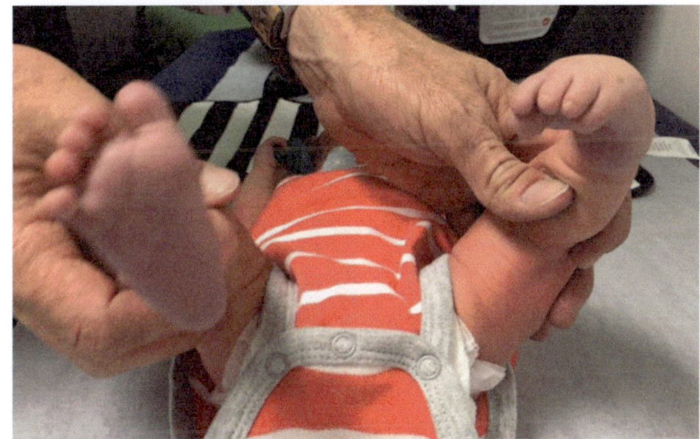

deformity. It is important to be aware of any knee or hip disorders when treating atypical clubfoot and making proper adjustments. Casting should be done with minimal padding to prevent motion and slipping, but care should be taken to protect skin especially in the atypical clubfeet that have sensory deficits. A thorough dermatological exam is performed after every cast change to prevent further complications.

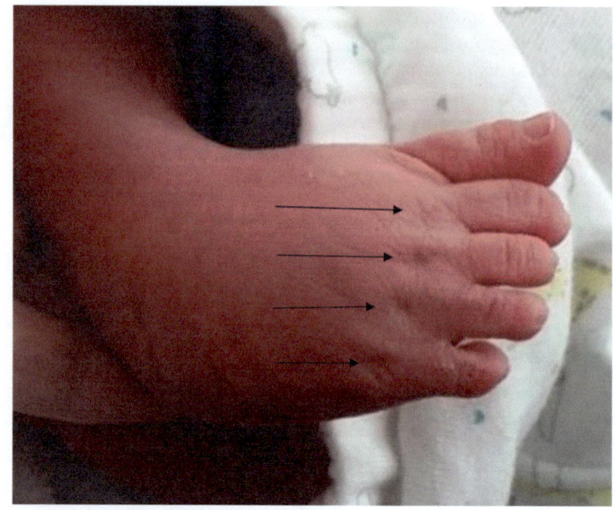

**Fig. 5.8** The photograph shows an atypical clubfoot illustrating the "dimpling" of the dorsal aspect of the metatarsophalangeal joints

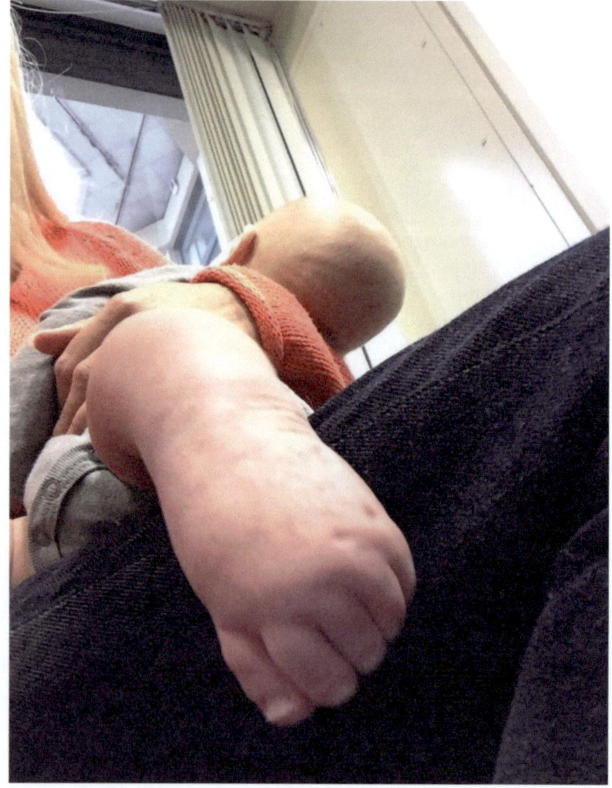

**Fig. 5.9** This is a 2½ month-old male with a tethered cord. Note the "glossy" appearance of the skin and dimpling at the fourth and fifth metatarsophalangeal joints

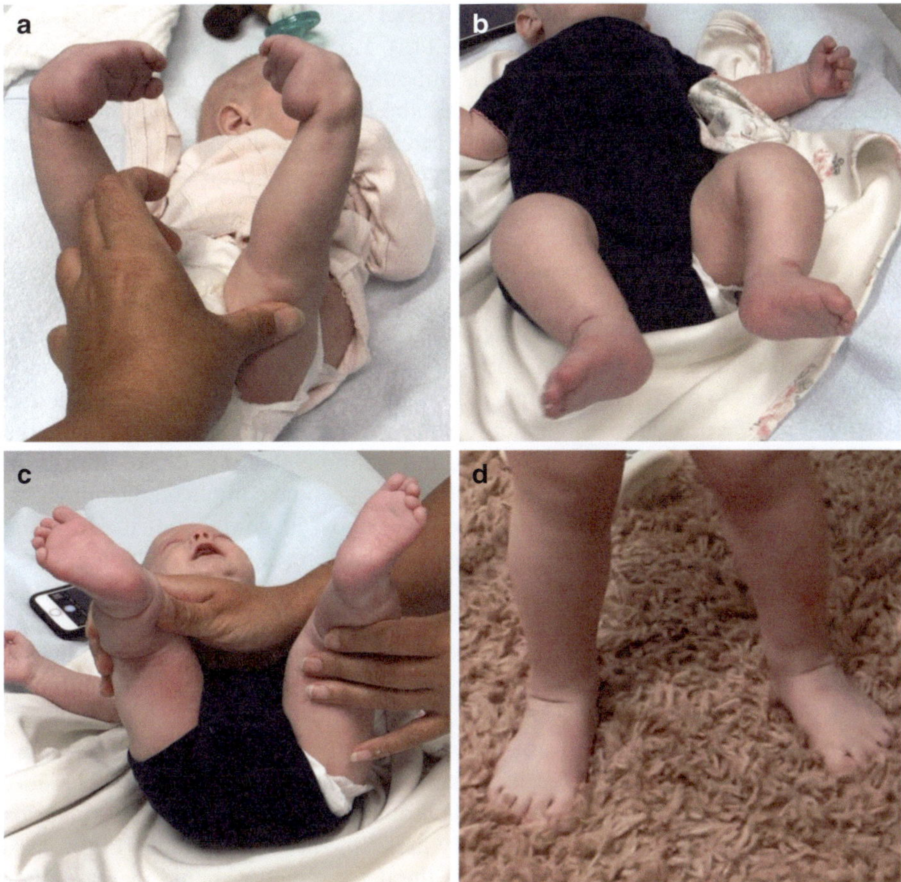

**Fig. 5.10** Patient with atypical bilateral clubfoot. (**a**) 1-month-old female with prominent plantar and posterior creases prior to treatment. (**b**, **c**) 3 months old after modified Ponseti casting technique. (**d**) Patient at 3 years old with maintained correction and no history of relapse

## Modified Ponseti Technique

It is recommended that atypical clubfoot be treated with the modified Ponseti technique as described by Ponseti et al. in 2006 [9, 14]. Ponseti et al. detailed a subset of clubfeet as being resistant to the traditional Ponseti method calling them "complex" and described a modified casting protocol for treatment [9]. Complex clubfoot is defined as a subset of isolated clubfeet that are short and stubby with severe equinus and plantarflexion of all metatarsals, a short hyperextended first toe and prominent plantar medial and posterior crease. Complex clubfeet are resistant to the standard Ponseti casting technique or iatrogenic as the result of improper casting.

The terms atypical and complex clubfoot have been discussed together and used interchangeably in the literature [76, 113–115]. However, as we learn more about clubfoot and its different categories, it is important to distinguish between atypical and complex clubfoot. Despite the fact that the Ponseti "complex clubfoot" study excluded syndromic feet, it supports the idea of adapting the Ponseti technique to include atypical clubfeet. Since this publication, there have been some studies supporting the use of the modified Ponseti technique for atypical clubfeet [14, 111]. Although the casting technique performed would be similar, regarding them as separate entities will inform proper management. The bracing treatment, relapse rates, and expected outcomes in atypical clubfeet are different and additional considerations are taken. Modifying the treatment regimen for atypical clubfoot usually results in correction with the least amount of surgical intervention [14, 111].

It is advised to delay casting until the infant reaches a normal birth weight and size allowing the practitioner to better identify the appropriate anatomic landmarks or allowing any other medical or surgical interventions that might take priority in stabilizing the patient. If the atypical clubfoot has become complicated from previous treatment with soft-tissue edema and/or wounds, it is important to allow the sores to heal and soft-tissue swelling to resolve before casting is reinitiated. Once the soft tissues heal, better manipulation is achieved preventing further complications.

The modified Ponseti technique consists of first identifying the subtalar joint by holding the toes and metatarsals with one hand while feeling the malleoli anteriorly with the thumb and index finger of the second hand (Fig. 5.11a). The thumb and index finger are then positioned anteriorly to grasp the head of the talus and feel the navicular on one side and the anterior tuberosity of the calcaneus on the other side. Motion is felt at the subtalar joint when the foot is slowly abducted, and the anterior tuberosity of the calcaneus moves laterally under the head of the talus (Fig. 5.11b, c). Motion is dependent on the severity of the deformity and should increase after the initial castings if proper technique has been performed. Clear identification of the head of the talus is paramount but may be difficult as it can be less prominent than the anterior tuberosity of the calcaneus. During cast application, the index finger rests over the posterior aspect of the lateral malleolus while the thumb of the same hand applies counter pressure over the lateral aspect of the head of the talus, not on the very prominent tuberosity of the calcaneus as this can inhibit calcaneal reduction (Fig. 5.12).

Next, hyperflexion of the metatarsals and rigid equinus are corrected simultaneously to prevent slippage. A posterior splint is applied behind the calf, heel, and sole and incorporated into a well-molded plaster cast immobilizing the foot in the correct position and avoiding the need for excessive plaster (Fig. 5.13a). The "four-finger technique" is performed by grasping the foot and ankle with both hands while the thumbs are placed under the metatarsals pushing the foot into dorsiflexion as an assistant stabilizes the knee in flexion (Fig. 5.13b). It is important not to hyperabduct the metatarsals and hindfoot. The knee is immobilized in flexion by applying another anterior splint from the thigh to the anterior leg and reinforcing it with plaster around the thigh (Fig. 5.13c, d). Using splints avoids excessive plaster behind

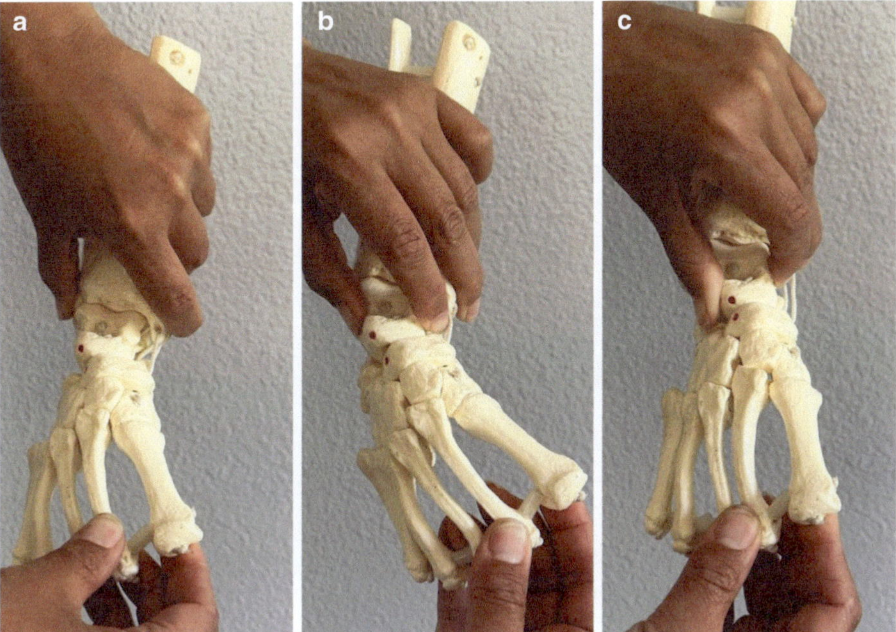

**Fig. 5.11** Model showing position of the talus and identification of the subtalar joint motion. (**a**) Identification of the subtalar joint starts with grasping the forefoot with one hand and with the second hand feeling anteriorly the lateral malleolus with the thumb and medial malleolus with the index finger. (**b**, **c**) The thumb and index finger are moved forward to palpate the head of the talus and feel the navicular on one side and the anterior tuberosity of the calcaneus on the other side. Motion is felt at the subtalar joint when the foot is slowly abducted, and the anterior tuberosity of the calcaneus moves laterally under the head of the talus

the knee and in front of the ankle. Typically, these patients are casted to their end range of motion. If any knee and hip extensions and/or flexions are remaining, they can be addressed later if they are problematic. Patients with clubfoot associated with myelomeningocele who also have congenital knee dislocations are managed with a modified casting protocol to address both deformities simultaneously [116].

It is recommended not to abduct more than 40°. Care is taken not to over abduct the foot to prevent tightening of the flexor tendons and the quadratus plantae muscle resulting in an increase of the cavus deformity. Casts are changed every 5–7 days similar to the traditional Ponseti protocol [117].

Most atypical clubfoot patients require an Achilles tenotomy to address the equinus and achieve full correction. The Achilles tenotomy is performed 1.5 cm above the posterior skin crease of the heel. The posterior tuberosity of the calcaneus is typically very high given the severe contracture of the Achilles. The goal is to achieve a plantigrade braceable foot. The authors have observed that ankle dorsiflexion can be less in this group of patients when compared to isolated clubfeet. In patients with prior treatment, a second tenotomy may be required to achieve correction. When repeating an Achilles tenotomy, a mini-open procedure is preferred to

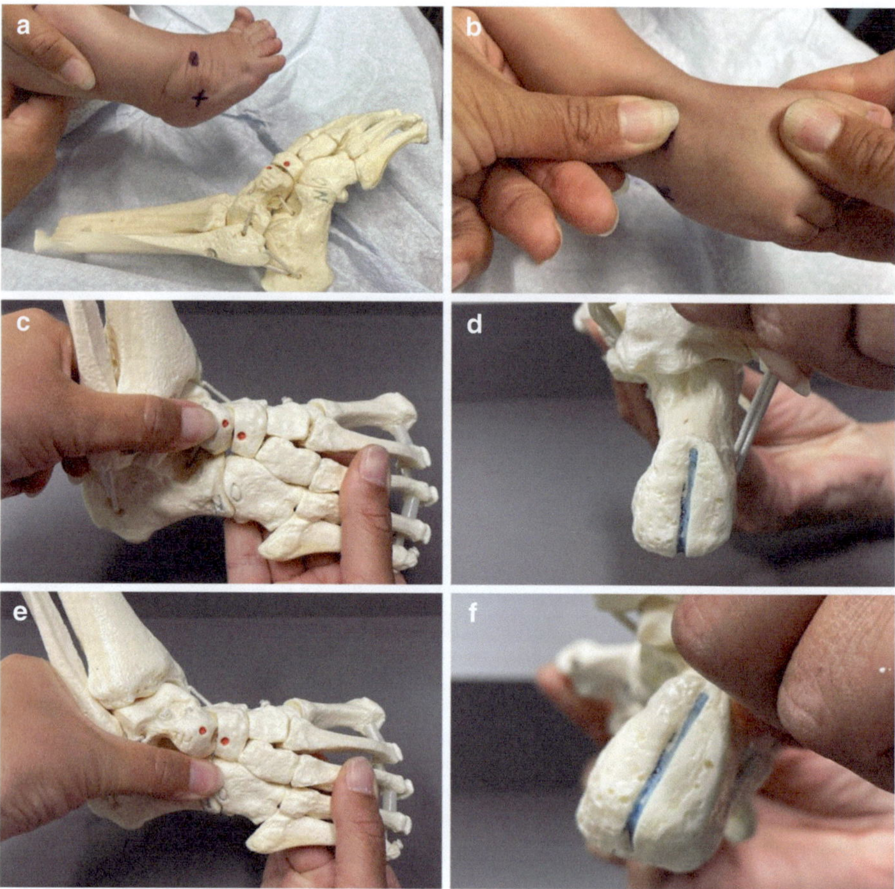

**Fig. 5.12** Hand placement for manipulation of atypical clubfoot. (**a**) Photograph demonstrating anatomical placement with the dots depicting the correct position at the lateral aspect of the talar head versus the "X" indicating the calcaneal cuboid joint and where not to place the thumb. (**b**) The index finger resting over the posterior aspect of the lateral malleolus while the thumb of the same hand applies counter pressure over the lateral aspect of the head of the talus. (**c**, **d**) Anatomical model showing correct manipulation technique with the index finger resting over the lateral malleolus while the thumb of the same hand applies counter pressure over the lateral aspect of the head of the talus allowing the calcaneus to glide under the talus correcting the varus deformity (blue line now perpendicular). (**e**, **f**) Calcaneal reduction is inhibited when counter pressure is applied to the calcaneal cuboid joint instead of the head of the talus. (Blue line showing the calcaneus remains in varus)

visualize complete transection of the tendon and release of any scar tissue. In severe cases, if the foot does not get to neutral after the tenotomy, a limited posterior release is considered as detailed in the Dobbs adaptation technique below. The post-tenotomy cast is applied in maximum dorsiflexion and no more than 40° of abduction and remains on for 3–4 weeks.

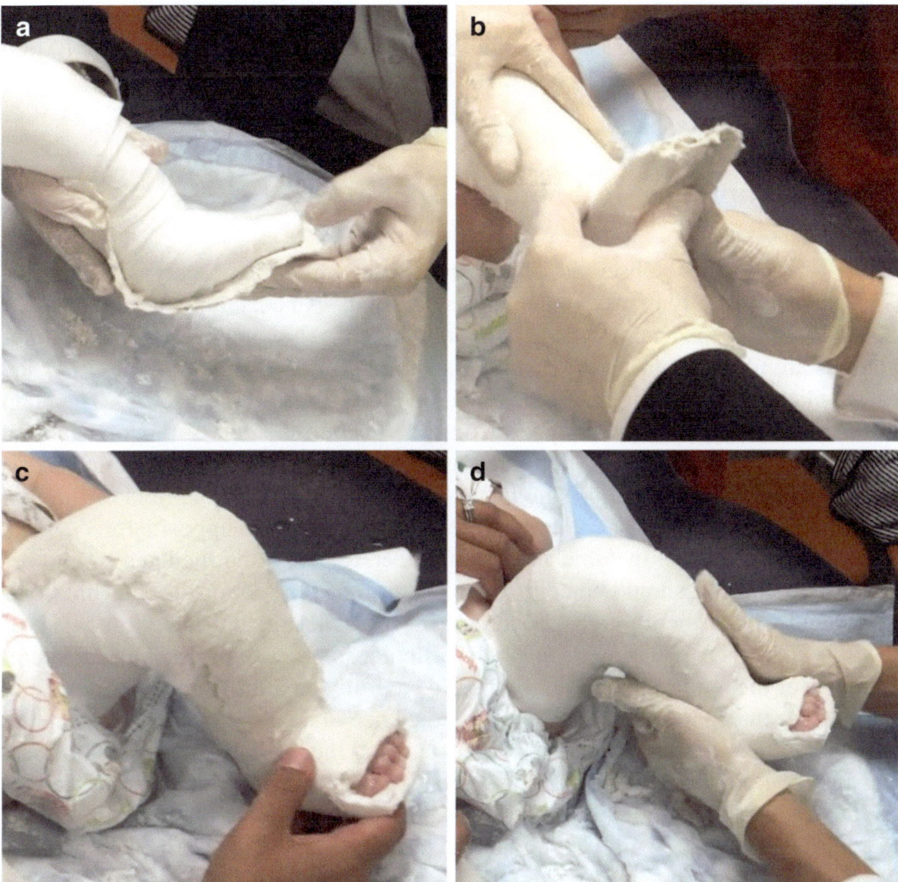

**Fig. 5.13** Modified Ponseti casting technique. (**a**) A posterior splint is applied behind the calf, heel, and sole of the foot and incorporated into a well-molded plaster cast. (**b**) Photograph showing the "four-finger technique". This is performed by grasping the foot and ankle with both hands while the thumbs are placed under the metatarsals pushing the foot into dorsiflexion as an assistant stabilizes the knee in flexion. (**c**) The knee is immobilized (110° of flexion if permissible or to the end of range of motion) using an anterior splint from the upper thigh to the anterior leg and reinforcing it with plaster. (**d**) Finished cast after completing the modified Ponseti casting technique

Expectations for atypical clubfeet are different from isolated clubfeet. The goal is to attain a neutral, plantigrade, and braceable foot. Attempting to gain too much correction by aggressive surgical procedures can lead to scarring contractures leading to poor outcomes long term [50, 55, 110]. Atypical clubfeet are generally more stiff and may require a greater number of casts [14, 15, 63, 79, 87, 118]. De Mulder et al. performed a systematic review of 11 studies and found that atypical clubfeet required an average of 7.2 casts when compared 5.4 casts in the isolated clubfoot [79]. In the treatment of atypical clubfoot, repeat neurological exams are important to assure the treatment plan is complete and all necessary studies and referrals have been made. After the last cast is removed, bracing or ankle foot orthosis (AFO) protocol is initiated, as well as any therapies required.

## Dobb's Adaptation Technique

Tibial bowing can be observed as a complication when treating atypical clubfoot (Fig. 5.14) especially in myelomeningocele patients. An adaptation to the modified Ponseti technique is recommended to address the tibial bowing. Customized manipulations are used to correct the distorted anatomy. In this adaptation, the lower-leg cast application is the same as in the modified Ponseti method (Fig. 5.15). The main difference in the technique is hyperflexing the knee to the end of range of motion and applying pressure on the proximal aspect of the tibia while the other hand is pulling anteriorly from behind the leg instead of at the end of the tibia or the foot (Fig. 5.16). This maneuver creates counter pressure with two opposite forces while hyperflexing the knee. In some atypical clubfeet, hyperflexing the knee is not possible, so the flexion should be done to the end of range of motion. This technique is performed so that the tight gastrocnemius muscle will not contribute to bowing of the tibia since its origin is proximal to the articular surfaces of the medial and lateral condyles of the femur. The plaster is applied carefully creating a smooth mold along the anterior tibia and posterior leg locking the knee in flexion. If care is not taken in cast application, motion of the knee will occur, and the leg will abut against the cast causing the tibial bowing. As the knee extends in a loose cast, it applies pressure to the proximal aspect of the tibia and allows the deforming force of the tight Achilles to contribute to the bowing. With hyperflexion of the knee, the gastrocnemius muscle relaxes decreasing tension distally.

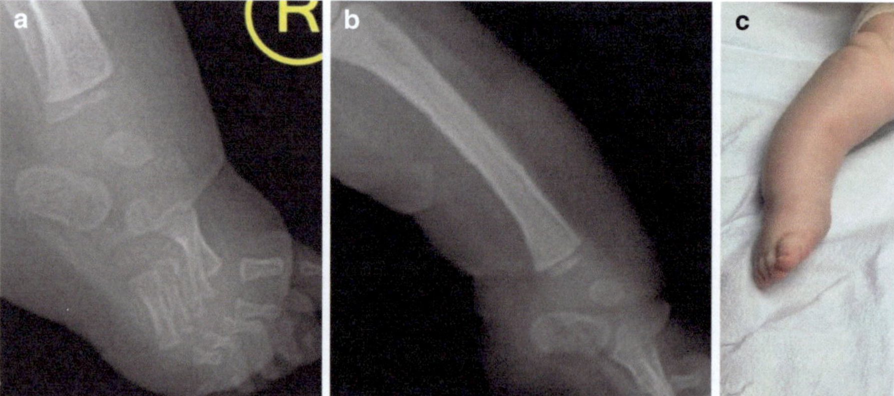

**Fig. 5.14** 4½ month old infant with tibial bowing. (**a**) All of the metatarsals, especially the first metatarsal, are in severe plantarflexion. (**b**) X-ray demonstrating tibial bowing. (**c**) Clinical picture with tibial bowing

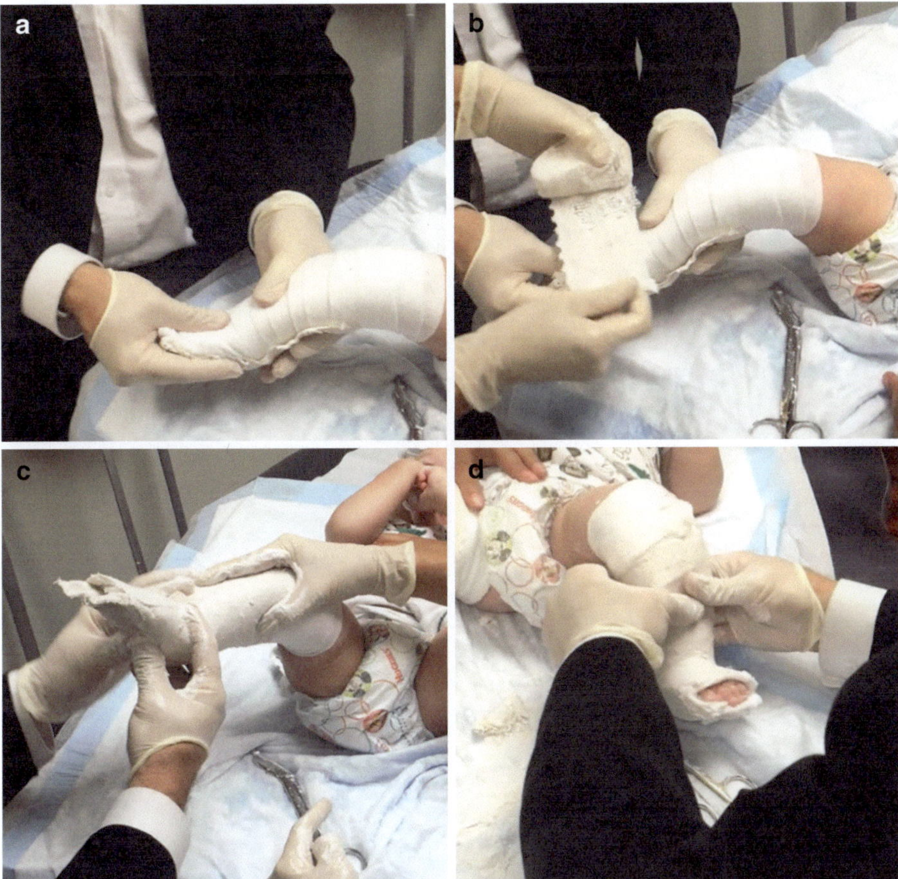

**Fig. 5.15** Dobbs adaptation technique lower leg application: (**a**) A posterior splint is applied behind the calf, heel, and sole of the foot to avoid excessive plaster use. (**b**) The posterior splint is incorporated into a well-molded plaster cast. (**c**) The "four-finger technique" is performed. (**d**) The plaster is applied carefully creating a smooth mold along the anterior tibia making sure to remove any dead space

All atypical clubfeet with tibial bowing require tenotomies, and some require further minimal posterior releases. This is done through a 1 cm longitudinal incision along the Achilles tendon. A right-angle clamp is used to protect the subcutaneous tissue and isolate the Achilles tendon, and a complete tenotomy is performed. Range of motion is performed to determine if adequate dorsiflexion was achieved after the tenotomy. If the ankle does not dorsiflex to neutral after tenotomy, then small retractors are inserted to protect the medial and lateral neurovascular bundles, and a limited posterior ankle and subtalar capsulotomy are performed in an "a la carte" fashion. Most of the tibial bowing is corrected with casting prior to the tenotomy, but there might be some residual bowing due to the tight gastrocnemius muscle. In most cases, full correction of the tibial

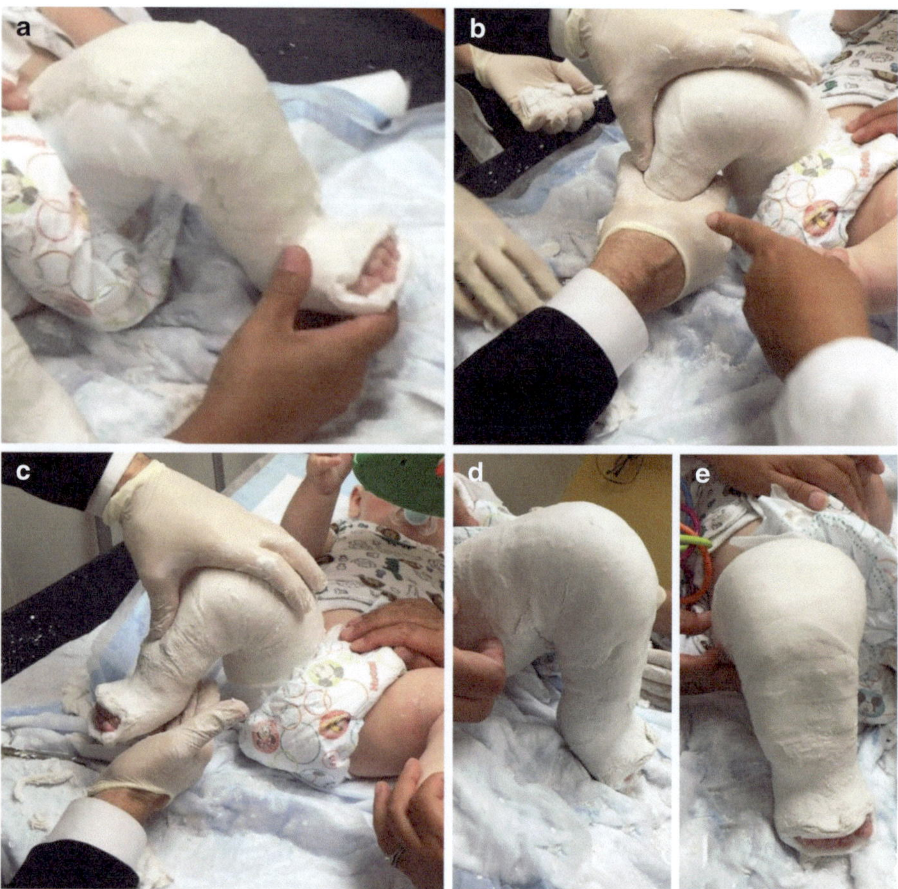

**Fig. 5.16** Dobbs adaptation technique upper leg application: (**a**) The knee is immobilized (at 110°–120° if possible if not to end of range of motion of flexion) by using an anterior splint from the upper thigh to the anterior leg and reinforcing it with plaster. (**b**) Hyperflexing the knee and applying pressure on the proximal aspect of the tibia while the other hand is pulling anteriorly from behind the leg instead of at the end of the tibia or the foot. (**c**) This maneuver creates counter pressure with two opposite forces while hyperflexing the knee. (**d**, **e**) Lateral and anterior view of the finished cast demonstrating a smooth mold along the anterior tibia and posterior leg locking the knee in flexion

bowing will be achieved after the final cast is removed. Following the Achilles tenotomy and/or minimal posterior release, the cast remains on for 3–4 weeks. After the last cast removal, the child will initiate physical therapy and bracing with the foot abduction brace (FAB) or ankle foot orthosis (AFO) of choice as described in the sections below.

# Imaging

Imaging is important when treating atypical clubfoot. Ultrasound (US) is a useful tool in diagnosing most clubfeet prenatally and helpful in the diagnosis of some atypical clubfeet (Fig. 5.1a). A spinal US should be considered in infants with atypical clubfoot as an initial test to rule out spinal cord anomalies. The indications for a spinal ultrasound include but are not limited to weak evertors or "drop toe sign," cutaneous findings such as a sacral dimple, a hairy patch of the lower back, hemangioma, and/or soft-tissue mass [119, 120]. However, it is important to recognize some of these findings early as spinal ultrasounds after 3 months are challenging since the spinal processes ossify [119]. In these cases, MRI may be needed for diagnosis. Ultrasounds can aid in ruling out other various associated conditions such as tethered cord, syrinx, spinal lipomas, and congenital hip dysplasia [119].

Radiographs of the foot and ankle are not routinely performed in the treatment of isolated clubfoot. However, in the atypical clubfoot, radiographs may be necessary for assessing other conditions and joints or if complications are encountered during treatment. Some atypical clubfeet have similar radiographic findings as seen in complex clubfoot. In these atypical clubfeet, the calcaneus and talus are usually in severe plantar flexion [2, 9, 121]. The cuboid may be displaced medially with all of the metatarsals in plantarflexion. Many atypical clubfeet are more rigid and severe, which predispose them to secondary bony changes, metaphyseal fractures, or pseudo corrections due to aggressive manipulation [111, 122]. If bruising or swelling is observed, radiographs may be utilized to rule out any fractures. Radiographs also assist in the evaluation and management of older patients who experience relapse or have had prior surgical interventions.

Radiographs are also used when assessing bowing of the tibia, foot anomalies, or rocker bottom deformity (Fig. 5.17). Rocker bottom deformity is created by improper adherence to the Ponseti casting principles. A plantar convexity of the foot is developed due to dorsiflexion of the forefoot without appropriate correction of the hindfoot equinus [123]. Clinical examination can be misleading, yielding an increase in dorsiflexion that comes from the forefoot and not the hindfoot. Examination of the lateral radiograph will aid in diagnosis of the rocker bottom deformity. It is important to address the sagittal plane with a tenotomy and/or minimally invasive posterior release in these cases. In rare occasions, if the atypical clubfoot has developed a severe rocker bottom deformity, the Dobbs method as used in vertical talus is performed [124].

Tarsal coalitions can be associated with atypical clubfeet on rare occasions [105, 125–128]. In infants, radiographs may not be helpful due to the bones not being fully ossified. In older patients, radiographs may be used to rule out any coalitions that might be impeding movement and correction. Diagnosing a tarsal coalition in the presence of a rigid equinovarus deformity can be difficult. These patients may require further evaluation and imaging including computerized tomography (CT) studies or magnetic resonance imaging (MRI) [127]. It is recommended to monitor the tarsal coalitions in infants if they do not inhibit adequate correction and allow a

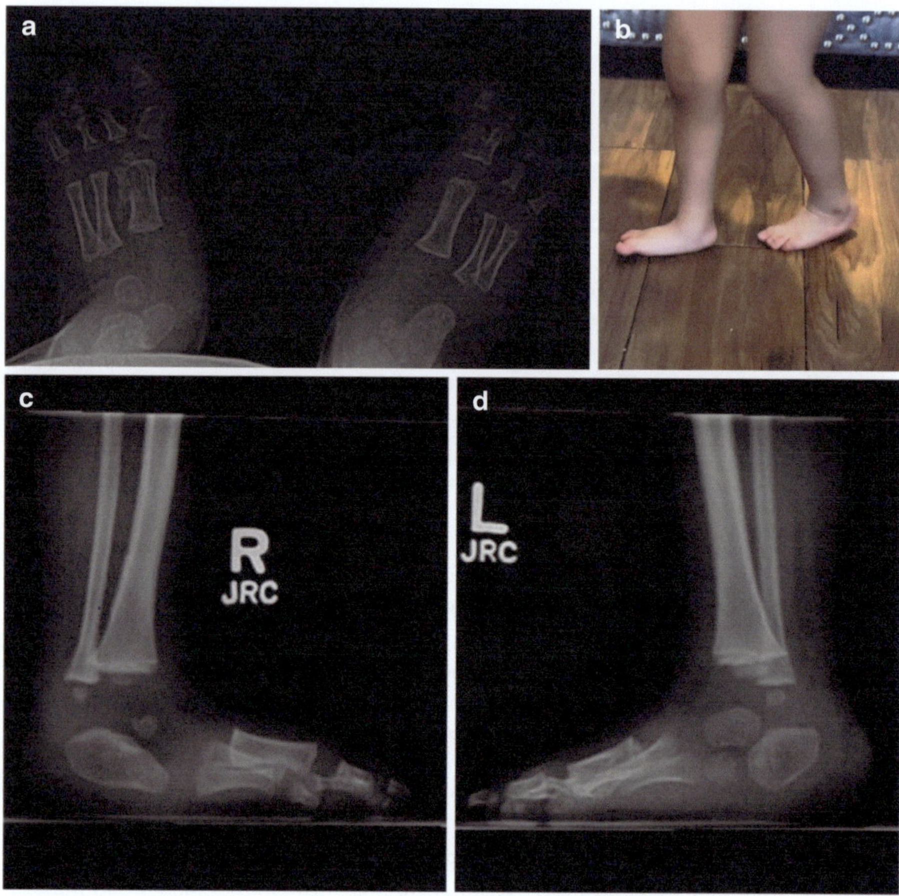

**Fig. 5.17** Rocker bottom deformity in a 2½ year old child with clubfoot and missing rays and toes as well as polysyndactyly. (**a**) Notice missing rays and polysyndactyly of first and second digit. (**b**) Side view of patient walking (**c**, **d**) Lateral view of right ankle and foot notice the rocker bottom deformity with heel not contacting the ground

plantigrade braceable foot. In these patients, treatment of the coalition is delayed until symptoms occur as long as the coalition is not impeding correction. Tarsal coalitions may not be found until surgical correction [129]. When assessing tarsal coalitions, it is important to remember that they often occur with fibular hemimelia [130, 131]. Atypical clubfeet can also be seen in association with polydactyly and/ or syndactyly and missing rays, which can also be evaluated on radiographs (Fig. 5.17a).

MRI has proven beneficial in the management of some atypical clubfeet including the diagnosis of possible associated neuromuscular abnormalities. MRIs are also useful in diagnosis and treatment of tarsal coalitions that may be present in a small subset of atypical clubfeet [127, 132]. MRI may be the most detailed

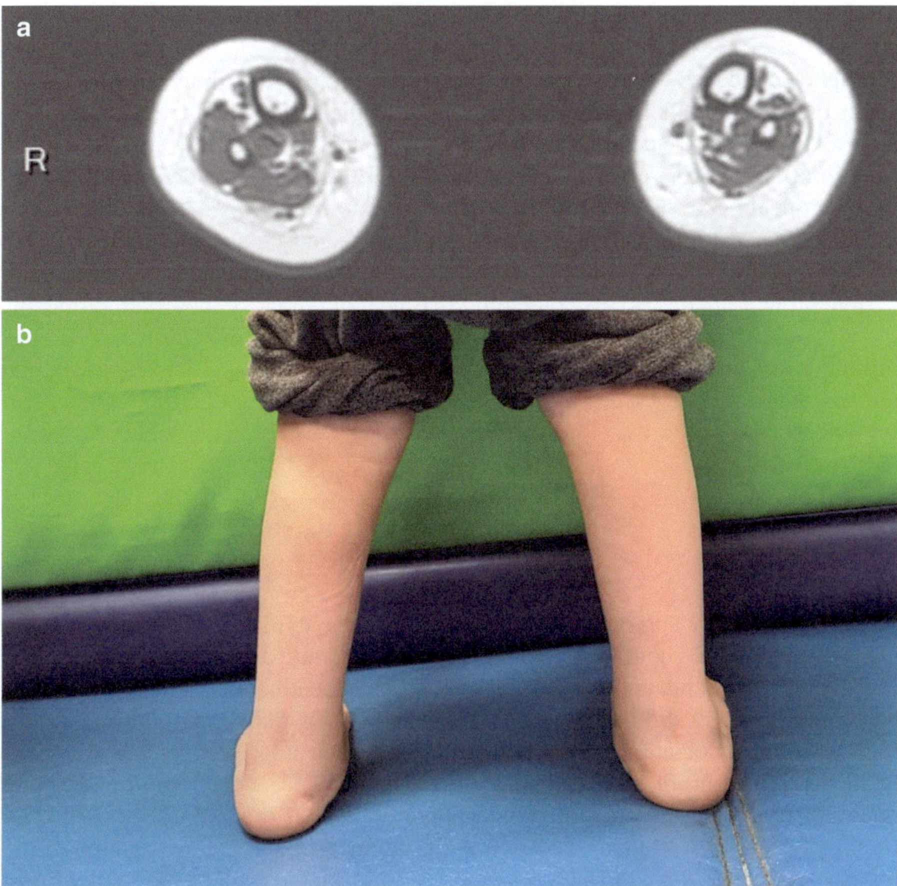

**Fig. 5.18** A 1.5 year old female with bilateral atypical clubfoot with soft tissue anomalies (**a**) MRI demonstrating excess epimysial fat deposition, intramuscular fat deposition, and muscle compartment hypoplasia similar to the findings of Moon et al. (**b**) Same patient standing. Note the thin appearance of the calves

examination that can be ordered for many of these conditions; however, it can be expensive and requires sedation to keep a child still during the procedure. Since there are risks involved, the provider has to consider the patient's age, benefits, and complications and collaborate with other specialties to decide how to proceed.

Recent articles used MRIs to predict a Ponseti treatment-resistant clubfoot. These atypical treatment-resistant clubfeet demonstrated soft-tissue anomalies [17]. Obtaining MRIs to identify hypoplastic limbs with a loss of muscle bulk in patients may explain some relapses (Fig. 5.18). Identification of deficient muscles can aid in developing individualized treatment plans including bracing needs or electrical stimulation, which may lead to better outcomes and fewer relapses. Further research is still required to prove the usefulness of MRIs long term, and a detailed physical exam is critical in figuring out who would benefit from MRI studies.

Higher incidence of neurological deficits are seen in recurrent clubfoot [133]. Other diagnostic tools that have been used in atypical clubfeet are electromyography (EMG) and nerve conduction velocity (NCV) tests. EMGs may also be used in ruling out a diagnosis of nerve palsy [134–137]. It has been shown that clubfoot with peroneal nerve dysfunction is very difficult to treat [16, 21, 133]. NCV tests identify issues with the nerve, whereas EMG detects muscular issues in response to nerve stimuli, therefore muscular disorders. EMGs may be helpful in determining peripheral neuropathy versus congenital peroneal nerve palsy; however, clinically, there is no difference in treatment, just diagnostic. Nerve stimulation and specific muscle group strengthening exercises can be designed for a particular patient and the possible benefits of a certain type of AFO or the need for continued bracing to prevent relapse.

## Consultations

A multidisciplinary approach is essential for treating atypical clubfeet, which usually continues throughout the patient's childhood and into adulthood. The treatment plan for these patients may require modifications depending on the exact diagnosis and their needs and abilities. Consulting a pediatric geneticist is helpful in diagnosing syndromic associations. Atypical clubfoot has been associated with a long list of malformations, chromosomal abnormalities, or known genetic syndromes; more than half of which are associated with abnormalities of the nervous system [12]. Rapid progress in sequencing technology has made affordable interrogation of the human genome possible [13]. Despite these efforts, there is still a subset of clubfeet that demonstrate the physical features associated with atypical clubfoot and may have other medical diagnoses but have not yet been associated with a known syndrome [17].

A referral to a pediatric neurologist is beneficial in atypical clubfoot cases. They will aid in establishing a neurological diagnosis and assist with developing a treatment plan. Depending on the severity and neurological involvement, they will follow the patient and monitor for any progressive changes as the child grows. Some spinal cord abnormalities or soft-tissue masses are referred to a pediatric neurosurgeon for possible surgical interventions.

A referral to a pediatric orthotist that has experience with clubfoot is a crucial part of their management. In many clinics, they will be fitting the child with any braces used. They can be invaluable with helping manage any pressure areas and making the AFOs, supramalleolar orthosis (SMOs), orthotics, or prosthetics the child may need to assist with improving their gait, function, and quality of life.

A physical therapy consultation is recommended for all atypical clubfeet. Physical therapists will help strengthen the lower extremities and core and maintain the flexibility of muscles and tissues, which will aid in mobility and function long term [111]. They can evaluate strengths and weaknesses and obtain baseline objective measurements. They play a vital role in the early detection of subtle muscle imbalances [72]. Physical therapists may incorporate neuromuscular electrical stimulation (NMES) in their treatment of some atypical clubfoot patients. NMES is the electrical stimulation of muscles through motor and sensory nerves applied at a given intensity to cause a muscle to contract and gain strength. This gain in strength may allow patients to maintain better correction and/or minimize the risk of relapse. This treatment has been used for many years to improve muscle quantity and quality in patients with significant muscle deficiency. In a few studies, it was found that electrical stimulation may have the potential to maintain or improve evertor muscle activity and ankle range of motion in isolated and atypical clubfeet [138–141]. This modality is beneficial as it improves muscle strength without pain or discomfort [141]. More research is necessary to fully grasp the benefits of all electrical stimulation modalities on atypical clubfoot patients.

Another modality physical therapists use is Kinesiology Therapeutic Tape (KT Tape). KT tape is an elastic, cloth tape with a paper backing that can be used to support and relieve pain in muscles, joints, and/or ligaments. KT tape provides support without limiting range of motion and is used to promote dorsiflexion and eversion. It is imperative to remember that a child's foot needs to have good mobility in order for the KT tape to have an effect. The authors have found this treatment to be useful; however, research in treatment of atypical clubfoot is needed.

Physical therapy is also crucial for patients who experience recurrences and/or require surgery. After treatment with serial casting with or without the addition of surgical intervention, patients should participate in physical therapy as often as three times a week after the last cast is removed [142, 143]. Therapists will develop a plan that is appropriate given the child's function and abilities. In order to help prevent a recurrent equinus contracture, all clubfoot caregivers are instructed on how to effectively perform range-of-motion exercises after removal of their last cast. These exercises are reviewed every visit.

Patients with atypical clubfeet may also benefit from occupational therapy and speech therapy as many of the other associated conditions can lead to developmental delays. Early intervention is a service and resource that is available to infants and children with developmental delays and disabilities. This may include physical therapy, speech therapy, occupational therapy, and other types of services based on the specific needs of the child. A team approach can help these children achieve the best physical, social, and cognitive development long term.

Studies have demonstrated that a percentage of infants with clubfoot will eventually carry other diagnoses that may take time to be identified including but not limited to syndromes, attention-deficit hyperactivity disorder (ADHD), autism, speech delay, and genetic abnormalities [12, 144, 145]. Other studies have reported delays in motor milestones when compared to their counterparts. Some have postulated that the clubfoot could be a marker for an underlying mild motor development abnormality [145–147]. Many of these other diagnoses could affect the treatment protocols as bracing may be more difficult in this patient population, and early intervention can potentially improve physical and social skills, likely improving their outcomes and quality of life.

## Bracing Protocol

Bracing is vital for successful clubfoot treatment and particularly important in atypical clubfoot. Although the casting period for treatment is relatively short and has the most visible result on the correction of the deformity, the bracing phase is crucial for maintaining correction and preventing relapse of deformity. The bracing in atypical clubfoot is usually longer than what is recommended for isolated clubfoot and in some cases may be indefinite.

Bracing the atypical clubfoot can be challenging and can often lead to brace intolerance. This usually is encountered at the early stages of brace initiation. Close caregiver education and communication has been shown to increase brace adherence and success [6]. A high recurrence rate has been associated with bracing noncompliance [148]. If issues with bracing are addressed and resolved within the first 6 months, continued brace compliance is higher [6, 14, 149]. Close follow-up is recommended to monitor the development of blisters on the heel or dorsum of the foot especially in the insensate patient. This is done by the provider or a dedicated clubfoot educator who instructs parents on brace wear and helps manage any bracing issues. When there are concerns that cannot be addressed over the phone, the child is brought back into the clinic until issues are resolved.

An important reason why caregivers have a hard time adhering with the bracing protocols is patient brace intolerance, which can be commonly experienced in the atypical clubfoot. Close follow-ups are crucial to ensure caregivers are understanding the application of the brace and making any modifications to aid with developing pressure sores. Inability to brace may be a result of attempting to brace an uncorrected clubfoot. Evaluating whether full correction has been achieved and maintained is essential to assure the child still fits in the brace well and has not experienced gradual recurrence over time.

Heel and foot blistering can occur throughout the bracing period in a corrected atypical clubfoot or even the non-clubfoot. This complication is commonly seen in isolated clubfeet but can become more problematic in atypical clubfeet due to the possible neurological deficits involved. Monitoring for any skin irritation is crucial as these sensory deficits predispose them to serious skin complications, which could require cessation of bracing for a period of time to allow the skin to heal [20]. Removal of the brace every 3–4 h in the first couple of weeks to check for pressure sores is beneficial to prevent deep blisters from forming as these children may not cry or resist bracing. If pressure areas occur, modifications can be made to the brace by adding varying types of padding, assuring socks are adequate and verifying fit. If the pressure sore continues and develops into a blister, cessation of the brace with possible application of a holding cast is considered. If some correction is lost, serial casting may need to be initiated to regain full correction. Once the blister heals and full correction is verified, the child will be placed back into the brace. Various braces are available and should be considered if problems continue despite adequate correction.

The standard foot abduction brace (FAB) can be used in most atypical clubfeet, but the abduction angle is reduced to 40° or to the amount of external rotation of the foot achieved in the last cast [14, 20]. In unilateral cases, the non-clubfoot is placed in 30° or 40° of external rotation. The width of the bar is usually set to the approximate shoulder width of the child. The FAB is measured and ordered during the last cast application allowing the child to transition into the brace immediately after cast removal. If the brace is not ready by the time of removal, then a holding cast is applied until the brace is available to maintain full correction.

The braces are usually worn full time (22–23 h/day) for the first 3 months then transitioned to part time (16–18 h/day) generally nights and naps until they are wearing them only at nighttime. The neurological involvement of the atypical clubfoot in conjunction with their functional ability, growth spurts, and history of recurrence over time will help dictate how long the child should brace. Some atypical clubfeet will need to brace indefinitely.

Bracing may need to be modified based on the different levels of neurological involvement especially in patients with myelomeningocele. Standard bracing can become a challenge making the standard FAB difficult to tolerate due to coexisting contractures of the hips and knees. The use of a daytime ankle foot orthosis (AFO) may be indicated in some atypical clubfoot patients indefinitely. The range of motion in some atypical clubfeet will be limited compared to isolated clubfeet since active lower extremity movements are more restricted in these patients. A daytime AFO can provide the structural support necessary for ambulation. Some atypical clubfeet may benefit from the use of an articulated AFO or active stimulators. Patients with knee contractures may benefit from using knee-ankle-foot orthoses (KAFOs) with ratcheting knees at nighttime. Different bracing options should be explored for each patient as the goal is to maintain the correction with a brace that is realistic and manageable by the family.

Close follow-up is necessary even when bracing is going well. If bracing continues without issues, patients can be transitioned to be seen at a longer interval to ensure they are maintaining their correction and the child is progressing well.

## Relapse

*Relapse* is defined as the recurrence of any of the components of a previously well-corrected clubfoot [2, 149, 150]. *Residual deformity* is different from relapse as these are clubfeet that were never fully corrected leaving behind deformities. These residual deformities may be more commonly seen in atypical clubfoot due to their severity and rigidity [148]. Initial adequate reduction of the talus is essential in preventing these residual deformities. These residual clubfeet can show improvements in one or more components of the deformity and may even tolerate bracing initially. However, the residual deformity predisposes the patient to brace intolerance and further deformity, which can be mistakenly classified as a relapse since the clubfoot starts to resemble its original appearance.

Although relapses may occur despite full correction and brace compliance, evaluation of possible other contributing factors should be considered especially in the atypical clubfoot. Lovel and Morcuende found that relapses in isolated clubfoot after the age of 6 were rare and that some of these recurrences were later diagnosed with neuromuscular diseases [151]. This study suggests that there may be unrecognized atypical clubfeet being treated as isolated clubfeet.

Relapses have been reported to be higher in atypical clubfeet [12, 14, 15, 20, 148]. Relapses in arthrogrypotic clubfeet have been shown not only to be higher in general but significantly higher (up to 75%) after aggressive surgical correction was performed [39]. In atypical clubfoot, casting periodically may be necessary to maintain a plantigrade braceable foot, which helps to avoid early surgical interventions that are associated with poor outcomes. Surgical interventions if necessary should be reserved for when the patient is older. Clubfoot associated with myelomeningocele has also been associated with a higher rate and frequency of recurrences and increases with higher lesions [72]. Poor evertor muscle function has been shown as a risk factor for relapse in both isolated and atypical clubfeet [139, 152]. Little et al. showed a 68% recurrence rate with isolated clubfoot patients who showed signs of poor evertor muscle function. Evertor muscle function must continually be assessed during treatment [152]. Patients with weak lateral compartments but functional tibialis anterior tendons may be candidates for early tibialis anterior tendon transfer. The authors recommend a split anterior tibialis tendon transfer (SPLATT) in the myelomeningocele patient if recurrence occurs.

Frequent evaluations are imperative to address early signs of relapse. High recurrence rates are associated with brace intolerance and noncompliance [148]. As mentioned above, if the problems and issues are addressed early and modifications are made with bracing, recurrences can be minimized with higher brace compliance [6, 14, 149]. Caregivers should also be instructed at each visit on how to effectively perform range-of-motion exercises of the ankle to minimize the chance of recurrent equinus contracture. Education about the high recurrence rate is helpful, so they can be proactive with their communication of any changes in their child's brace tolerance, flexibility, or gait pattern.

When relapses are encountered in atypical clubfeet, they should be initially managed with a second series of manipulations and castings with a possible repeat Achilles tenotomy or selective posterior releases and aggressive physical therapy. The deformity generally improves with re-casting in most cases. In arthrogrypotic feet, the frequency of castings diminish as the patient ages and ultimately stabilizes.

A tibialis anterior tendon transfer (TATT) should be considered when the child is at least 3–4 years of age, and there is dynamic supination of the forefoot noted during the swing phase [2, 153]. This should only be performed if the patient has a 4/5 muscle strength. It is important to note that many atypical clubfeet do not fall in this category. However, patients with weak lateral compartments but a functional tibialis anterior muscle might be candidates for an early tibialis anterior tendon transfer. The transfer is still beneficial in these cases as it can eliminate part of the deforming force causing the relapse. Consideration should be given to splitting the tendon based on the patient's clinical picture. It should be noted that if a TATT/SPLATT is performed, this should be done after most of the correction of the transverse, and frontal planes are achieved with serial casting. This procedure is performed to maintain correction as a "biologic brace" and not only as a corrective procedure. If these are performed without any prior serial casting, the deformity may not be fully corrected. The sagittal plane is usually addressed with a repeat open Achilles tenotomy and a possible selective posterior release. After the TATT/SPLATT is performed, the patient should be casted with an above knee nonweight-bearing cast for 4 weeks and then transition into a below-the-knee weight bearing cast for 2 weeks. After the casting is complete, the child will benefit from a daytime AFO to allow strengthening and ease of return to ambulation. The AFO outer leaf is slowly weaned with transition into an SMO if possible. The SMO also is discontinued over time if the child has the strength and ability to walk on their own. Some children with atypical clubfoot will remain in a daytime AFO indefinitely depending on function. The child will use some form of nighttime brace dictated by their tolerance and circumstance.

More research is still necessary in understanding relapses especially in atypical clubfeet. In the future, we may be able to perform diagnostic studies on clubfoot patients and obtain prognostic knowledge. With this information in combination with the patient's other diagnosis and genetic risk factors, we may be able to predict relapses before they occur and customize individual treatment plans. For example, if the MRI demonstrates healthy muscle in all compartments of the lower leg, that patient may be at low risk of relapse, and treatment could be individualized to allow that patient to stop bracing earlier. On the other hand, if the MRI demonstrated little or no muscle in the lateral compartment, one may predict this patient has a greater risk of relapse and be a candidate for an early tendon transfer or potential use of a daytime AFO.

## Conclusion

Clubfoot is a developmental lower-limb anomaly affecting all of the structures in the lower leg including the nerves, vessels, muscles, tendons, ligaments, and bone. From early research including Dr. Ponseti's work, the abnormal anatomy and structural changes of the muscles, tendons, and ligaments in a clubfoot have been well described. This is easily observed in a physical exam in an isolated unilateral clubfoot patient. The most obvious difference is the circumference of the legs. An isolated clubfoot has all the structures needed to make the foot and ankle function properly even with the noted anatomical differences, which is not the case in atypical clubfeet. Atypical clubfoot is a separate entity and should be treated differently than isolated clubfoot. The associated conditions or syndromes and underlying anatomical differences make them more difficult to treat since they may require more casts and have higher recurrence rates and potential complications. These differences are important to identify as they are prognostic giving the provider and parents more information on expectations of outcomes and long-term correction and function. The goal is to perform a detailed exam that will identify these atypical clubfeet early so that personalization of treatment can be initiated.

All types of clubfeet benefit from the Ponseti casting method and its modifications. Historically, the atypical clubfoot displayed inadequate responses to treatment with the traditional Ponseti method and resulted in extensive surgical interventions. Modifications to the Ponseti method have broadened the spectrum of successful outcomes for these patients. Bracing is necessary for successful treatment often longer than what is recommended for isolated clubfoot and may be indefinite. Bracing the atypical clubfoot can be challenging and can often lead to brace intolerance. Monitoring for any skin irritation is crucial as sensory deficits predispose them to skin complications, which could require cessation of bracing for a period of time to allow the skin to heal. This usually is encountered at the early stages of brace initiation, when moving to a new brace, or if correction has been lost.

A multidisciplinary approach is essential for these patients as the treatment plan requires modification depending on their diagnosis, needs, and abilities. Most atypical clubfoot patients will benefit from therapies. Physical therapists will help strengthen the lower extremities and core and maintain the flexibility of muscles and tissues, which will aid in greater mobility and better long-term function. It is important to try to diagnose any associated conditions to develop the proper treatment plan and predict the patient's prognosis. Although a successful correction of the clubfoot deformity can be achieved following the modified Ponseti method, the long-term outcome and function will be determined by the other pathologies associated with the atypical clubfoot. As we learn more about atypical clubfeet, we can use the Ponseti method with its modifications to treat and maintain correction allowing for better foot and ankle function and improving not only the patient's quality of life but also those of their caregivers and loved ones.

# References


1. Ponseti IV, Smoley EN. Congenital clubfoot: the results of treatment. J Bone Joint Surg Am. 1963;45:261–75.
2. Ponseti I. Congenital clubfoot. Fundamentals of treatment. 2nd ed. Oxford University Press; 1996.
3. Laaveg SJ, Ponseti IV. Long-term results of treatment of congenital club foot. J Bone Joint Surg Am. 1980;62(1):23–31.
4. Cooper DM, Dietz FR. Treatment of idiopathic clubfoot. A thirty-year follow-up note. J Bone Joint Surg Am. 1995;77(10):1477–89.
5. Scher DM, Feldman DS, van Bosse HJP, Sala DA, Lehman WB. Predicting the need for tenotomy in the Ponseti method for correction of clubfeet. J Pediatr Orthop. 2004;24(4):349–52.

6. Dobbs MB, Rudzki JR, Purcell DB, Walton T, Porter KR, Gurnett CA. Factors predictive of outcome after use of the Ponseti method for the treatment of idiopathic clubfeet. J Bone Joint Surg Am. 2004;86(1):22–7.

7. Shabtai L, Specht SC, Herzenberg JE. Worldwide spread of the Ponseti method for clubfoot. World J Orthop. 2014;5(5):585–90.

8. Herzenberg JE, Radler C, Bor N. Ponseti versus traditional methods of casting for idiopathic clubfoot. J Pediatr Orthop. 2002;22(4):517–21.

9. Ponseti IV, Zhivkov M, Davis N, Sinclair M, Dobbs MB, Morcuende JA. Treatment of the complex idiopathic clubfoot. Clin Orthop. 2006;451:171–6.

10. Lourenço AF, Morcuende JA. Correction of neglected idiopathic clubfoot by the Ponseti method. J Bone Joint Surg Br. 2007;89(3):378–81.

11. Funk JF, Lebek S, Seidl T, Placzek R. [Comparison of treatment results of idiopathic and non-idiopathic congenital clubfoot: prospective evaluation of the Ponseti therapy]. Orthopade. 2012;41(12):977–83.

12. Gurnett CA, Boehm S, Connolly A, Reimschisel T, Dobbs MB. Impact of congenital talipes equinovarus etiology on treatment outcomes. Dev Med Child Neurol. 2008;50(7):498–502.

13. Dobbs MB, Gurnett CA. The 2017 ABJS Nicolas Andry Award: advancing personalized medicine for clubfoot through translational research. Clin Orthop. 2017;475(6):1716–25.

14. Boehm S, Limpaphayom N, Alaee F, Sinclair MF, Dobbs MB. Early results of the Ponseti method for the treatment of clubfoot in distal arthrogryposis. J Bone Joint Surg Am. 2008;90(7):1501–7.

15. Janicki JA, Narayanan UG, Harvey B, Roy A, Ramseier LE, Wright JG. Treatment of neuromuscular and syndrome-associated (non idiopathic) clubfeet using the Ponseti method. J Pediatr Orthop. 2009;29(4):393–7.

16. Edmonds EW, Frick SL. The drop toe sign: an indicator of neurologic impairment in congenital clubfoot. Clin Orthop. 2009;467(5):1238–42.

17. Moon DK, Gurnett CA, Aferol H, Siegel MJ, Commean PK, Dobbs MB. Soft-tissue abnormalities associated with treatment-resistant and treatment-responsive clubfoot: findings of MRI analysis. J Bone Joint Surg Am. 2014;96(15):1249–56.

18. Stoll C, Alembick Y, Dott B, Roth MP. Associated anomalies in cases with congenital clubfoot. Am J Med Genet A. 2020;182(9):2027–36.

19. Sadler B, Gurnett CA, Dobbs MB. The genetics of isolated and syndromic clubfoot. J Child Orthop. 2019;13(3):238–44.

20. Gerlach DJ, Gurnett CA, Limpaphayom N, Alaee F, Zhang Z, Porter K, et al. Early results of the Ponseti method for the treatment of clubfoot associated with myelomeningocele. J Bone Joint Surg Am. 2009;91(6):1350–9.

21. Song KS, Kang CH, Min BW, Bae GC, Cho CH, Lee JH. Congenital clubfoot with concomitant peroneal nerve palsy in children. J Pediatr Orthop B. 2008;17(2):85–9.

22. de Carvalho NJ, Dias LS, Gabrieli AP. Congenital talipes equinovarus in spina bifida: treatment and results. J Pediatr Orthop. 1996;16(6):782–5.

23. Hennigan SP, Kuo KN. Resistant talipes equinovarus associated with congenital constriction band syndrome. J Pediatr Orthop. 2000;20(2):240–5.

24. Flynn JM, Herrera-Soto JA, Ramirez NF, Fernandez-Feliberti R, Vilella F, Guzman J. Clubfoot release in myelodysplasia. J Pediatr Orthop B. 2004;13(4):259–62.

25. Widmann RF, Do TT, Burke SW. Radical soft-tissue release of the arthrogrypotic clubfoot. J Pediatr Orthop B. 2005;14(2):111–5.

26. Nguyen Khac V, Desroches A, Bouchaïb J, Padovani JP, Wicart P. Results of talectomy for inveterate or recurrent clubfoot. Orthop Traumatol Surg Res. 2021;109:103146.

27. Turco VJ. Resistant congenital club foot--one-stage posteromedial release with internal fixation. A follow-up report of a fifteen-year experience. J Bone Joint Surg Am. 1979;61(6A):805–14.

28. Crawford AH, Marxen JL, Osterfeld DL. The Cincinnati incision: a comprehensive approach for surgical procedures of the foot and ankle in childhood. J Bone Joint Surg Am. 1982;64(9):1355–8.

29. Simons GW. Complete subtalar release in club feet. Part II--comparison with less extensive procedures. J Bone Joint Surg Am. 1985;67(7):1056–65.

30. Letts M, Davidson D. The role of bilateral talectomy in the management of bilateral rigid clubfeet. Am J Orthop (Belle Mead NJ). 1999;28(2):106–10.

31. Wei SY, Sullivan RJ, Davidson RS. Talo-navicular arthrodesis for residual midfoot deformities of a previously corrected clubfoot. Foot Ankle Int. 2000;21(6):482–5.

32. Dobbs MB, Nunley R, Schoenecker PL. Long-term follow-up of patients with clubfeet treated with extensive soft-tissue release. J Bone Joint Surg Am. 2006;88(5):986–96.

33. Church C, McGowan A, Henley J, Donohoe M, Niiler T, Shrader MW, et al. The 5-year outcome of the Ponseti method in children with idiopathic clubfoot and arthrogryposis. J Pediatr Orthop. 2020;40(7):e641–6.

34. Church C, Bourantas C, Butler S, Salazar-Torres JJ, Henley J, Donohoe M, et al. The effectiveness of serial casting in the treatment of recurrent equinovarus in children with arthrogryposis. J Pediatr Orthop. 2023;43(2):117–22.

35. Yoshioka S, Huisman NJ, Morcuende JA. Peroneal nerve dysfunction in patients with complex clubfeet. Iowa Orthop J. 2010;30:24–8.

36. Morcuende JA, Dobbs MB, Frick SL. Results of the Ponseti method in patients with clubfoot associated with arthrogryposis. Iowa Orthop J. 2008;28:22–6.

37. Dobbs MB, Gurnett CA. Update on clubfoot: etiology and treatment. Clin Orthop. 2009;467(5):1146–53.

38. Dobbs MB, Gurnett CA. Genetics of clubfoot. J Pediatr Orthop B. 2012;21(1):7–9.

39. Drummond DS, Cruess RL. The management of the foot and ankle in arthrogryposis multiplex congenita. J Bone Joint Surg Br. 1978;60(1):96–9.

40. Bamshad M, Jorde LB, Carey JC. A revised and extended classification of distal arthrogryposis. Am J Med Genet. 1996;65(4):277–81.

41. Bamshad M, Van Heest AE, Pleasure D. Arthrogryposis: a review and update. J Bone Joint Surg Am. 2009;91(Suppl 4):40–6.

42. Hall JG, Kimber E, Dieterich K. Classification of arthrogryposis. Am J Med Genet C Semin Med Genet. 2019;181(3):300–3.

43. Whittle J, Johnson A, Dobbs MB, Gurnett CA. Models of distal arthrogryposis and lethal congenital contracture syndrome. Genes. 2021;12(6):943.

44. Niles KM, Blaser S, Shannon P, Chitayat D. Fetal arthrogryposis multiplex congenita/fetal akinesia deformation sequence (FADS)-aetiology, diagnosis, and management. Prenat Diagn. 2019;39(9):720–31.

45. Hall JG, Reed SD, Greene G. The distal arthrogryposis: delineation of new entities--review and nosologic discussion. Am J Med Genet. 1982;11(2):185–239.

46. Sells JM, Jaffe KM, Hall JG. Amyoplasia, the most common type of arthrogryposis: the potential for good outcome. Pediatrics. 1996;97(2):225–31.

47. Hall JG. Arthrogryposis multiplex congenita: etiology, genetics, classification, diagnostic approach, and general aspects. J Pediatr Orthop B. 1997;6(3):159–66.

48. Toydemir RM, Bamshad MJ. Sheldon-Hall syndrome. Orphanet J Rare Dis. 2009;4:11.

49. Lloyd-Roberts CC, Lettin A. Arthrogryposis multiplex congenita. J Bone Joint Surg Br. 1970;52(B(3)):494–508.

50. Menelaus MB. Talectomy for equinovarus deformity in arthrogryposis and spina bifida. J Bone Joint Surg Br. 1971;53(3):468–73.

51. Zimbler S, Craig CL. The arthrogrypotic foot plan of management and results of treatment. Foot Ankle. 1983;3(4):211–9.

52. Hall JG, Reed SD, Driscoll EP, Part I. Amyoplasia: a common, sporadic condition with congenital contractures. Am J Med Genet. 1983;15(4):571–90.

53. Carlson WO, Speck GJ, Vicari V, Wenger DR. Arthrogryposis multiplex congenita. A long-term follow-up study. Clin Orthop Relat Res. 1985;(194):115–23.
54. Södergård J, Ryöppy S. Foot deformities in arthrogryposis multiplex congenita. J Pediatr Orthop. 1994;14(6):768–72.
55. Legaspi J, Li YH, Chow W, Leong JC. Talectomy in patients with recurrent deformity in clubfoot. A long-term follow-up study. J Bone Joint Surg Br. 2001;83(3):384–7.
56. Guidera KJ, Drennan JC. Foot and ankle deformities in arthrogryposis multiplex congenita. Clin Orthop Relat Res. 1985;(194):93–8.
57. Niki H, Staheli LT, Mosca VS. Management of clubfoot deformity in amyoplasia. J Pediatr Orthop. 1997;17(6):803–7.
58. Hahn G. Arthrogryposis. Pediatric review and habilitative aspects. Clin Orthop. 1985;194:104–14.
59. Khan MA, Chinoy MA. Treatment of severe and neglected clubfoot with a double zigzag incision: outcome of 21 feet in 15 patients followed up between 1 and 5 years. J Foot Ankle Surg. 2006;45(3):177–81.
60. Palmer PM, MacEwen GD, Bowen JR, Mathews PA. Passive motion therapy for infants with arthrogryposis. Clin Orthop. 1985;194:54–9.
61. Williams P. The management of arthrogryposis. Orthop Clin North Am. 1978;9(1):67–88.
62. Segal LS, Mann DC, Feiwell E, Hoffer MM. Equinovarus deformity in arthrogryposis and myelomeningocele: evaluation of primary talectomy. Foot Ankle. 1989;10(1):12–6.
63. van Bosse HJP, Marangoz S, Lehman WB, Sala DA. Correction of arthrogrypotic clubfoot with a modified Ponseti technique. Clin Orthop. 2009;467(5):1283–93.
64. Swaroop VT, Dias L. Orthopedic management of spina bifida. Part I: hip, knee, and rotational deformities. J Child Orthop. 2009;3(6):441–9.
65. Ntimbani J, Kelly A, Lekgwara P. Myelomeningocele - a literature review. Interdiscip Neurosurg. 2020;19:100502.
66. Sharrard WJ, Grosfield I. The management of deformity and paralysis of the foot in myelomeningocele. J Bone Joint Surg Br. 1968;50(3):456–65.
67. Adzick NS. Fetal myelomeningocele: natural history, pathophysiology, and in-utero intervention. Semin Fetal Neonatal Med. 2010;15(1):9–14.
68. Fieggen K, Stewart C. Aetiology and antenatal diagnosis of spina bifida. S Afr Med J. 2014;104:218.
69. Deak KL, Boyles AL, Etchevers HC, Melvin EC, Siegel DG, Graham FL, et al. SNPs in the neural cell adhesion molecule 1 gene (NCAM1) may be associated with human neural tube defects. Hum Genet. 2005;117(2–3):133–42.
70. Padmanabhan R. Etiology, pathogenesis and prevention of neural tube defects. Congenit Anom. 2006;46(2):55–67.
71. Westcott MA, Dynes MC, Remer EM, Donaldson JS, Dias LS. Congenital and acquired orthopedic abnormalities in patients with myelomeningocele. Radiographics. 1992;12(6):1155–73.
72. Swaroop VT, Dias L. Orthopaedic management of spina bifida-part II: foot and ankle deformities. J Child Orthop. 2011;5(6):403–14.
73. Sharrard WJ, Webb J. Supra-malleolar wedge osteotomy of the tibia in children with myelomeningocele. J Bone Joint Surg Br. 1974;56B(3):458–61.
74. Trumble T, Banta JV, Raycroft JF, Curtis BH. Talectomy for equinovarus deformity in myelodysplasia. J Bone Joint Surg Am. 1985;67(1):21–9.
75. Dias LS, Stern LS. Talectomy in the treatment of resistant talipes equinovarus deformity in myelomeningocele and arthrogryposis. J Pediatr Orthop. 1987;7(1):39–41.
76. Matar HE, Beirne P, Bruce CE, Garg NK. Treatment of complex idiopathic clubfoot using the modified Ponseti method: up to 11 years follow-up. J Pediatr Orthop B. 2017;26(2):137–42.
77. Moroney PJ, Noël J, Fogarty EE, Kelly PM. A single-center prospective evaluation of the Ponseti method in non idiopathic congenital talipes equinovarus. J Pediatr Orthop. 2012;32(6):636–40.

78. Abo El-Fadl S, Sallam A, Abdelbadie A. Early management of neurologic clubfoot using Ponseti casting with minor posterior release in myelomeningocele: a preliminary report. J Pediatr Orthop B. 2016;25(2):104–7.

79. De Mulder T, Prinsen S, Van Campenhout A. Treatment of non-idiopathic clubfeet with the Ponseti method: a systematic review. J Child Orthop. 2018;12(6):575–81.

80. Ferrando Meseguer E, Roig Sánchez S, Pino Almero L, Romano Bataller A, Mínguez Rey MF. Syndromic clubfoot beyond arthrogryposis and myelomeningocele: orthopedic treatment with Ponseti method. Rev Esp Cir Ortop Traumatol. 2021;65(3):180–5.

81. Marreiros H, Loff C, Calado E. Osteoporosis in paediatric patients with spina bifida. J Spinal Cord Med. 2012;35(1):9–21.

82. Safavi-Abbasi S, Mapstone TB, Archer JB, Wilson C, Theodore N, Spetzler RF, et al. History of the current understanding and management of tethered spinal cord. J Neurosurg Spine. 2016;25(1):78–87.

83. Archibeck MJ, Smith JT, Carroll KL, Davitt JS, Stevens PM. Surgical release of tethered spinal cord: survivorship analysis and orthopedic outcome. J Pediatr Orthop. 1997;17(6):773–6.

84. Muthukumar N, Subramaniam B, Gnanaseelan T, Rathinam R, Thiruthavadoss A. Tethered cord syndrome in children with anorectal malformations. J Neurosurg. 2000;92(4):626–30.

85. Yamada S, Lonser RR. Adult tethered cord syndrome. J Spinal Disord. 2000;13(4):319–23.

86. Haro H, Komori H, Okawa A, Kawabata S, Shinomiya K. Long-term outcomes of surgical treatment for tethered cord syndrome. J Spinal Disord Tech. 2004;17(1):16–20.

87. Jackson T, Jones A, Miller N, Georgopoulos G. Clubfoot and tethered cord syndrome: results of treatment with the Ponseti method. J Pediatr Orthop. 2019;39(6):318–21.

88. Chan BWH, Chan KS, Koide T, Yeung SM, Leung MBW, Copp AJ, et al. Maternal diabetes increases the risk of caudal regression caused by retinoic acid. Diabetes. 2002;51(9):2811–6.

89. Bray JJH, Crosswell S, Brown R. Congenital talipes equinovarus and congenital vertical talus secondary to sacral agenesis. BMJ Case Rep. 2017;2017:bcr2017219786.

90. Renshaw TS. Sacral agenesis. J Bone Joint Surg Am. 1978;60(3):373–83.

91. Patterson TJ. Congenital ring-constrictions. Br J Plast Surg. 1961;14:1–31.

92. Zionts LE, Habell B. The use of the Ponseti method to treat clubfoot associated with congenital annular band syndrome. J Pediatr Orthop. 2013;33(5):563–8.

93. Carpiaux AM, Hosseinzadeh P, Muchow RD, Iwinski HJ, Walker JL, Milbrandt TA. The effectiveness of the Ponseti method for treating clubfoot associated with amniotic band syndrome. J Pediatr Orthop. 2016;36(3):284–8.

94. Kino Y. Clinical and experimental studies of the congenital constriction band syndrome, with an emphasis on its etiology. J Bone Joint Surg Am. 1975;57(5):636–43.

95. Tada K, Yonenobu K, Swanson AB. Congenital constriction band syndrome. J Pediatr Orthop. 1984;4(6):726–30.

96. Askins G, Ger E. Congenital constriction band syndrome. J Pediatr Orthop. 1988;8(4):461–6.

97. Foulkes GD, Reinker K. Congenital constriction band syndrome: a seventy-year experience. J Pediatr Orthop. 1994;14(2):242–8.

98. Walter JH, Goss LR, Lazzara AT. Amniotic band syndrome. J Foot Ankle Surg. 1998;37(4):325–33.

99. Ozkan K, Unay K, Goksan B, Akan K, Aydemir N, Ozkan NK. Congenital constriction ring syndrome with foot deformity: two case reports. Cases J. 2009;2:6696.

100. Unger S, Superti-Furga A. Diastrophic dysplasia. In: Adam MP, Everman DB, Mirzaa GM, Pagon RA, Wallace SE, Bean LJ, et al. editors. GeneReviews®. Seattle: University of Washington; 1993 [cited 2023 Feb 25]. http://www.ncbi.nlm.nih.gov/books/NBK1350/.

101. Al Kaissi A, Kenis V, Melchenko E, Chehida FB, Ganger R, Klaushofer K, et al. Corrections of lower limb deformities in patients with diastrophic dysplasia. Orthop Surg. 2014;6(4):274–9.

102. Canavese F, Sussman MD. Orthopaedic manifestations of congenital myotonic dystrophy during childhood and adolescence. J Pediatr Orthop. 2009;29(2):208–13.

103. Renard D, Rivier F, Dimeglio A, Labauge P. Congenital talipes equinovarus associated with myotonic dystrophy type 2. Muscle Nerve. 2010;42(3):457.

104. Schilling L, Forst R, Forst J, Fujak A. Orthopaedic disorders in myotonic dystrophy type 1: descriptive clinical study of 21 patients. BMC Musculoskelet Disord. 2013;14:338.
105. Caskey PM, Lester EL. Association of fibular hemimelia and clubfoot. J Pediatr Orthop. 2002;22(4):522–5.
106. Merrill LJ, Gurnett CA, Siegel M, Sonavane S, Dobbs MB. Vascular abnormalities correlate with decreased soft tissue volumes in idiopathic clubfoot. Clin Orthop. 2011;469(5):1442–9.
107. Gurnett CA, Alaee F, Kruse LM, Desruisseau DM, Hecht JT, Wise CA, et al. Asymmetric lower-limb malformations in individuals with homeobox PITX1 gene mutation. Am J Hum Genet. 2008;83(5):616–22.
108. Ester AR, Weymouth KS, Burt A, Wise CA, Scott A, Gurnett CA, et al. Altered transmission of HOX and apoptotic SNPs identify a potential common pathway for clubfoot. Am J Med Genet A. 2009;149A(12):2745–52.
109. Levin MN, Kuo KN, Harris GF, Matesi DV. Posteromedial release for idiopathic talipes equinovarus. A long-term follow-up study. Clin Orthop Relat Res. 1989;242:265–8.
110. Green AD, Lloyd-Roberts GC. The results of early posterior release in resistant club feet. A long-term review. J Bone Joint Surg Br. 1985;67(4):588–93.
111. Kowalczyk B, Lejman T. Short-term experience with Ponseti casting and the Achilles tenotomy method for clubfeet treatment in arthrogryposis multiplex congenita. J Child Orthop. 2008;2(5):365–71.
112. Dunkley M, Gelfer Y, Jackson D, Parnell E, Armstong J, Rafter C, et al. Mid-term results of a physiotherapist-led Ponseti service for the management of non-idiopathic and idiopathic clubfoot. J Child Orthop. 2015;9(3):183–9.
113. Chu A, Nachamie H, Lehman W. Management of the complex clubfoot: current concept review. JPOSNA® 2019;1(1). https://www.jposna.org/index.php/jposna/article/view/39.
114. van Bosse HJP. Challenging clubfeet: the arthrogrypotic clubfoot and the complex clubfoot. J Child Orthop. 2019;13(3):271–81.
115. Patel A, Mongia AK, Sharma RK, Saini R, Chaudhary C, Singh S. Outcome of atypical & complex clubfoot managed by modified Ponseti method-a prospective study. J Foot Ankle Surg. 2022;61(5):1081–5.
116. Dobbs MB, Boehm S, Grange DK, Gurnett CA. Case report: Congenital knee dislocation in a patient with Larsen syndrome and a novel filamin B mutation. Clin Orthop. 2008;466(6):1503–9.
117. Ponseti IV, Smoley EN. The classic: congenital club foot: the results of treatment. 1963. Clin Orthop Relat Res. 2009;467(5):1133–45.
118. Matar HE, Beirne P, Garg N. The effectiveness of the Ponseti method for treating clubfoot associated with arthrogryposis: up to 8 years follow-up. J Child Orthop. 2016;10(1):15–8.
119. Fitzgerald K. Ultrasound examination of the neonatal spine. Australas J Ultrasound Med. 2011;14(1):39–41.
120. Vanderhave KL, Brighton B, Casey V, Montijo H, Scannell B. Applications of musculoskeletal ultrasonography in pediatric patients. J Am Acad Orthop Surg. 2014;22(11):691–8.
121. Turco V. Recognition and management of the atypical idiopathic clubfoot. In: The clubfoot: the present and a view of the future. New York: Springer; 1994. p. 76–7.
122. Volz R, Paulsen M, Morcuende J. Distal tibia/fibula fractures following clubfoot casting--report of four cases. Iowa Orthop J. 2009;29:117–20.
123. Koureas G, Rampal V, Mascard E, Seringe R, Wicart P. The incidence and treatment of rocker bottom deformity as a complication of the conservative treatment of idiopathic congenital clubfoot. J Bone Joint Surg Br. 2008;90(1):57–60.
124. Dobbs MB, Purcell DB, Nunley R, Morcuende JA. Early results of a new method of treatment for idiopathic congenital vertical talus. J Bone Joint Surg Am. 2006;88(6):1192–200.
125. Grant AD, Rose D, Lehman W. Talocalcaneal coalition in arthrogryposis multiplex congenita. Bull Hosp Jt Dis Orthop Inst. 1982;42(2):236–41.
126. Herzenberg JE, Goldner JL, Martinez S, Silverman PM. Computerized tomography of talocalcaneal tarsal coalition: a clinical and anatomic study. Foot Ankle. 1986;6(6):273–88.

127. Spero CR, Simon GS, Tornetta P. Clubfeet and tarsal coalition. J Pediatr Orthop. 1994;14(3):372–6.
128. Rao BS, Joseph B. Varus and equinovarus deformities of the foot associated with tarsal coalition. Foot. 1994;4(2):95–9.
129. Van Rysselberghe NL, Souder CD, Mubarak SJ. Unsuspected tarsal coalitions in equinus and varus foot deformities. J Pediatr Orthop B. 2020;29(4):370–4.
130. Searle CP, Hildebrand RK, Lester EL, Caskey PM. Findings of fibular hemimelia syndrome with radiographically normal fibulae. J Pediatr Orthop B. 2004;13(3):184–8.
131. Eberhardt O, Langendörfer M, Fernandez FF, Wirth T. [Clubfoot associated with tibial and fibular hemimelia]. Z Orthopadie Unfallchirurgie. 2012;150(5):525–32.
132. Patel CV. The foot and ankle: MR imaging of uniquely pediatric disorders. Magn Reson Imaging Clin N Am. 2009;17(3):539–47, vii.
133. Thometz J, Sathoff L, Liu XC, Jacobson R, Tassone JC. Electromyography nerve conduction velocity evaluation of children with clubfeet. Am J Orthop (Belle Mead NJ). 2011;40(2):84–6.
134. Brown RE, Storm BW. "Congenital" common peroneal nerve compression. Ann Plast Surg. 1994;33(3):326–9.
135. Macnicol MF, Nadeem RD. Evaluation of the deformity in clubfoot by somatosensory evoked potentials. J Bone Joint Surg Br. 2000;82(5):731–5.
136. Nadeem RD, Brown JK, Lawson G, Macnicol MF. Somatosensory evoked potentials as a means of assessing neurological abnormality in congenital talipes equinovarus. Dev Med Child Neurol. 2000;42(8):525–30.
137. Feldbrin Z, Gilai AN, Ezra E, Khermosh O, Kramer U, Wientroub S. Muscle imbalance in the aetiology of idiopathic club foot. An electromyographic study. J Bone Joint Surg Br. 1995;77(4):596–601.
138. Dagenais LM, Lahay ER, Stueck KA, White E, Williams L, Harris SR. Effects of electrical stimulation, exercise training and motor skills training on strength of children with meningomyelocele: a systematic review. Phys Occup Ther Pediatr. 2009;29(4):445–63.
139. Gelfer Y, Durham S, Daly K, Shitrit R, Smorgick Y, Ewins D. The effect of neuromuscular electrical stimulation on congenital talipes equinovarus following correction with the Ponseti method: a pilot study. J Pediatr Orthop B. 2010;19(5):390–5.
140. Son J, Lee D, Kim Y. Effects of involuntary eccentric contraction training by neuromuscular electrical stimulation on the enhancement of muscle strength. Clin Biomech (Bristol, Avon). 2014;29(7):767–72.
141. Morales-Osorio G, Lomeli-Gonzalez J, Hernandez-Valadez NI, Saldana EA, Arenas-Sordo ML. Electrostimulation to increase peroneal muscle strength in pediatric patients with post-surgical clubfoot. J Pediatr Rev. 2016 [cited 2023 Feb 26];In Press. http://jpediatricsreview.com/en/articles/2852.html.
142. Dimeglio A, Canavese F. The French functional physical therapy method for the treatment of congenital clubfoot. J Pediatr Orthop B. 2012;21(1):28–39.
143. Bernstein RM. Arthrogryposis and amyoplasia. J Am Acad Orthop Surg. 2002;10(6):417–24.
144. Bacino CA, Hecht JT. Etiopathogenesis of equinovarus foot malformations. Eur J Med Genet. 2014;57(8):473–9.
145. Lööf E. Additional challenges in children with idiopathic clubfoot: is it just the foot? J Child Orthop. 2019;13(3):245–51.
146. Garcia NL, McMulkin ML, Tompkins BJ, Caskey PM, Mader SL, Baird GO. Gross motor development in babies with treated idiopathic clubfoot. Pediatr Phys Ther. 2011;23(4):347–52.
147. Andriesse H, Westbom L, Hägglund G. Motor ability in children treated for idiopathic clubfoot. A controlled pilot study. BMC Pediatr. 2009;9:78.
148. Azarpira MR, Emami MJ, Vosoughi AR, Rahbari K. Factors associated with recurrence of clubfoot treated by the Ponseti method. World J Clin Cases. 2016;4(10):318–22.
149. Morcuende JA, Dolan LA, Dietz FR, Ponseti IV. Radical reduction in the rate of extensive corrective surgery for clubfoot using the Ponseti method. Pediatrics. 2004;113(2):376–80.

150. Eidelman M, Kotlarsky P, Herzenberg JE. Treatment of relapsed, residual and neglected clubfoot: adjunctive surgery. J Child Orthop. 2019;13(3):293–303.
151. Lovell ME, Morcuende JA. Neuromuscular disease as the cause of late clubfoot relapses: report of 4 cases. Iowa Orthop J. 2007;27:82–4.
152. Little Z, Yeo A, Gelfer Y. Poor evertor muscle activity is a predictor of recurrence in idiopathic clubfoot treated by the Ponseti method: a prospective longitudinal study with a 5-year follow-up. J Pediatr Orthop. 2019;39(6):e467–71.
153. Zhao D, Liu J, Zhao L, Wu Z. Relapse of clubfoot after treatment with the Ponseti method and the function of the foot abduction orthosis. Clin Orthop Surg. 2014;6(3):245–52.

# Chapter 6
# Management of Complex Clubfoot: Challenges and Solutions

Nitza N. Rodriguez, Robert J. Spencer, and Matthew B. Dobbs

## Introduction

Congenital talipes equinovarus (CTEV), commonly known as clubfoot, is one of the most common orthopedic birth defects affecting approximately 1 in 1000 children worldwide [1–5]. Clubfoot is unilateral in 50% of cases, affecting the right side more frequently [5, 6]. The standard treatment for clubfoot is manipulation with serial casting as originally described by Dr. Ponseti [7]. The Ponseti method is currently considered the gold standard for treating all clubfeet [7–15]. The treatment is simple, effective, and inexpensive and has gained popularity around the world [8].

Although clubfoot is easily recognizable at birth, the degree of severity varies from mild to rigid and difficult to manipulate and treat. Most CTEV (~80%) occurs as an individual birth defect and is referred to as **isolated clubfoot** (idiopathic) [13, 14, 16, 17]. The remaining are **atypical clubfeet** and defined as a clubfoot in patients with additional malformations, chromosomal abnormalities, known genetic syndromes, or minor neurological manifestations without associated conditions or syndromes [15, 17–21]. **Complex clubfoot** is defined as a subset of isolated clubfeet that are short and stubby with severe equinus and plantarflexion of all metatarsals, a short hyperextended first toe and prominent plantar medial and posterior crease (Figs. 6.1, 6.2 and 6.3). Complex clubfeet are resistant to the standard Ponseti casting technique or iatrogenic as the result of improper casting. The modified Ponseti

N. N. Rodriguez (✉) · R. J. Spencer
Southern California Foot and Ankle Specialists, Ladera Ranch, CA, USA

M. B. Dobbs
Paley Institute, St. Mary's Medical Center, West Palm Beach, FL, USA
e-mail: mdobbs@paleyinstitute.org



M. B. Dobbs et al. (eds.), *Clubfoot and Vertical Talus*,
https://doi.org/10.1007/978-3-031-34788-7_6

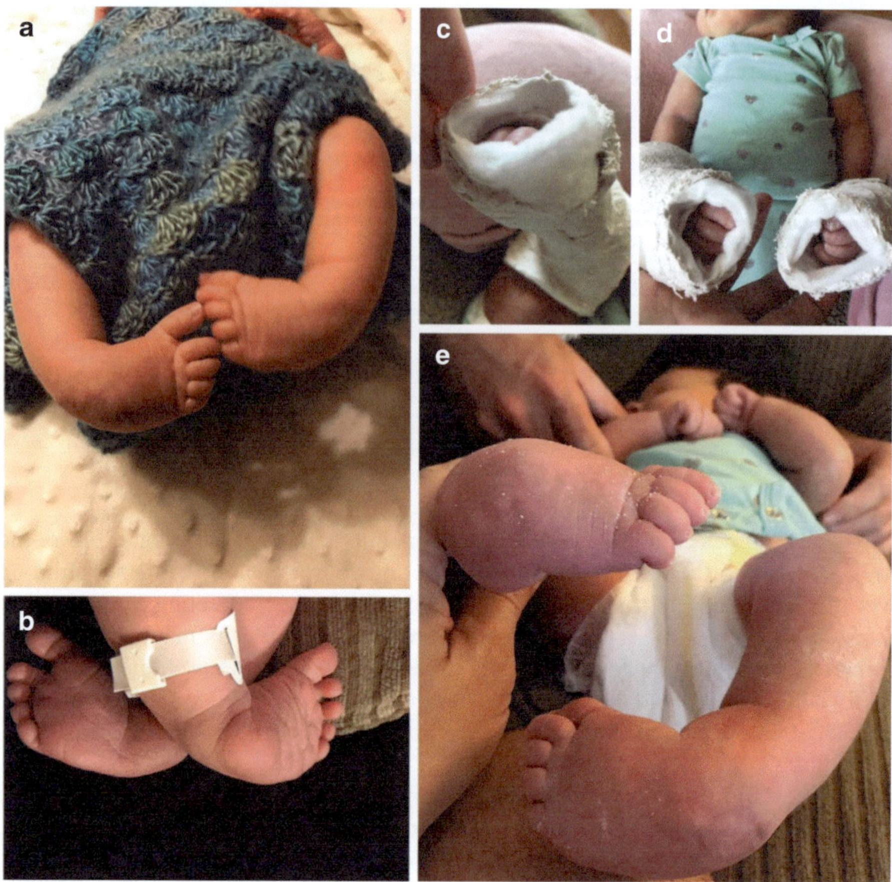

**Fig. 6.1** Early development of complex clubfoot features. (**a**) Infant before cast application. Notice there is no swelling present. (**b**) Plantar view with minimal creases and mild cavus deformity. (**c**) Photograph of first loosely fitting plaster cast application. (**d**) Bilateral casts with noted slipping. (**e**) After removal of the slipping cast. Notice the swelling and worsening of the equinus and cavus deformity

casting technique was developed to address these difficult feet. Utilizing the modified Ponseti casting technique allows for a plantigrade foot and flexible, fully functional foot and ankle without the need for extensive surgery (Figs. 6.2 and 6.4). In this chapter, challenges and solutions for treatment of complex clubfoot including relapse and management are discussed.

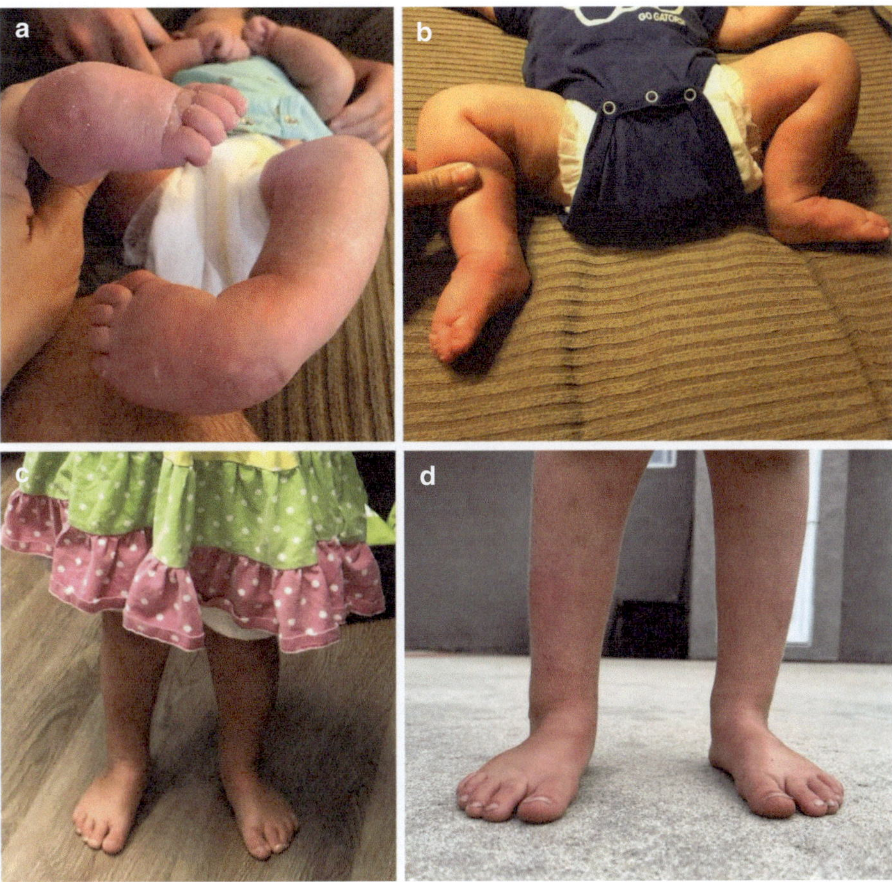

**Fig. 6.2** Same patient from Fig. 6.1 demonstrating the results of using the modified Ponseti technique. (**a**) Infant after removal of loosely fitting slipped casts demonstrating the appearance of short downward pointing feet with severe equinus and cavus developing. (**b**) Patient at 10 weeks old after transfer of care and completing the modified ponseti technique. (**c**) Correction maintained at age 2 1/2 years old. (**d**) Patient at 5 years old with no history of relapse

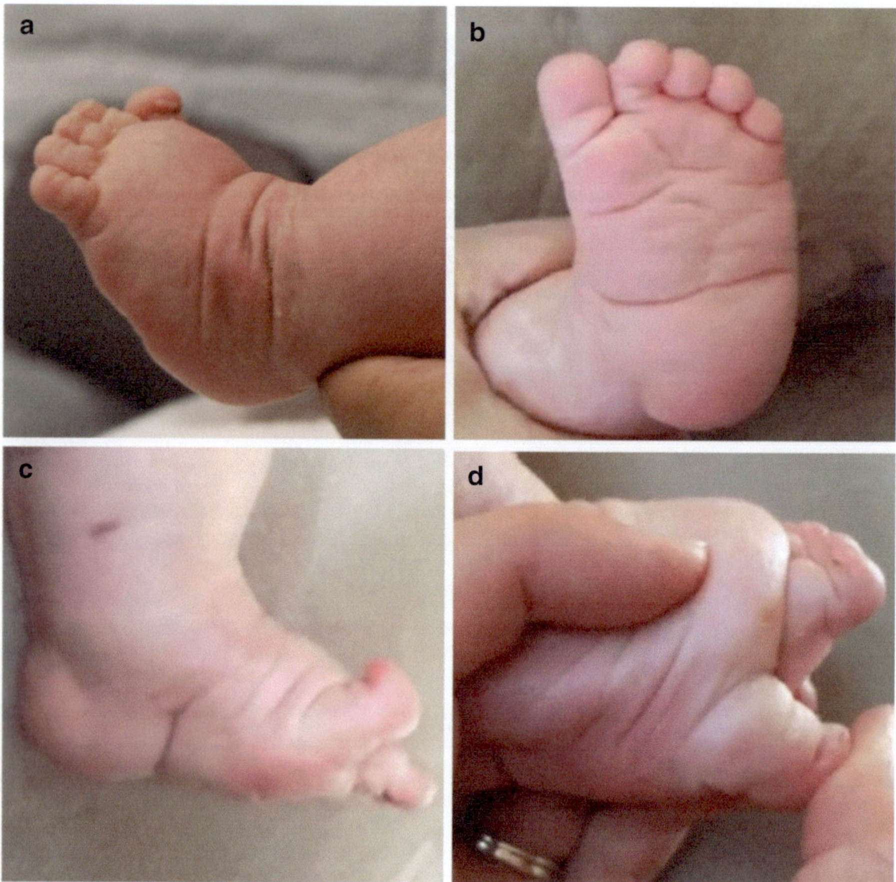

**Fig. 6.3** A 3 1/2 month old male with complex clubfoot after seven plaster casts and tenotomies with history of multiple slipped casts. (**a**) Notice the short and stubby foot in equinus. (**b**) Note the deep plantar transverse crease. (**c**) Demonstrating the short hyperextended 1st digit and prominent plantar medial crease. (**d**) Note the edema dorsally with a small wound caused from hyperextended first digit with the nail abutting against the skin

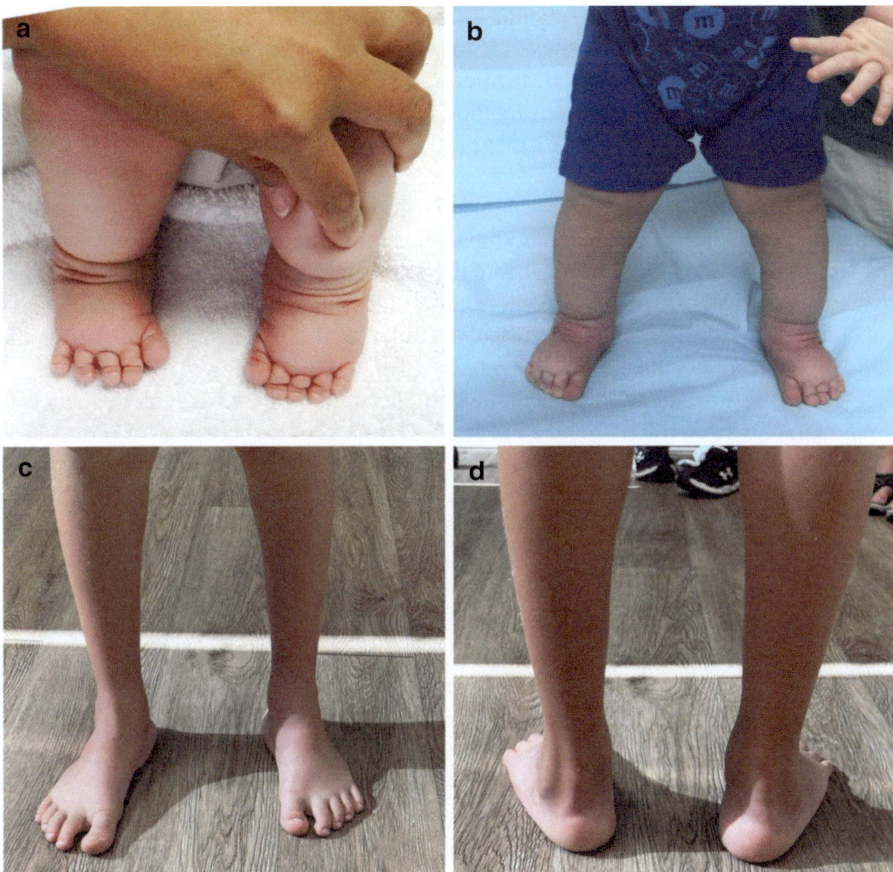

**Fig. 6.4** Same patient from Fig. 6.3 demonstrating the results of using the modified Ponseti technique. (**a**) 3 1/2 month old male after seven plaster casts and tenotomies with history of multiple slipped casts. (**b**) Patient at 8 months old after transfer of care and completing the modified Ponseti technique and repeat tenotomies. (**c**) Anterior view of patient at 7 years of age without history of relapse. (**d**) Posterior view

## Complex Clubfoot

From the early stages of clubfoot treatment, authors have described varying severities of clubfoot [7, 22–24]. Historically, the majority of clubfoot literature has addressed isolated clubfoot treatment. In 1994, Turco first described a small subset of isolated clubfeet as being "atypical" and refractory to treatment. He reported these to appear as a typical idiopathic clubfoot at birth without any associated neurological condition or syndromes. He observed an Achilles tendon that appeared wide and very tight resulting in a deep crease just proximal to the heel. The feet were in adduction and the metatarsals in plantarflexion causing a severe cavus foot with a deep crease across the plantar aspect of the foot. Turco warned specifically against surgical correction in these feet as this resulted in grotesque, overcorrected severe flatfeet [25]. Ponseti et al. further detailed these subset of clubfeet as being resistant to the traditional Ponseti method calling them "complex" and described a modified casting protocol for treatment [26]. The terms atypical and complex clubfoot have been discussed together and used interchangeably in the literature [27–30]. However, as we learn more about clubfoot and its different categories, it is important to distinguish between atypical and complex clubfoot. Although the casting technique used is similar, regarding them as separate entities will inform proper management. The bracing treatment, relapse rates, and expected outcomes in atypical clubfeet are different, and additional considerations are taken as described in the atypical clubfoot chapter.

Due to the limited literature about complex clubfoot, the actual incidence is unknown. However, the incidence has been estimated to be between 6.5% and 17% of isolated clubfeet [26, 28, 29, 31–35]. It was initially uncertain and questioned whether complex clubfeet were idiopathic or iatrogenic [26, 34, 35]. Joseph Hiram Kite wrote in his paper in 1970, "A clubfoot that has been partially corrected by casts is often harder to correct than an untreated clubfoot. This is true when the foot has been carried through improper maneuvers as the casts are applied" [23]. Ponseti et al. were uncertain whether their referred patients were complex at birth or as a result of improper casting [26]. Dragoni et al. later concluded that their series of complex clubfeet were created as a result of improper manipulation and casting technique [34]. However as more literature is published, it is accepted that complex clubfoot features can be present at birth or iatrogenic [27, 29, 34, 36]. Whether the complex clubfoot is present at birth or iatrogenic in nature, the treatment is the same.

In complex clubfoot, a thorough history and physical exam is an integral component of treatment. Obtaining a history of treatment including the number of previous casting attempts, prior surgical interventions, family history of clubfoot, and ruling out any congenital defects or neuromuscular disorders is essential. A comprehensive physical exam is performed with the patient completely undressed and examined from head to toe. The head, neck, and face are assessed for signs of torticollis or other indications of a syndrome. The spine is examined from top to bottom for any masses, birthmarks, skin tags, tuft of hair, or sacral dimple to rule out spinal issues (Fig. 6.5). The upper and lower limbs are assessed for range of motion, tone, and deformity. A hip examination is performed ruling out hip dysplasia. Observations of the length of the legs and girth of the thighs and calves are performed. It is important to assess the neurological function of the lower extremities and rule out an atypical clubfoot. Plantar stimulation is performed on all clubfeet assuring the child dorsiflexes their toes and ankle and splays their toes (Fig. 6.6). Evaluation of evertor muscle function is performed and repeated at all subsequent office visits.

During the physical exam, the foot may be difficult to examine as the joints are stiff, and the landmarks may be challenging to identify (Fig. 6.7e). The anterior tuberosity of the calcaneus is prominent dorsally, and the head of the talus may be hard to palpate. Range of motion should be performed on all the joints and documented. There is usually minimal motion in the severely supinated tarsal joints

**Fig. 6.5**  Photograph shows a 2-month-old infant with a sacral dimple

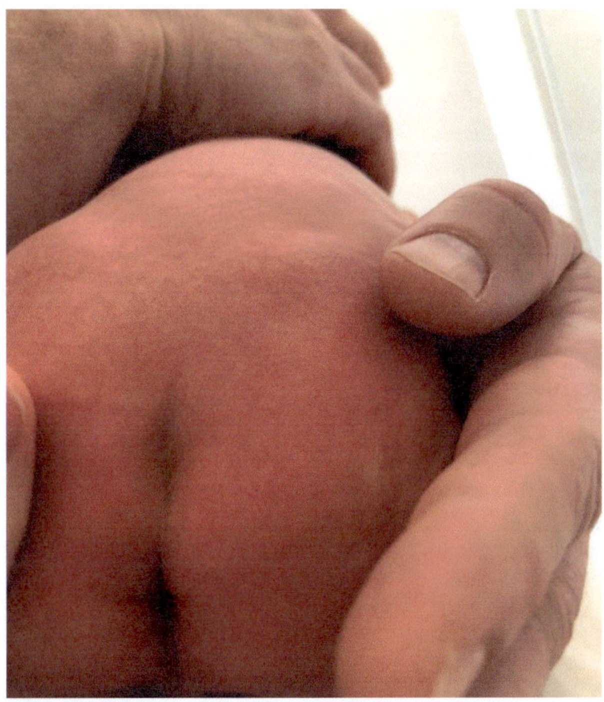

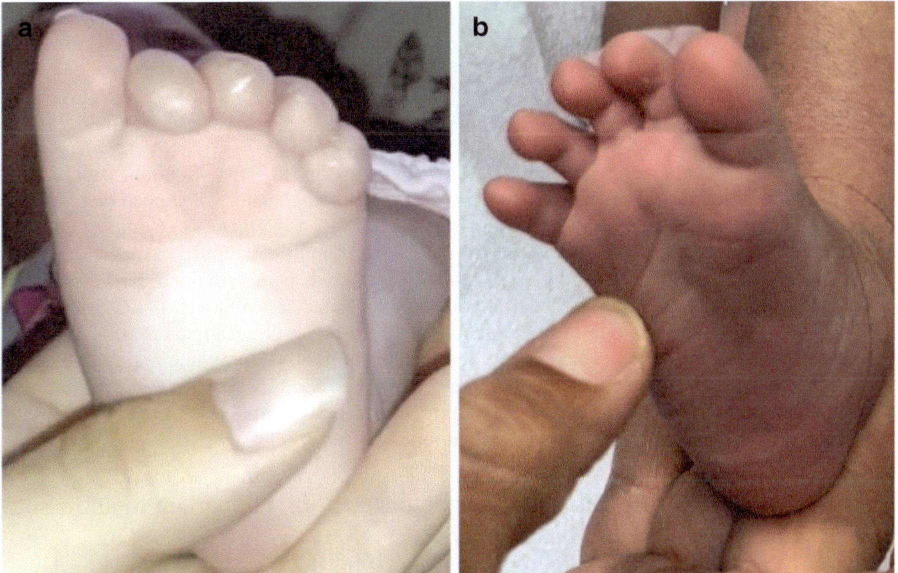

**Fig. 6.6**  Plantar stimulation of foot. (**a**) Persistent plantarflexion of toes in a 3-month-old female with atypical clubfoot. Note the drop toe sign. (**b**) Note the dorsiflexion of the ankle and splaying of toes in a 3-month-old female with isolated clubfoot

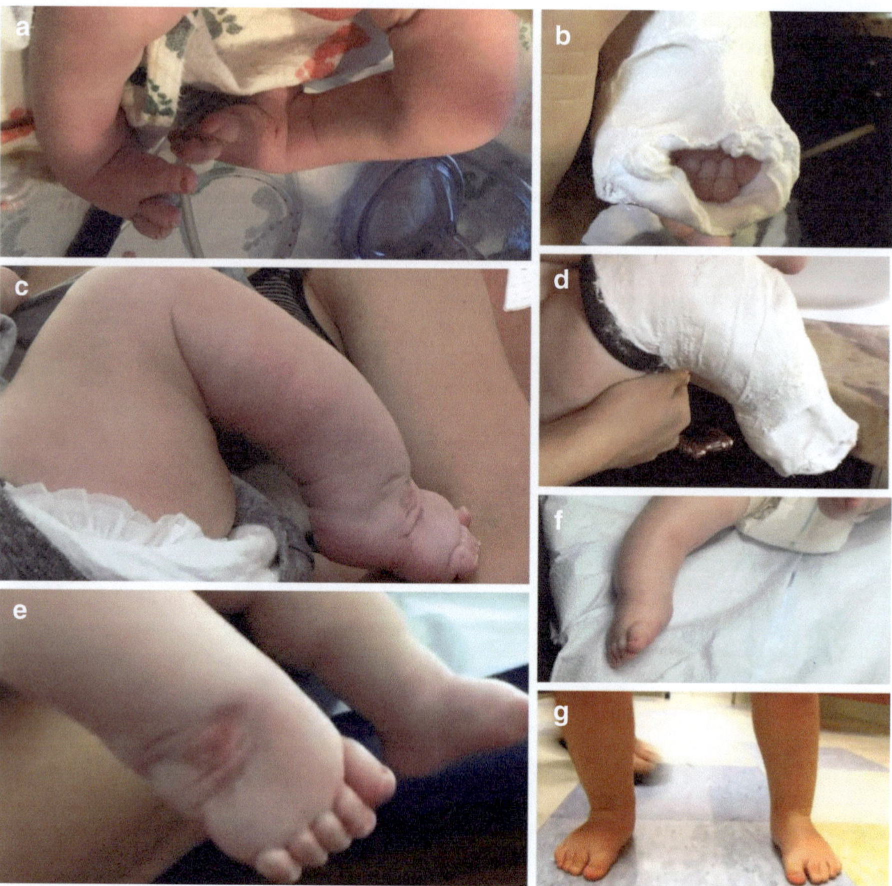

**Fig. 6.7** Development of a complex clubfoot with tibial bowing (**a**) Newborn infant with isolated clubfoot before casting. (**b**) Patient at 6 months old with significant history of slipped casts. Notice the poorly molded heavy cast resulting in slipping and "disappearing toes". (**c**) Complex clubfoot development with tibial bowing after 14 casts and history of multiple slipped casts. (**d**) Last cast before transfer of care demonstrating short, heavily plastered, poorly molded cast. Notice the prominent large thumbprint to the dorsal lateral foot. (**e**) After cast removal, notice inability to identify anatomic landmarks due to severe edema and grotesque deformity caused by improper casting technique causing the development of a complex clubfoot. (**f**) Only minimal improvement noted in the foot after one cast using the modified Ponseti method. Notice the persistent anterior tibial bow. (**g**) Patient at 3 years of age with correction achieved after using Dobb's adaptation technique and a repeat Achilles tenotomy with minimal posterior release

making manipulation and casting more complicated. It is important to allow soft-tissue edema to resolve before initiating recasting.

Some of the clinical features seen in complex clubfeet are distinct features developed during the casting process due to faulty casting. However, some of these features may be present before casting is initiated. It is imperative to detect and recognize a complex clubfoot before or during treatment to avoid further

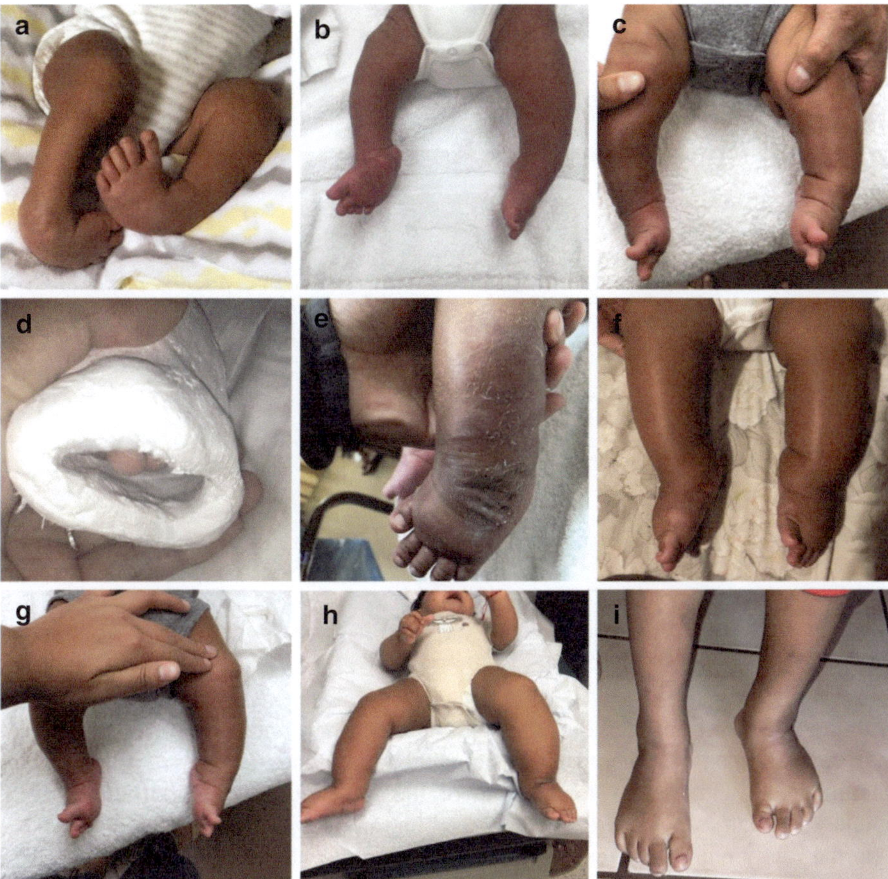

**Fig. 6.8**  Series of photographs demonstrating development of a complex clubfoot. (**a**) Patient at 12 days old with bilateral clubfoot before treatment. (**b**) After the first cast was removed. (**c**) Initial stage of the development of complex features after slipped casts. Notice the swelling especially of the left, the crease formation developing and the short hyperextended 1st digits. (**d**) Slipped third cast with "disappearing toes". (**e**) Left leg with extensive soft-tissue complications; noted edema, bruising, short and hyperextended first digit. (**f**) After bilateral tenotomies the patient still has noted residual swelling and continued complex clubfoot features. (**g**) Four weeks after allowing soft tissue swelling to decrease before casting is reinitiated. Note the patient's residual deformity. (**h**) After transfer of care and treatment with the modified Ponseti technique with three serial casts and repeat open tenotomies. (**i**) Patient at 4 years old with adequate correction but clinical signs of weakness of the lateral compartment

complications and employ the proper treatment modifications. A complex clubfoot demonstrates most of the following physical features: rigid equinus, severe plantarflexion of all the metatarsals, a deep crease above the heel, a transverse crease in the sole of the foot, and a short and hyperextended first toe [26] (Figs. 6.1, 6.3, and 6.10). Other characteristics may include edema and ecchymosis due to loose casts causing abnormal pressures to the lower extremity (Fig. 6.8e). "Disappearing toes"

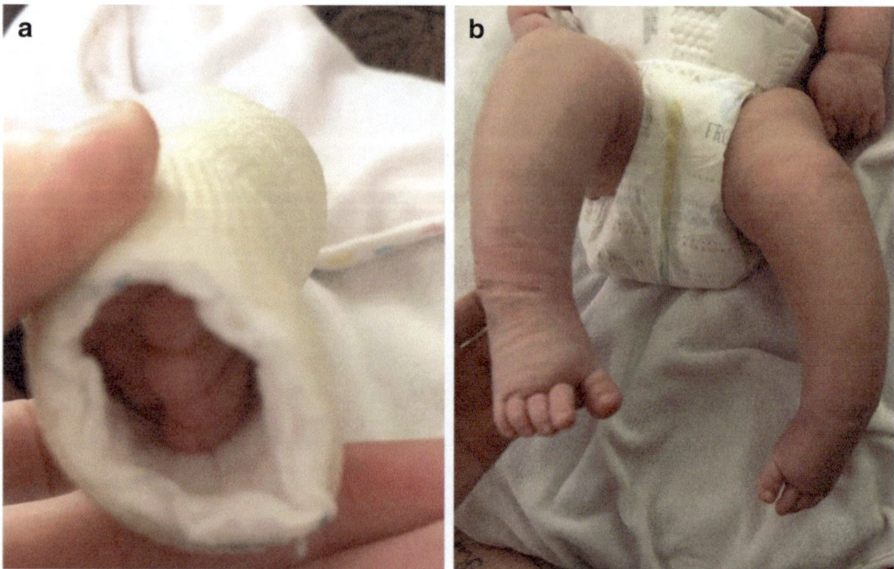


**Fig. 6.9** Complex clubfoot in soft roll cast. (**a**) Infant with soft roll casts that have slipped. (**b**) Infant after removal of slipped casts causing "disappearing toes" with edema and the dorsal skin pushed distally

with the dorsal skin pushed distally is another common finding (Fig. 6.9). The heel may be pushed against the posterior tibia and appear flattened (Fig. 6.10b). A deep lateral crease with lateral subluxation of the forefoot on the hindfoot (midfoot abduction break) may be present due to pronating or everting the foot or excessive external rotation using the calcaneocuboid joint rather than the talus as the fulcrum (Fig. 6.11e–f). Pronation of the forefoot will worsen the deformity by locking the adducted calcaneus under the talus while the midfoot and forefoot are twisted into eversion causing the appearance of a "bean-shaped" foot [37] (Fig. 6.11f). Anterior bowing of the tibia can result from slipping in the cast (Fig. 6.7c). The Achilles tendon is also extremely tight and fibrotic up to the central portion of the calf [26]. The foot may have the appearance of being short and arched downward.

Early identification of a complex clubfoot and utilization of the modified Ponseti technique is crucial to avoid failure of treatment. Dragoni et al. described risk factors for developing a complex iatrogenic deformity as a severe clubfoot according to the Pirani score, a short stubby clubfoot, and an unmolded plaster cast that slips [34]. Duman et al. discussed that the shortness of the first metatarsal of a complex clubfoot is the most resistant component of the treatment [38]. Bozkurt et al. reported a higher incidence of complex clubfoot in their referred patients compared with their initial patients, which is consistent with the authors' experience [39]. Ponseti et al. also had a higher percentage of complex clubfeet from referred patients [26]. Deviation from the Ponseti method increases the likelihood of treatment failure [40, 41]. Ponseti discussed that casting should be done by an experienced

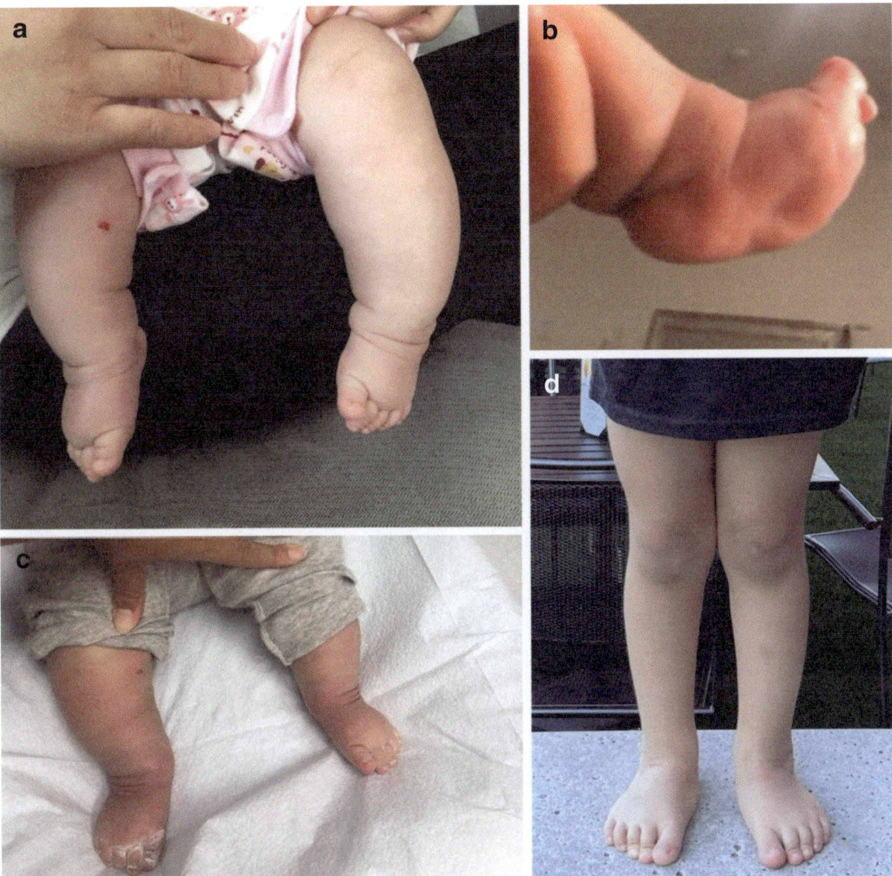

**Fig. 6.10** Bilateral complex clubfeet with history of multiple slipped casts. (**a**) A 2-month-old after four slipped casts. (**b**) Note the flattened heel abutting up against the tibia and prominent posterior creases. (**c**) After modified Ponseti technique and bilateral tenotomies, 1 month after being in braces without issues. (**d**) At 4 years of age without history of relapse

practitioner who understands the pathologic anatomy of the foot and not designated to an unsupervised assistant [37]. Miller et al. compared institutions with multiple providers who used nonuniform Ponseti cast applications to another institution using a single provider with strict adherence to the Ponseti principles. The results showed the nonuniform Ponseti cast applications led to 46% of the cases requiring major surgical intervention compared to 1.7% following the strict Ponseti protocols [41]. Mayne et al. showed that a dedicated Ponseti clinic had superior results with their outcomes of clubfoot treatment when compared to a general clinic [40]. Strict adherence to the Ponseti principles has demonstrated a decrease in failure rates [40–42].

The materials used for clubfoot treatment are important. We recommend the use of plaster of Paris, a material that allows shaping and molding, which is essential in

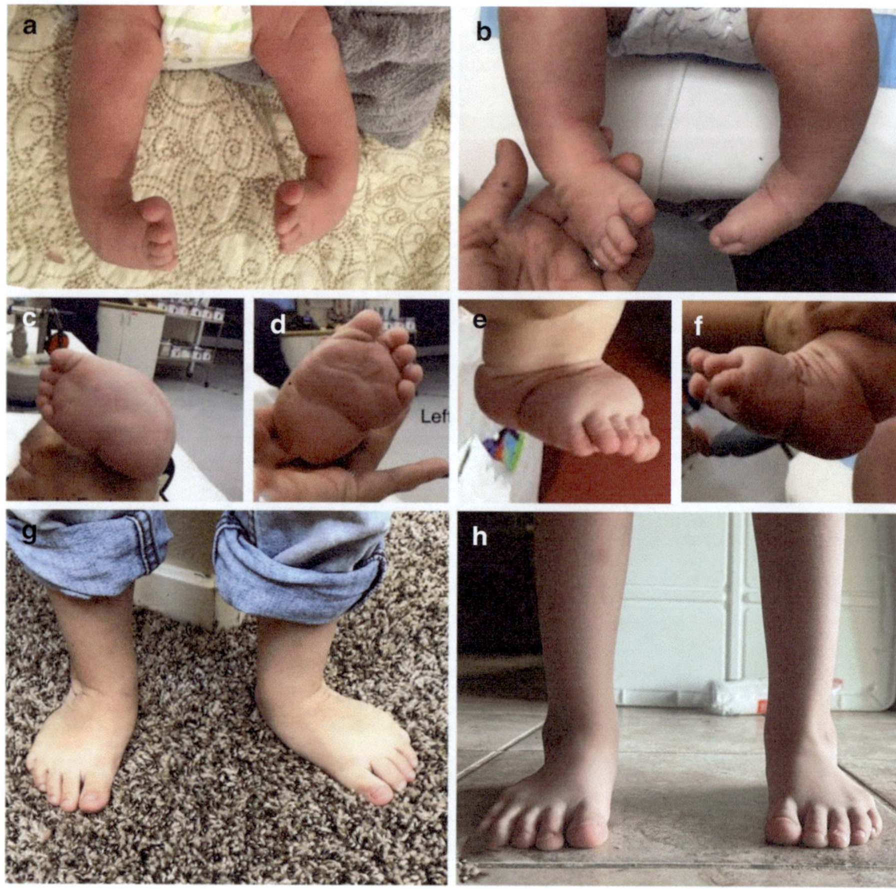

**Fig. 6.11** Patient with development of a complex clubfeet. (**a**) 3-week-old infant before treatment. (**b**) Patient at 6 weeks old after first cast removed. (**c–f**) 5 months old after 4 months of casting and Right side tenotomy and two tenotomies of the left side. (**c**) Noted lateral crease forming on the right foot. (**d**) Note the increase of the cavus with significant plantar crease of the left foot. (**e**) Notice the increase in the midfoot break of the right foot with a lateral crease formation. (**f**) "Bean-shape" foot appearance of the left foot. (**g**) Patient at 2 years old after transfer of care and correction using the modified Ponseti technique with serial casts, repeat tenotomies, and minimal posterior release. After this visit, the brace angle was decreased further to 30° on the left side due to the noted pronation in stance and physical therapy was initiated. (**h**) Patient at 4 years and 10 months old with good function and maintenance of correction without a history of relapse

identification of anatomic landmarks crucial for clubfoot correction. This is especially important when treating complex clubfeet since the landmarks are more difficult to find due to the complexities. Soft rolls and fiberglass casts do not allow the precise molding that is done with plaster and make these small anatomical landmarks even more difficult to identify. Soft rolls are generally too soft allowing motion and bending of the knee increasing the chance of slipping (Fig. 6.12).

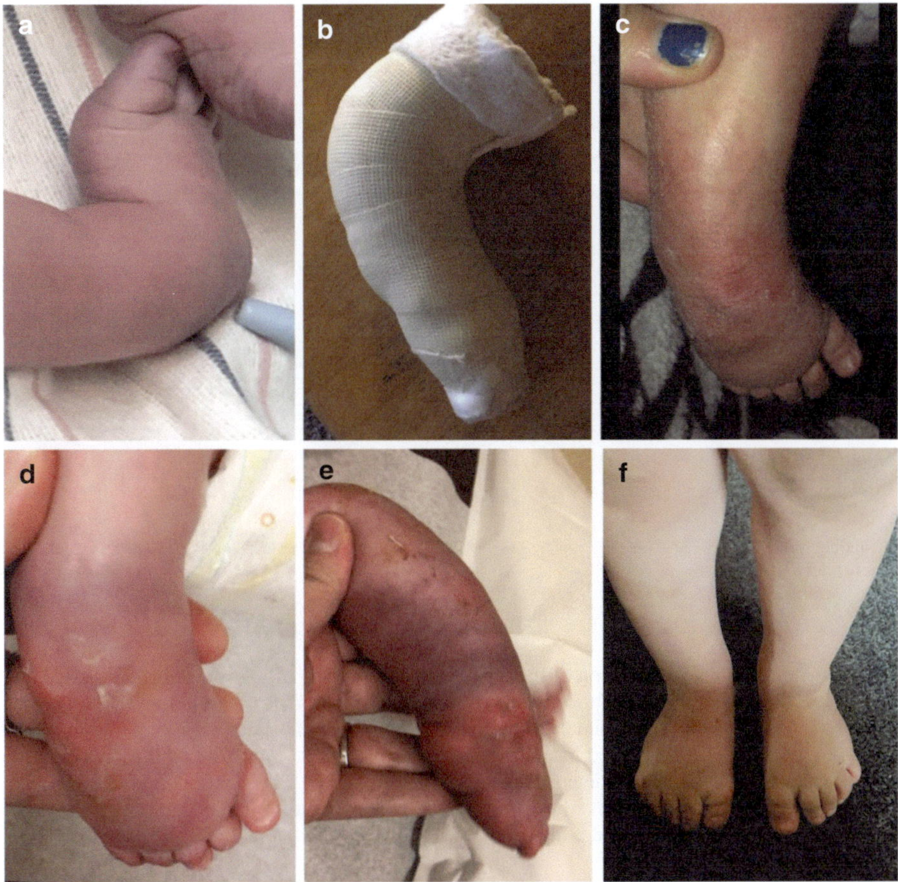

**Fig. 6.12** Development of complex clubfoot with significant soft-tissue complications. (**a**) Newborn Infant with isolated clubfoot before casting. (**b**) Photograph of one of the many casts that slipped completely off the infant's leg. (**c**) Initial stages of complex clubfoot features with anterior and lateral edema developing. (**d**) Further development of complex features with increased edema and erythema noted. (**e**) Severe deformity and bruising with open wounds developed after months of slipped casts. (**f**) Patient at 3 years old after transfer of care treated with the modified Ponseti method and Achilles tenotomy

However, it is important to recognize that if plaster casts are used but not molded correctly, the efforts are futile and can lead to further slipping and grotesque deformities [34] (Fig. 6.7). The key is the physician must know the approach to manipulation and feel comfortable with materials being used.

Casting is done with minimal padding to prevent motion and slipping and allowing maximum control. It is essential to use above-the-knee casts from toe to groin to prevent the ankle and talus from rotating. Above-the-knee casts allow for the best correction, considering the gastrocnemius muscle originates above the knee allowing for better control of the deforming forces. If application is far below the groin,

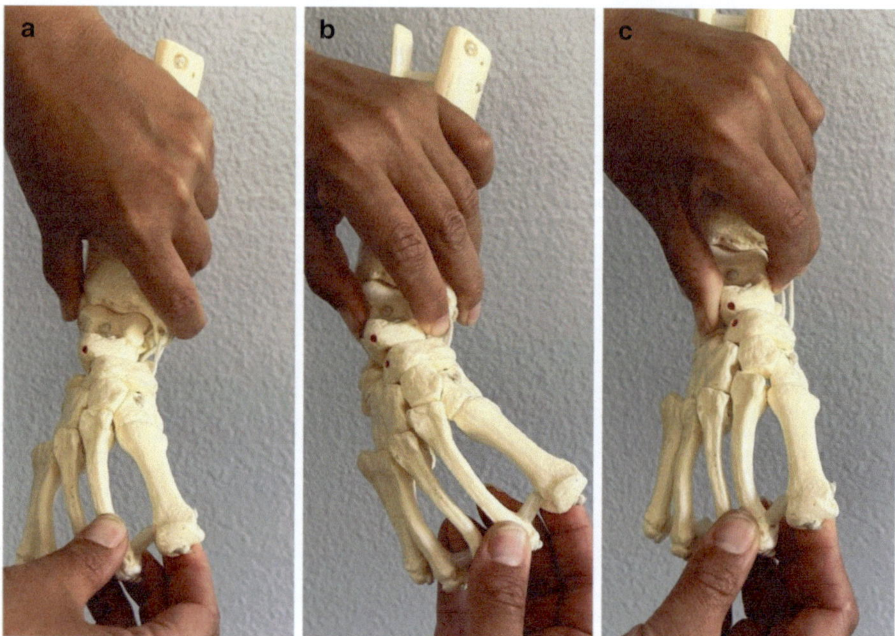

**Fig. 6.13** Model showing position of the talus and identification of the subtalar joint motion. (**a**) Identification of the subtalar joint starts with grasping the forefoot with one hand and with the second hand feeling anteriorly the lateral malleolus with the thumb and medial malleolus with the index finger. (**b**, **c**) The thumb and index finger are moved forward to palpate the head of the talus and feel the navicular on one side and the anterior tuberosity of the calcaneus on the other side. Motion is felt at the subtalar joint when the foot is slowly abducted and the anterior tuberosity of the calcaneus moves laterally under the head of the talus

the gastrocnemius muscle will not be immobilized, and treatment can be compromised due to the cast slipping causing various degrees of deformity. Another cause for slipping is not achieving enough bend in the knee during cast application leading to motion and possible further deformity.

## Modified Ponseti Technique

Complex clubfoot is a separate entity and should be treated differently than isolated clubfoot. Modifying the treatment regimen for these patients results in correction of the deformities [26–28, 36, 38, 43]. When treating complex clubfoot, it is recommended to use the modified Ponseti method described by Ponseti et al. in 2006 [26]. When encountering complex clubfoot, it is imperative to allow severe edema, bruising, and/or sores to heal before casting is reinitiated (Fig. 6.12). Once the soft tissues heal, better manipulation is achieved preventing further complications and correct identification of the subtalar joint.

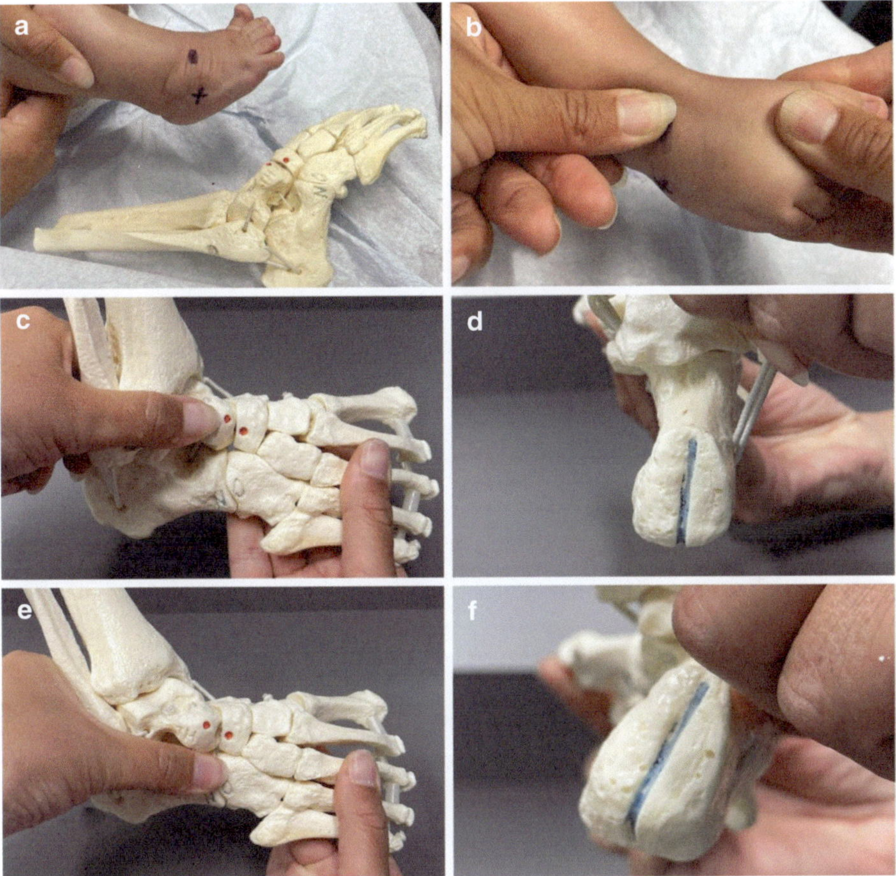

**Fig. 6.14** Hand placement for manipulation of complex clubfoot. (**a**) Photograph demonstrating anatomical placement with the dots showing the correct position at the lateral aspect of the talar head versus the "X" indicating the calcaneal cuboid joint and where not to place the thumb. (**b**) The index finger resting over the posterior aspect of the lateral malleolus while the thumb of the same hand applies counter pressure over the lateral aspect of the head of the talus. (**c**, **d**) Anatomical model showing correct manipulation technique with the index finger resting over the lateral malleolus while the thumb of the same hand applies counter pressure over the lateral aspect of the head of the talus allowing the calcaneus to glide under the talus correcting the varus deformity (blue line now perpendicular). (**e**, **f**) Calcaneal reduction is inhibited when counter pressure is applied to the calcaneal cuboid joint instead of the head of the talus. (Blue line showing the calcaneus remains in varus)

The modified Ponseti technique consists of first identifying the subtalar joint by holding the toes and metatarsals with one hand while feeling the malleoli anteriorly with the thumb and index finger of the second hand (Fig. 6.13a). The thumb and index finger are then positioned anteriorly to grasp the head of the talus and feel the navicular on one side and the anterior tuberosity of the calcaneus on the other side (Fig. 6.13b, c). Motion is felt at the subtalar joint when the foot is slowly abducted,

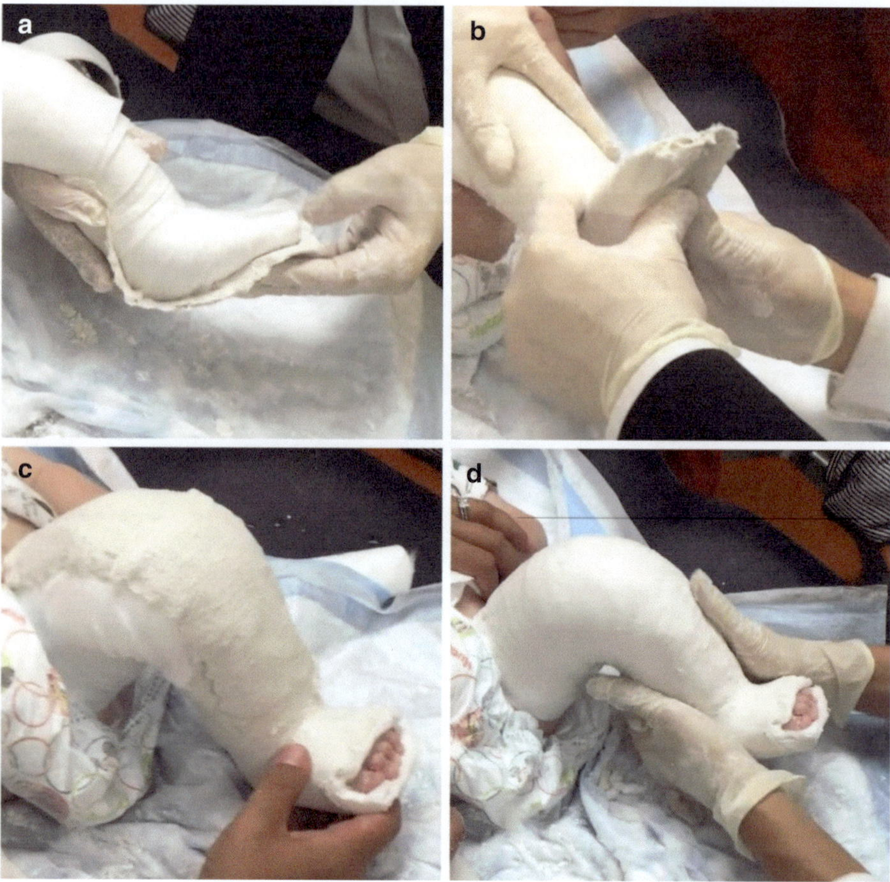

Fig. 6.15 Modified Ponseti casting technique. (a) A posterior splint is applied behind the calf, heel, and sole of the foot and incorporated into a well-molded plaster cast. (b) Photograph showing the "four-finger technique." This is performed by grasping the foot and ankle with both hands while the thumbs are placed under the metatarsals pushing the foot into dorsiflexion as an assistant stabilizes the knee in flexion. (c) The knee is immobilized at 110° of flexion by using an anterior splint from the upper thigh to the anterior leg and reinforcing it with plaster. (d) Finished cast after completing the modified Ponseti casting technique

and the anterior tuberosity of the calcaneus moves laterally under the head of the talus (Fig. 6.13c). Motion is dependent on the severity of the deformity and should increase after the initial castings if proper technique has been performed. Clear identification of the head of the talus is paramount but may be difficult as it can be less prominent than the anterior tuberosity of the calcaneus. During cast application, the index finger rests over the posterior aspect of the lateral malleolus while the thumb of the same hand applies counter pressure over the lateral aspect of the head of the talus, not on the very prominent tuberosity of the calcaneus as this can inhibit calcaneal reduction (Fig. 6.14).

Next, hyperflexion of the metatarsals and rigid equinus are corrected simultaneously to prevent slippage. A posterior splint is applied behind the calf, heel, and sole and incorporated into a well-molded plaster cast immobilizing the foot in the correct position and avoiding the need for excessive plaster (Fig. 6.15a). The "four-finger technique" is performed by grasping the foot and ankle with both hands while the thumbs are placed under the metatarsals pushing the foot into dorsiflexion as an assistant stabilizes the knee in flexion (Fig. 6.15b). It is important not to hyperabduct the metatarsals and hindfoot. The knee is immobilized at 110° of flexion by applying another anterior splint from the thigh to the anterior leg and reinforcing it with plaster around the thigh (Fig. 6.15c). Using splints will avoid excessive plaster behind the knee and in front of the ankle.

Adduction of the forefoot is typically corrected after one or two cast applications. It is recommended not to abduct more than 40° [26]. Care is taken not to over abduct the foot to prevent tightening of the flexor tendons and the quadratus plantae muscle resulting in an increase of the cavus deformity. Casts are changed every 5–7 days similar to the traditional Ponseti protocol [7].

Most complex clubfoot patients require an Achilles tenotomy to address the equinus and achieve full correction [26]. The Achilles tenotomy is performed 1.5 cm above the posterior skin crease of the heel. The posterior tuberosity of the calcaneus is typically very high given the severe contracture of the Achilles [26]. It is important to ensure a complete tenotomy is achieved as the tendon is very deep and wide. The goal is to achieve at least 5° of dorsiflexion. It has been observed that ankle dorsiflexion can be less in this group of patients when compared to isolated clubfeet [26]. In patients with prior treatment, a second tenotomy may be required to achieve full correction. When repeating an Achilles tenotomy, a mini-open procedure is preferred to visualize complete transection of the tendon and release of any scar tissue. In severe cases, if 5° of dorsiflexion is not achieved after the tenotomy, a limited posterior release is considered as detailed in the Dobbs adaptation technique below. The post tenotomy cast is applied in maximum dorsiflexion and no more than 40° of abduction. This cast remains on for 3–4 weeks.

It is essential to remember that these feet are unusually more stiff and may require a greater number of casts. In the treatment of complex clubfoot, continued neurological exams are critical in order to ensure the clubfoot is occurring in isolation [31]. After the last cast is removed, bracing or ankle foot orthosis (AFO) protocol is initiated as described in the respective sections below.


## Dobb's Adaptation Technique


Tibial bowing can be observed when treating a severe complex clubfoot. We recommend adjusting the modified Ponseti technique to address tibial bowing. This technique is an adaptation to the modified Ponseti technique. Customized manipulations are used to correct the distorted anatomy. In this adaptation, the lower-leg cast application is the same as in the modified Ponseti method (Fig. 6.16). The main

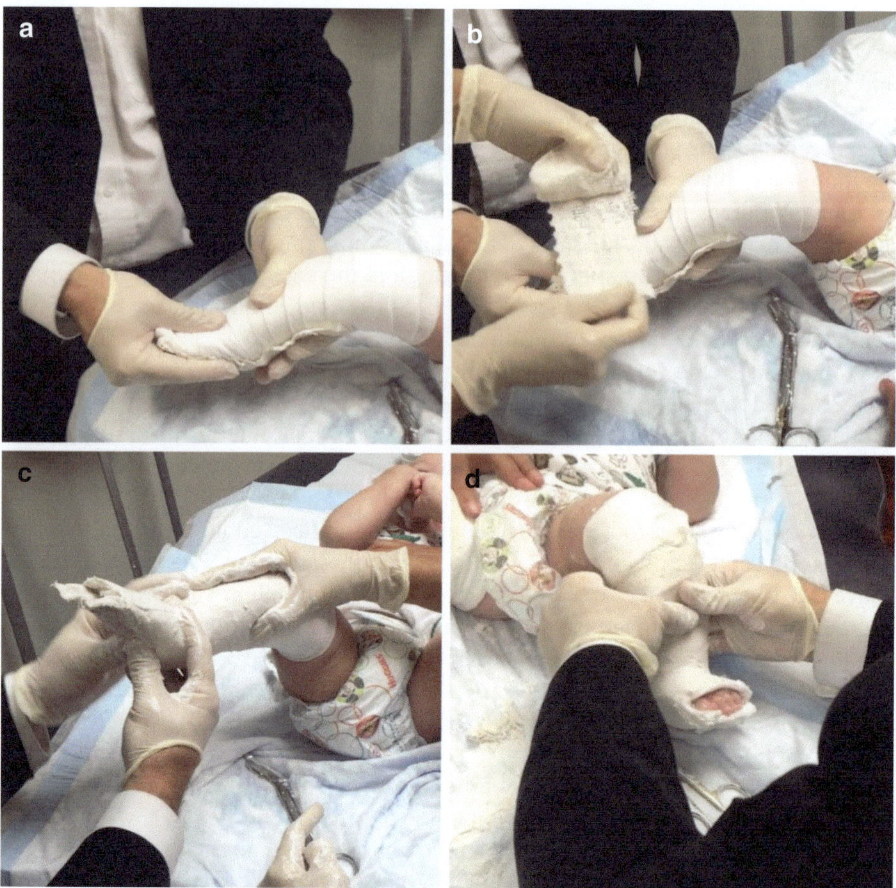

**Fig. 6.16** Dobbs adaptation technique lower leg application: (**a**) A posterior splint is applied behind the calf, heel, and sole of the foot to avoid excessive plaster use. (**b**) The posterior splint is incorporated into a well-molded plaster cast. (**c**) The "four-finger technique" is performed. (**d**) The plaster is applied carefully creating a smooth mold along the anterior tibia making sure to remove any dead space

difference in the technique is hyperflexing the knee and applying pressure on the proximal aspect of the tibia while the other hand is pulling anteriorly from behind the leg instead of at the end of the tibia or the foot (Fig. 6.17). This maneuver creates counter pressure with two opposite forces while hyperflexing the knee to 110°–120°. If this is not performed, the tight gastrocnemius muscle will contribute to bowing of the tibia since its origin is proximal to the articular surfaces of the medial and lateral condyles of the femur. The plaster is applied carefully creating a smooth mold along the anterior tibia and posterior leg locking the knee in flexion. If care is not taken in cast application, motion of the knee will occur, and the leg will abut against the cast causing the tibial bowing. As the knee extends in a loose cast, it applies pressure to the proximal aspect of the tibia and allows the deforming force of the tight Achilles

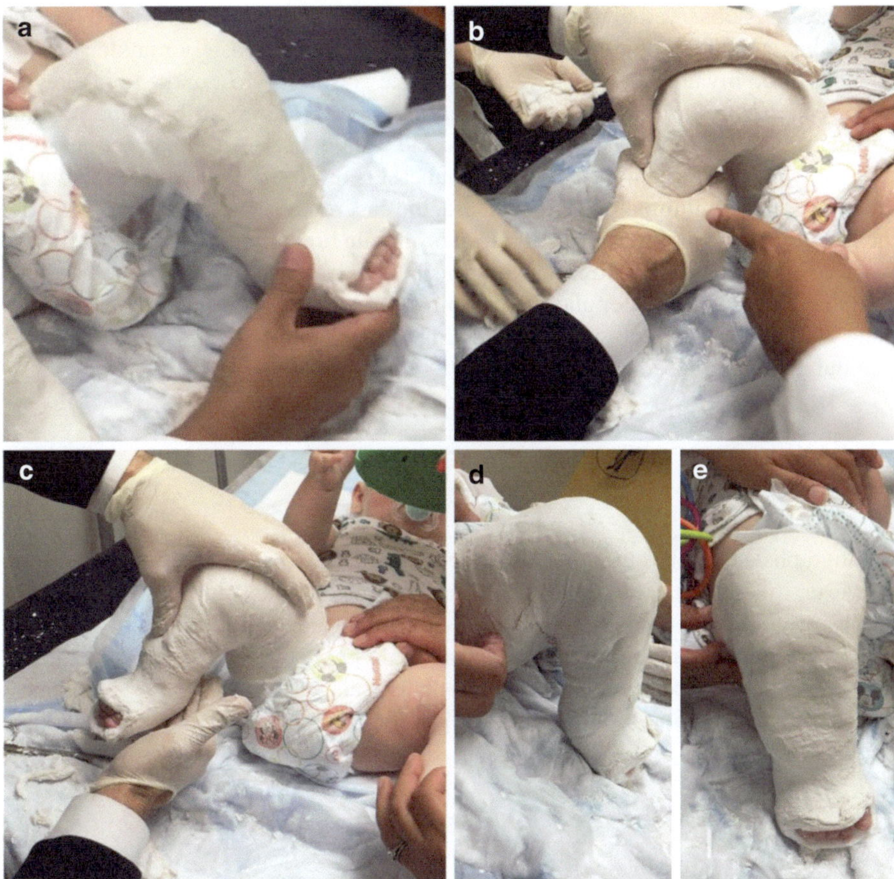

**Fig. 6.17** Dobbs adaptation technique upper leg application: (**a**) The knee is immobilized at 110°–120° of flexion by using an anterior splint from the upper thigh to the anterior leg and reinforcing it with plaster. (**b**) Hyperflexing the knee and applying pressure on the proximal aspect of the tibia while the other hand is pulling anteriorly from behind the leg instead of at the end of the tibia or the foot. (**c**) This maneuver creates counter pressure with two opposite forces while hyperflexing the knee to 110°–120°. (**d**, **e**) Lateral and anterior view of the finished cast demonstrating a smooth mold along the anterior tibia and posterior leg locking the knee in flexion

to contribute to the bowing. With hyperflexion of the knee, the gastrocnemius muscle relaxes decreasing tension distally.

All severely complex clubfeet with tibial bowing require tenotomies, and some require further minimal posterior releases. In these cases, an open technique is recommended to perform the Achilles tenotomy and minimal posterior release. This is done through a 1-cm longitudinal incision along the Achilles tendon. A right-angle clamp is used to protect the subcutaneous tissue and isolate the Achilles tendon, and a complete tenotomy is performed. Range of motion is performed to determine if adequate dorsiflexion was achieved after the tenotomy. If less than 5° of dorsiflexion is observed after tenotomy, then small retractors are inserted to protect the medial and lateral neurovascular bundles, and a limited posterior ankle and subtalar capsulotomy are performed in an "a la carte" fashion. Most of the tibial bowing is corrected with casting prior to the tenotomy, but there might be some residual bowing due to the tight gastrocnemius muscle. In most cases, full correction of the tibial bowing will be achieved after the final cast is removed. Following the Achilles tenotomy and/or minimal posterior release, the cast remains on for 3–4 weeks. After the last cast removal, the child will return or initiate bracing with the foot abduction brace of choice as described in the sections below. It is important to remember that complex clubfeet are stiffer and may require a greater number of casts. In the treatment of complex clubfeet with tibial bowing, repeat neurological exams are vital to rule out an undiagnosed atypical clubfoot.

## Imaging

Radiographs are not routinely performed in the treatment of isolated clubfoot. However, imaging may be considered when treating complex clubfoot. When radiographs are obtained in a complex clubfoot, the calcaneus and talus are in severe plantarflexion with a parallel talocalcaneal angle [25, 26] (Fig. 6.18a). The cuboid may be displaced medially with all of the metatarsals, especially the first metatarsal, in severe plantarflexion. Some complex clubfeet are hyperabducted at the LisFranc

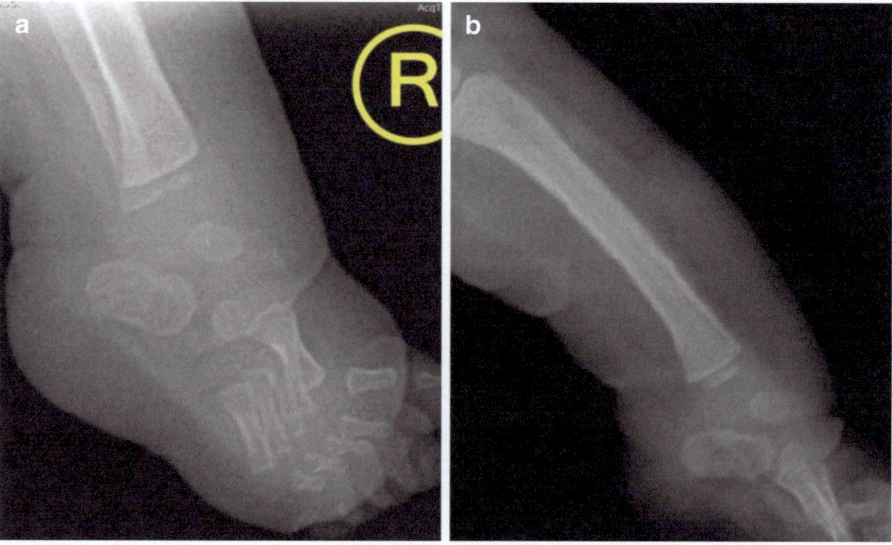


**Fig. 6.18** 4 1/2 months old infant with complex clubfoot and tibial bowing. (**a**) All of the metatarsals, especially the first metatarsal, are in severe plantarflexion. (**b**) X-ray demonstrating tibial bowing

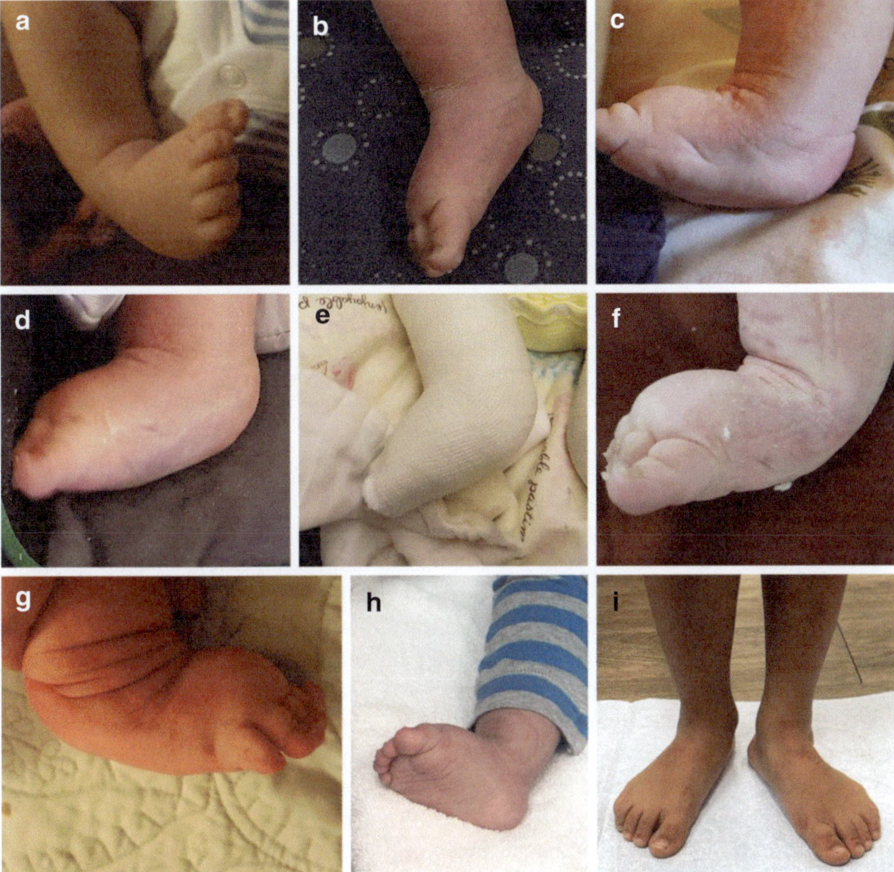

**Fig. 6.19** Development of rocker bottom deformity. (**a**) Newborn with isolated clubfoot before treatment. (**b**) After removal of the first cast. (**c**) After removal of the third cast. Note the rocker bottom deformity is starting to form. (**d**) After removal of the fifth cast with continued signs of deformity and dorsal edema. (**e**) Photograph of the 6th cast. Notice the plantar convexity of cast. (**f**) Full development of a rocker bottom due to dorsiflexion of the forefoot without appropriate correction of the hindfoot equinus. (**g**) Persistent rocker bottom after weeks out of casts. Parents were instructed to use a foot abduction brace that he was unable to keep on without slipping out of the braces. (**h**) Patient after transfer of care and treatment consisting of serial casts and tenotomy. (**i**) Patient at 5 years of age without a history of relapse

joint with as much as 90° of plantarflexion [26]. Radiographs may be used when specifically assessing bowing of the tibia and rocker bottom deformity and/or ruling out possible fractures. Rocker bottom deformity is created by improper adherence to the Ponseti casting principles (Fig. 6.19). A plantar convexity of the foot is developed due to dorsiflexion of the forefoot without appropriate correction of the hindfoot equinus [44]. Clinical examination can be misleading, yielding an increase in dorsiflexion that comes from the forefoot and not the hindfoot. Examination of the

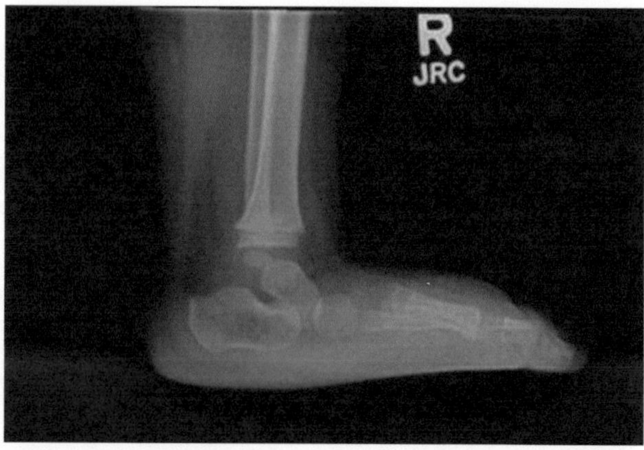

**Fig. 6.20** Rocker bottom deformity in a 2 1/2 year old child with clubfoot

lateral radiograph will aid in diagnosis of the rocker bottom deformity (Fig. 6.20). It is important to address the sagittal plane deformity with a tenotomy and/or minimally invasive posterior release in these cases.

Radiographs can also assist in the evaluation and management of older patients who have had prior surgical interventions. When encountering a severely rigid foot in older patients, radiographs can be used to rule out a tarsal coalition that may be impeding movement and correction. Studies have shown that tarsal coalitions can be associated with clubfeet on rare occasions [45–48]. Radiographs of infants may not be helpful due to the bones not being fully ossified. Diagnosing a tarsal coalition in the presence of a rigid equinovarus deformity can be difficult. These patients may require further evaluation and imaging including computerized tomography (CT) or magnetic resonance imaging (MRI) studies [46]. Monitoring the tarsal coalitions in infants is recommended as long as it does not prevent a plantigrade braceable foot. Treatment of the tarsal coalitions should be delayed until symptoms occur and the feet are larger.

Clubfoot is commonly diagnosed prenatally with ultrasound as early as the first trimester of pregnancy. Ultrasounds can also be useful in diagnosing congenital hip dysplasia. There are varying reports regarding the association of developmental dysplasia of the hip in children with CTEV [49–51]. However, there are consistent recommendations that risk factors exist in patients with a family history of hip dysplasia and/or breech births and first-born children [52].

## Consultations

Consultations are an important part of management in the treatment of all complex clubfeet. A **physical therapy** consultation is useful in the treatment of complex clubfoot. Physical therapy is considered after the last cast is removed especially if the child is of walking age or older when treatment is initiated. Due to the increased number of casts seen with complex clubfoot, physical therapy aids in recovering the strength in the muscles and helps with flexibility. Physical therapists play a crucial role in the early detection of subtle muscle imbalances by evaluating strengths and weaknesses and obtaining baseline objective measurements. This can be particularly useful in unilateral clubfoot to avoid compensating with the non-clubfoot. Another modality physical therapists use is Kinesiology Therapeutic Tape (KT Tape). KT tape is an elastic cloth tape used to support and relieve pain in muscles, joints, and/or ligaments. KT tape provides support without limiting range of motion and is used to promote dorsiflexion and eversion. Adequate mobility is necessary in order for the kinesiotape to have an effect.

Physical therapy is also vital in patients who experience recurrences and/or require surgery. After treatment with serial casts with or without the addition of surgical intervention, physical therapy is initiated as often as three to five times a week after the last cast is removed. Therapists will aid with age-appropriate gross motor skills and help with the return to normal activity. As the patient recovers and strengthens the lower extremity muscles, community-based sports and activities can be explored safely with the guidance of the provider and physical therapist.

Even if formal physical therapy is not explored, stretching and strengthening are important to maintain correction and improve long-term function in all clubfeet. In order to help prevent a recurrent equinus contracture, all clubfoot caregivers are instructed on how to effectively perform range-of-motion exercises as soon as children come out of their last cast. These exercises should be reviewed every visit (https://www.dobbsbrace.com/clubfoot-tutorials).

A referral to a **pediatric orthotist** that has experience with clubfoot is a crucial part of the treatment plan. In many clinics, they will be the one fitting the child with any braces used. They are invaluable with helping manage any pressure areas and making the ankle foot orthosis (AFO), supramalleolar orthosis (SMO), and/or orthotics the child might need to assist with gait and function and improve their quality of life during the various stages of treatment.

**Early intervention** is a service and resource that is considered when treating clubfoot. Studies have demonstrated that a percentage of infants with clubfoot will eventually carry other medical conditions that may require time in obtaining a definitive diagnosis [13, 53, 54]. Studies have also reported delays in motor milestones when compared to their counterparts [55]. Early intervention can potentially improve physical and social skills, improving their outcomes and quality of life. These services may include physical therapy, occupational therapy, speech therapy, and other types of services based on the specific needs of the child and family. A team approach can help these children achieve the best physical, social, and cognitive development long term. If there are concerns for secondary diagnosis, obtaining consultations with a **pediatric neurologist** or **geneticist** may be helpful for ruling out an atypical clubfoot.

## Bracing Protocol

Bracing is vital to the success in all clubfoot treatment. The casting period of clubfoot is usually short but has the most visible results on the correction of the deformity; however, the bracing phase that is crucial for maintenance is much longer typically lasting 4–6 years. A foot abduction brace (FAB) is used to prevent relapse of the deformity in most complex clubfeet [26]. The FAB should be measured and ordered during the last cast application allowing the child to transition directly into the brace after removal of the last cast. If the brace is not ready by the time of removal, then a holding cast is applied until the brace is available to maintain full correction.

If brace intolerance is encountered, it is usually at the early stages of brace initiation. Since the responsibility of the brace lies with the family, close communication with the caregivers has been shown to increase brace adherence and success [56]. A high recurrence rate is associated with bracing noncompliance [57]. If the issues with bracing are addressed and resolved within the first few months, continued brace compliance is higher [56, 58]. Many parents feel anxiety moving into the bracing stage as they now have the daily task of bracing the child. It is recommended to have close follow-up to monitor the development of pressure sores or blisters on the heel or dorsum of the foot. This is done by the provider or a dedicated clubfoot nurse educator who instructs parents on brace wear and helps manage any bracing issues. When there are concerns that cannot be addressed over the phone, the child is brought back into the clinic until issues are resolved.

Brace intolerance can be a major reason why caregivers have a hard time adhering with the bracing protocols. Continued clinical evaluation is crucial to ensure caregivers are understanding the application of the brace and making any modifications to aid with pressure sores. Nonadherence with brace wear may be a result of attempts to brace an uncorrected clubfoot. This is commonly seen in iatrogenic complex clubfeet as the foot may no longer fit well in the brace due to gradual recurrence over time from residual deformity.

Heel and foot blistering can occur throughout the bracing period in a corrected clubfoot or even the non-clubfoot. In the first couple of weeks, having the caregiver remove the brace every 3–4 hours to check for pressure sores is useful in prevention of deep blister formation. If pressure areas occur, modifications can be made to the shoes by adding varying types of padding. If the pressure sore continues and develops into a blister, cessation of the brace is necessary with possible application of a holding cast to prevent loss of correction. If some correction is lost during management of the blisters, serial casting may need to be initiated to regain full correction. Once the blister heals and full correction is verified, the child is placed back into the FAB with close follow-up. Various foot abduction braces are available and can be explored if skin issues continue.

The FAB is worn full time (23 h a day) for the first 3 months then transitioned to part time (14–18 h a day) generally nights and naps until they are wearing them only at nighttime until 4–6 years of age. The standard FAB can be used in most complex

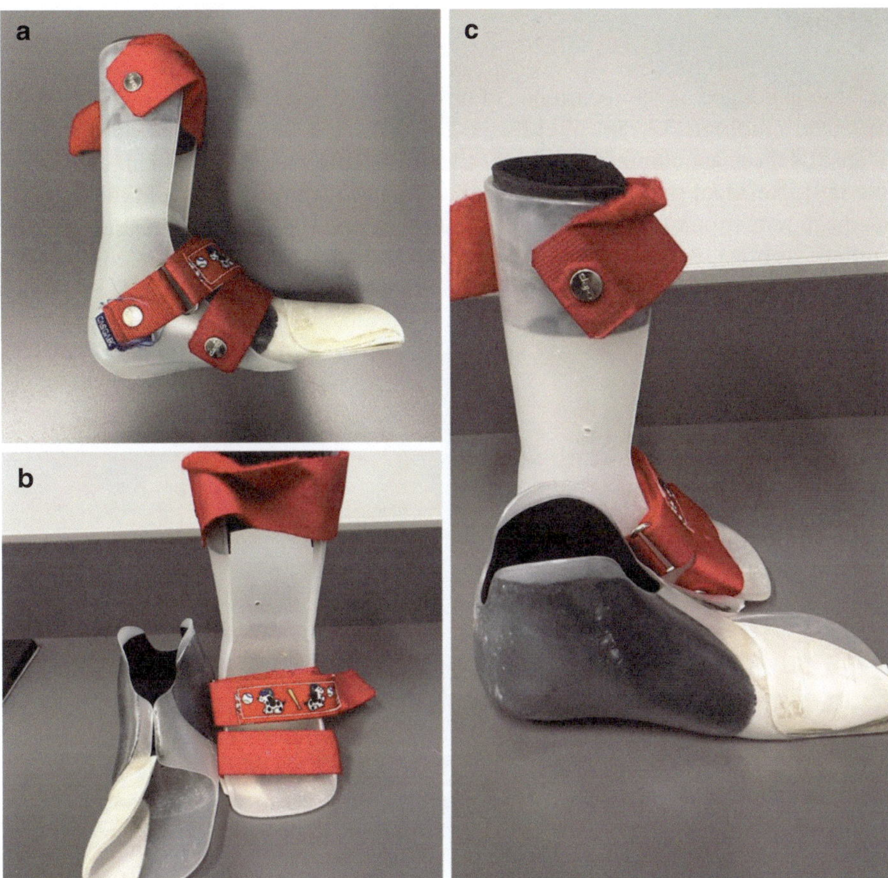

**Fig. 6.21** Ankle foot orthosis (AFO) used in walking patients. (**a**) Complete AFO used initially after treatment. (**b**) Supramalleolar orthosis (SMO) units can be removed from the outer leaf. (**c**) SMO can be used separately once the patient is strong enough to get rid of the AFO portion

clubfeet, but the abduction angle should be reduced to no greater than 40° [26]. In unilateral cases, the non-clubfoot is placed in 30° or 40° of external rotation [26]. The width of the bar is set to the approximate shoulder width of the child.

The bracing protocols may need to be modified in the case of relapse in complex clubfeet. A daytime AFO is helpful in assisting these children after treatment of a recurrence if they are of walking age. The goal is to wean these children out of the AFO after they have initiated physical therapy and regained their muscle strength. This is especially useful following Tibialis Anterior Tendon Transfer (TATT) with or without soft-tissue releases as discussed in the relapse section below. After the TATT, they wear the AFO for 6–8 weeks, then transition into a SMO for another 4–8 weeks depending on strength, which is guided by recommendations from the physical therapist (Fig. 6.21). Nighttime stretching braces are worn and continued until 4–6 years of age and during growth spurts or at least 6 months to 1 year after surgical interventions. Close follow up is necessary even when bracing is going well.

# Relapse

Relapse is defined as the recurrence of any of the components of a previously well-corrected clubfoot [37, 58, 59] (Fig. 6.22). Residual deformity is different from relapse as these are clubfeet that were never fully corrected leaving behind deformities [59]. Residual deformity is seen in some iatrogenic complex clubfoot. Initial adequate reduction of the talus is essential in preventing these residual deformities. In these clubfeet, the foot usually shows improvements in one or more components of the deformity and may even tolerate bracing initially. However, the residual

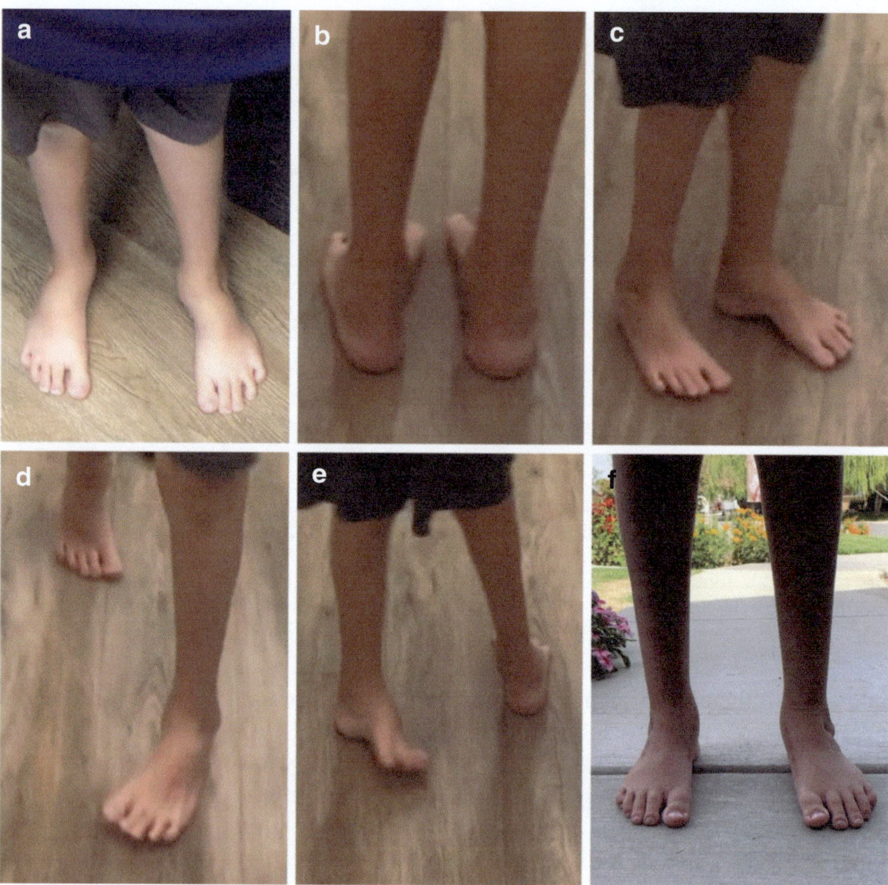

**Fig. 6.22** 8-year-old boy with a history of complex clubfoot as an infant who underwent casting with soft rolls without success leading to posteromedial release surgeries and presented with a relapse. (**a**) Patient in stance. Note the supination in his feet. (**b**) Posterior view demonstrating supination and forefoot adduction of the Left foot. (**c**) Side view demonstrating the cavus deformity of his Left foot. (**d**) Dynamic supination noted in gait. (**e**) Side view of dynamic supination while turning. (**f**) Patient at 9 years old after three serial casts and Achilles tenotomies, Tibialis Anterior Tendon Transfer (TATT) and minimally invasive posterior releases

deformity predisposes the patient to brace intolerance and further deformity, which can be mistakenly classified as a relapse since the clubfoot starts to resemble its original appearance. Relapse also can occur from weakness and decreased muscle strength. Evaluating everter muscle strength at each visit will help identify weaknesses or rule out an atypical clubfoot. If an identifiable weakness is assessed, initiation of physical therapy and consideration of an early TATT are helpful.

Frequent evaluations are necessary to address early signs of relapse. Higher recurrence rates have been associated with complex clubfeet [27, 34]. Matar et al. observed 17 complex clubfeet with an average of 7-year follow-up and noted an overall relapse rate of 53% [27]. Dragoni et al. evaluated nine complex clubfeet and noted a 55% recurrence rate with an average of 7.2 year follow-up [34]. High recurrence rates are also associated with brace intolerance and noncompliance [36]. If the problems with bracing are addressed early, recurrences can be minimized with higher brace compliance [56, 58]. Caregivers should be instructed at each visit on how to effectively perform range-of-motion exercises of the ankle to minimize the chance of recurrent equinus contracture. Education about the higher recurrence rates is helpful, so caregivers can be proactive with their communication of any changes in the child's brace tolerance, flexibility, or gait pattern.

When relapses are encountered in complex clubfeet, they are initially managed with a second series of manipulations and castings with a possible repeat Achilles tenotomy or selective posterior releases. The deformity generally improves with re-casting in most cases. A tibialis anterior tendon transfer is considered when the child is at least 2 1/2 years of age, and there is dynamic supination of the forefoot noted during the swing phase [37]. This is only performed if the patient has good function of the tendon with a minimum of 4/5 muscle strength. When a TATT is performed, most of the correction of the transverse and frontal planes are achieved with serial casting prior to surgery. This procedure is performed to maintain correction as a "biologic brace" and not only as a corrective procedure. If the TATT is performed without any prior serial casting, the deformity may not be fully corrected (Fig. 6.23). The sagittal plane is usually addressed with a repeat open Achilles tenotomy and selective minimally invasive posterior release. In severe relapses in older children, other ancillary procedures may be required. After the TATT is performed, the patient is casted with a nonweight-bearing above-knee cast for 4 weeks and then transition into a below-the-knee weight-bearing cast for 2 weeks. After the casting is complete, the child will benefit from a daytime AFO for 6–8 weeks to allow strengthening and help ease return to ambulation while also strengthening the proximal muscles and core. After the use of an AFO, the child will transition to a SMO for another 4–6 weeks depending on how quickly the child is able to return to normal activities. Brace cessation should be tailored to the patient's strength and clinical exam. Continued follow-up is done to assess any changes in gait pattern and functional abilities. The use of bracing and physical therapy may be needed through any growth spurts.

More research is still necessary in understanding relapses and the cause of clubfoot. In the future, a detailed physical exam in combination with the use of diagnostic studies will give us prognostic knowledge. With this information in combination

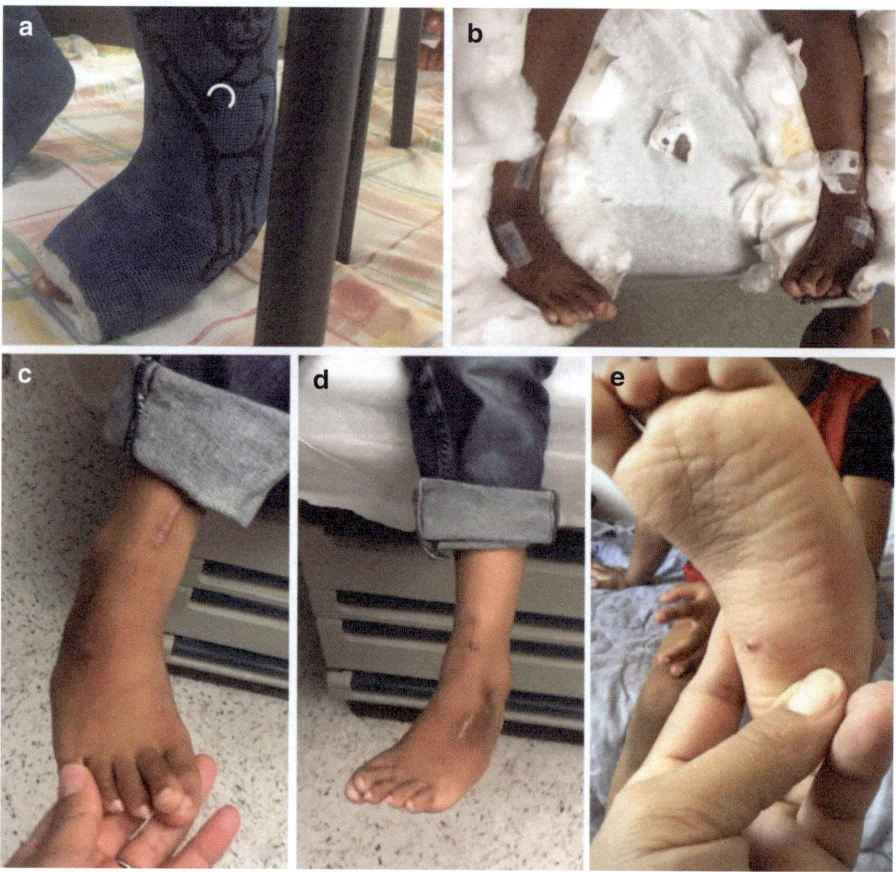

**Fig. 6.23** 3-year-old boy with history of complex clubfoot with residual deformity after a Tibialis Anterior Tendon Transfer (TATT). (**a**) Patient was placed in a below the knee walking cast after a TATT without serial casting prior to surgery. (**b**) Cast removal at 3 weeks after TATT, notice the position of the legs inside the casts. (**c**) Right foot with residual deformity after TATT. (**d**) Left foot also with noted residual deformity after TATT. (**e**) Plantar view of left foot demonstrating the adduction still present after surgery

with genetic risk factors, we may be able to predict relapses before they occur and customize individual treatment plans. For example, if an MRI demonstrates healthy muscle in all compartments of the lower leg, that patient may be at low risk of relapse, and treatment could be individualized to allow that patient to stop bracing earlier. In contrast, if the MRI demonstrated a smaller or absent muscle in the lateral compartment, one may predict this patient has a greater risk of relapse and be a candidate for an early tendon transfer [21]. Regardless of the patient's type of clubfoot, most children should remain active and strong and will benefit from a stretching and strengthening routine.

Relapse in the literature is often considered only as a patient who had treatment after initial correction; however, many patients have residual deformity that is not treated. Relapse is also subjective, and the actual diagnosis and treatment plan can vary depending on the healthcare provider and parents as there are currently no standardized relapse recommendations. Research in the future can assist with knowing how much flexibility and strength is needed at the time of brace cessation or what other factors contribute to the likelihood of relapse. When dealing with older children, follow-ups may become less frequent in many clinics, and some patients stop seeing their doctor altogether. It may be difficult to tell what exactly these patient's functional outcomes are if they stop following up with their particular doctor, and another provider takes over care. It is important to educate parents about functional limitations that can occur with growth spurts after bracing cessation especially when obvious residual deformity is present. Patients need to follow up with their healthcare provider if they experience pain or have changes in their gait pattern. Some of these patients do not have any signs of visible deformity. When they ambulate, they demonstrate a "normal" gait pattern. However, when examined, they demonstrate equinus and complain of pain in their ankles or have limitations with squatting and/or balance. Open communication with these families allows them to return to the clinic for evaluation and initiate bracing, physical therapy, or further treatment, if needed.

# References


1. Chung CS, Nemechek RW, Larsen IJ, et al. Genetic and epidemiological studies of clubfoot in Hawaii. General and medical considerations. Hum Hered. 1969;19:321–42.
2. Wynne-Davies R. Genetic and environmental factors in the etiology of talipes equinovarus. Clin Orthop. 1972;84:9–13.
3. Beals RK. Club foot in the Maori: a genetic study of 50 kindreds. N Z Med J. 1978;88(618):144–6.
4. Dobbs MB, Gurnett CA. Genetics of clubfoot. J Pediatr Orthop Part B. 2012;21(1):7–9.
5. Rieger MA, Dobbs MB. Clubfoot. Clin Podiatr Med Surg. 2022;39(1):1–14.
6. Wynne-Davies R. Family studies and the cause of congenital club foot. talipes equinovarus, talipes Calcaneo-valgus and Metatarsus varus. J Bone Joint Surg Br. 1964;46:445–63.
7. Ponseti IV, Smoley EN. Congenital clubfoot: the results of treatment. J Bone Joint Surg Am. 1963;45:261–75.
8. Shabtai L, Specht SC, Herzenberg JE. Worldwide spread of the Ponseti method for clubfoot. World J Orthop. 2014;5(5):585–90.
9. Lourenço AF, Morcuende JA. Correction of neglected idiopathic club foot by the Ponseti method. J Bone Joint Surg Br. 2007;89(3):378–81.
10. Funk JF, Lebek S, Seidl T, Placzek R. Comparison of treatment results of idiopathic and non-idiopathic congenital clubfoot: prospective evaluation of the Ponseti therapy. Orthopade. 2012;41(12):977–83.
11. Laaveg SJ, Ponseti IV. Long-term results of treatment of congenital club foot. J Bone Joint Surg Am. 1980;62(1):23–31.
12. Herzenberg JE, Radler C, Bor N. Ponseti versus traditional methods of casting for idiopathic clubfoot. J Pediatr Orthop. 2002;22(4):517–21.

13. Gurnett CA, Boehm S, Connolly A, Reimschisel T, Dobbs MB. Impact of congenital talipes equinovarus etiology on treatment outcomes. Dev Med Child Neurol. 2008;50(7):498–502.
14. Dobbs MB, Gurnett CA. The 2017 ABJS Nicolas Andry Award: advancing personalized medicine for clubfoot through translational research. Clin Orthop. 2017;475(6):1716–25.
15. Boehm S, Limpaphayom N, Alaee F, Sinclair MF, Dobbs MB. Early results of the Ponseti method for the treatment of clubfoot in distal arthrogryposis. J Bone Joint Surg Am. 2008;90(7):1501–7.
16. Dobbs MB, Gurnett CA. Update on clubfoot: etiology and treatment. Clin Orthop. 2009;467(5):1146–53.
17. Sadler B, Gurnett CA, Dobbs MB. The genetics of isolated and syndromic clubfoot. J Child Orthop. 2019;13(3):238–44.
18. Song KS, Kang CH, Min BW, Bae GC, Cho CH, Lee JH. Congenital clubfoot with concomitant peroneal nerve palsy in children. J Pediatr Orthop Part B. 2008;17(2):85–9.
19. Edmonds EW, Frick SL. The drop toe sign: an indicator of neurologic impairment in congenital clubfoot. Clin Orthop. 2009;467(5):1238–42.
20. Gerlach DJ, Gurnett CA, Limpaphayom N, Alaee F, Zhang Z, Porter K, et al. Early results of the Ponseti method for the treatment of clubfoot associated with myelomeningocele. J Bone Joint Surg Am. 2009;91(6):1350–9.
21. Moon DK, Gurnett CA, Aferol H, Siegel MJ, Commean PK, Dobbs MB. Soft-tissue abnormalities associated with treatment-resistant and treatment-responsive clubfoot: findings of MRI analysis. J Bone Joint Surg Am. 2014;96(15):1249–56.
22. Kite JH. The operative treatment of congenital clubfeet. Instr Course Lect. 1955;12:100–5.
23. Kite JH. Conservative treatment of the resistant recurrent clubfoot. Clin Orthop. 1970;70:93–110.
24. Kite JH. Nonoperative treatment of congenital clubfoot. Clin Orthop. 1972;84:29–38.
25. Turco V. Recognition and management of the atypical idiopathic clubfoot. In: The clubfoot: the present and a view of the future. New York: Springer; 1994. p. 76–7.
26. Ponseti IV, Zhivkov M, Davis N, Sinclair M, Dobbs MB, Morcuende JA. Treatment of the complex idiopathic clubfoot. Clin Orthop. 2006;451:171–6.
27. Matar HE, Beirne P, Bruce CE, Garg NK. Treatment of complex idiopathic clubfoot using the modified Ponseti method: up to 11 years follow-up. J Pediatr Orthop Part B. 2017;26(2):137–42.
28. Chu A, Nachamie H, Lehman W. Management of the complex clubfoot: current concept review. JPOSNA. 2019;1:1. Available from https://www.jposna.org/index.php/jposna/article/view/39.
29. van Bosse HJP. Challenging clubfeet: the arthrogrypotic clubfoot and the complex clubfoot. J Child Orthop. 2019;13(3):271–81.
30. Patel A, Mongia AK, Sharma RK, Saini R, Chaudhary C, Singh S. Outcome of atypical & complex clubfoot managed by modified Ponseti method-a prospective study. J Foot Ankle Surg. 2022;2022:4.
31. Yoshioka S, Huisman NJ, Morcuende JA. Peroneal nerve dysfunction in patients with complex clubfeet. Iowa Orthop J. 2010;30:24–8.
32. Ford-Powell VA, Barker S, Khan MSI, Evans AM, Deitz FR. The Bangladesh clubfoot project: the first 5000 feet. J Pediatr Orthop. 2013;33(4):40–4.
33. Perveen R, Evans AM, Ford-Powell V, Dietz FR, Barker S, Wade PW, et al. The Bangladesh clubfoot project: audit of 2-year outcomes of Ponseti treatment in 400 children. J Pediatr Orthop. 2014;34(7):720–5.
34. Dragoni M, Gabrielli A, Farsetti P, Bellini D, Maglione P, Ippolito E. Complex iatrogenic clubfoot: is it a real entity? J Pediatr Orthop Part B. 2018;27(5):428–34.
35. van Praag VM, Lysenko M, Harvey B, Yankanah R, Wright JG. Casting is effective for recurrence following Ponseti treatment of clubfoot. J Bone Joint Surg Am. 2018;100(12):1001–8.
36. Göksan SB, Bursali A, Bilgili F, Sivacioğlu S, Ayanoğlu S. Ponseti technique for the correction of idiopathic clubfeet presenting up to 1 year of age. A preliminary study in children with untreated or complex deformities. Arch Orthop Trauma Surg. 2006;126(1):15–21.

37. Ponseti I. Congenital clubfoot. Fundamentals of treatment. 2nd ed. Oxford: Oxford University Press; 1996.
38. Duman S, Camurcu Y, Cobden A, Ucpunar H, Karahan N, Bursali A. Clinical outcomes of iatrogenic complex clubfoot treated with modified Ponseti method. Int Orthop. 2020;44(9):1833–40.
39. Bozkurt C, Sarıkaya B, Sipahioğlu S, Altay MA, Çetin BV. Using the modified Ponseti method to treat complex clubfoot: early results. Jt Dis Relat Surg. 2021;32(1):170–6.
40. Mayne AIW, Bidwai AS, Beirne P, Garg NK, Bruce CE. The effect of a dedicated Ponseti service on the outcome of idiopathic clubfoot treatment. Bone Jt J. 2014;96(10):1424–6.
41. Miller NH, Carry PM, Mark BJ, Engelman GH, Georgopoulos G, Graham S, et al. Does strict adherence to the Ponseti method improve isolated clubfoot treatment outcomes? A two-institution review. Clin Orthop. 2016;474(1):237–43.
42. Dunkley M, Gelfer Y, Jackson D, Parnell E, Armstong J, Rafter C, et al. Mid-term results of a physiotherapist-led Ponseti service for the management of non-idiopathic and idiopathic clubfoot. J Child Orthop. 2015;9(3):183–9.
43. Mandlecha P, Kanojia RK, Champawat VS, Kumar A. Evaluation of modified Ponseti technique in treatment of complex clubfeet. J Clin Orthop Trauma. 2019;10(3):599–608.
44. Koureas G, Rampal V, Mascard E, Seringe R, Wicart P. The incidence and treatment of rocker bottom deformity as a complication of the conservative treatment of idiopathic congenital clubfoot. J Bone Joint Surg Br. 2008;90(1):57–60.
45. Herzenberg JE, Goldner JL, Martinez S, Silverman PM. Computerized tomography of talocalcaneal tarsal coalition: a clinical and anatomic study. Foot Ankle. 1986;6(6):273–88.
46. Spero CR, Simon GS, Tornetta P. Clubfeet and tarsal coalition. J Pediatr Orthop. 1994;14(3):372–6.
47. Seetharama Rao B, Joseph B. Varus and equinovarus deformities of the foot associated with tarsal coalition. Foot. 1994;4(2):95–9.
48. Van Rysselberghe NL, Souder CD, Mubarak SJ. Unsuspected tarsal coalitions in equinus and varus foot deformities. J Pediatr Orthop Part B. 2020;29(4):370–4.
49. Perry DC, Tawfiq SM, Roche A, Shariff R, Garg NK, James LA, et al. The association between clubfoot and developmental dysplasia of the hip. J Bone Joint Surg Br. 2010;92(11):1586–8.
50. Chou DT, Ramachandran M. Prevalence of developmental dysplasia of the hip in children with clubfoot. J Child Orthop. 2013;7(4):263–7.
51. Zhao D, Rao W, Zhao L, Liu J, Chen Y, Shen P, et al. Is it worthwhile to screen the hip in infants born with clubfeet? Int Orthop. 2013;37(12):2415–20.
52. Paton RW, Choudry QA, Jugdey R, Hughes S. Is congenital talipes equinovarus a risk factor for pathological dysplasia of the hip? A 21-year prospective, longitudinal observational study. Bone Jt J. 2014;96(11):1553–5.
53. Bacino CA, Hecht JT. Etiopathogenesis of equinovarus foot malformations. Eur J Med Genet. 2014;57(8):473–9.
54. Lööf E, Andriesse H, Broström EW, André M, Bölte S. Neurodevelopmental difficulties in children with idiopathic clubfoot. Dev Med Child Neurol. 2019;61(1):98–104.
55. Lööf E. Additional challenges in children with idiopathic clubfoot: is it just the foot? J Child Orthop. 2019;13(3):245–51.
56. Dobbs MB, Rudzki JR, Purcell DB, Walton T, Porter KR, Gurnett CA. Factors predictive of outcome after use of the Ponseti method for the treatment of idiopathic clubfeet. J Bone Joint Surg Am. 2004;86(1):22–7.
57. Azarpira MR, Emami MJ, Vosoughi AR, Rahbari K. Factors associated with recurrence of clubfoot treated by the Ponseti method. World J Clin Cases. 2016;4(10):318–22.
58. Morcuende JA, Dolan LA, Dietz FR, Ponseti IV. Radical reduction in the rate of extensive corrective surgery for clubfoot using the Ponseti method. Pediatrics. 2004;113(2):376–80.
59. Eidelman M, Kotlarsky P, Herzenberg JE. Treatment of relapsed, residual and neglected clubfoot: adjunctive surgery. J Child Orthop. 2019;13(3):293–303.

# Chapter 7
# Surgical Release for Clubfoot: Principles, Indications, and Evaluation


Ken N. Kuo, Peter A. Smith, and Adam Graf


## Introduction of Comprehensive Surgical Releases

Brockman published a monograph on Congenital Club Foot [1] and established the technique of surgical correction of clubfoot. In the ensuing four decades, a number of publications showed poor results, and it was standard to perform multiple surgeries over many years for each patient It was not until 1971 when Turco published an article on one stage posteromedial release with internal fixation [2] that comprehensive surgical procedures gradually gained popularity. In 1979, Turco published a follow-up article that reviewed 240 clubfeet with posteromedial releases, and he reported 83.8% good results according to his criteria [3]. He also concluded that the best results with the least complications occurred in children who were operated between 1 and 2 years old. For the incision, Turco used a posteromedial curved approach. In 1982, Crawford published an article on using the Cincinnati incision after Giannestras' original incision for correction of congenital vertical talus [4]. The Cincinnati approach rapidly gained acceptance and popularity among pediatric


K. N. Kuo (✉)
National Taiwan University Hospital, Taipei, Taiwan

Taipei Medical University, Taipei, Taiwan

Rush University Medical Center, Chicago, IL, USA

P. A. Smith
Rush University Medical Center, Chicago, IL, USA

Shriners Hospital for Children, Chicago, IL, USA
e-mail: psmith@shrinenet.org

A. Graf
Rush University Medical Center, Chicago, IL, USA
e-mail: agraf@shrinenet.org

orthopedic surgeons who treat clubfoot. In 1982–1983, McKay published three-part articles with detailed analysis of pathological anatomy and emphasized the importance of rotation of the calcaneus under the talus in correcting the clubfoot deformity [5–7]. In 1985, Simons published a series of two articles on complete subtalar release as part of posterior medial releases with good results in comparison to the traditional posterior medial releases [8, 9]. He did mention the possibility of overcorrection in complete subtalar releases and emphasized the importance of precise reposition at the end of the procedure. With the evidence of overcorrection in some cases, Bensahel in 1987 used the term "à la carte" to address the need to limit the procedure only to the necessary structures [10].

Although his results were first published in 1963 [11], it was not until the 1990s that the Ponseti method of treatment became adopted by many pediatric orthopedic surgeons. The results are much better especially with range of motion and pain. In a 30-year follow-up study, Dobbs reported patients treated with combined posterior, medial, and lateral extensive release at different times by different surgeons had generally poor functional results and arthritic changes [12]. In a comparison study of the Ponseti method and extensive soft-tissue release method by Smith, Kuo et al., with detailed analysis of physical function, foot biomechanics, and quality-of-life metrics, at more than 20 years follow-up, concluded that although individuals in each treatment group experienced some pain, weakness, and reduced range of motion (ROM), they were highly functional into early adulthood [13]. At adulthood the Ponseti group fared somewhat better than the surgically treated group in ROM at the physical examination and during gait. That group had greater strength and, more importantly, less pain reported on outcomes scores (SF-36). It is apparent that the Ponseti method is a preferable means of correcting clubfoot, both in a general applicability to a population of children that may not have access to surgery, but moreover, the long term results are preferable if there is no scar on the foot.

In spite of better results and popularity of the Ponseti method, there are still some cases of failure that require soft-tissue surgery. Among different centers, it varies from 2% to 20%. Familiarity with soft-tissue procedures and à la carte nature of the treatment are important to practicing pediatric orthopedic surgeons.


## Surgical Principles and Technique

**Indications and Surgical Principles** The initial management of clubfoot deformity is the Ponseti method of manipulation and casting. Only those with persistent relapse where the practitioner is unable to correct the foot by use of the Ponseti method are candidates for posterior medial releases. The person who performs the surgery should be familiar with normal anatomy of the foot and ankle and the pathoanatomy of the clubfoot. In surgery, it is most important not to overcorrect the deformity, especially the subtalar joint. One should pay attention to the cartilage and not to damage it. The cartilage is soft, and the contracted soft tissues are tight.

## Surgical Technique

**Position**  Under general anesthesia, the patient is placed in the prone position with soft rolls under the chest and pelvis. It is essential to protect the airway. The procedure can be performed with a tourniquet.

**Incision**  A Cincinnati incision is carried out (Fig. 7.1). It starts at the midpoint of the first metatarsal through the talonavicular junction on the medial side, curves below the medial malleolus, proceeds posteriorly through the area 1 cm proximal to the heel skin crease, and continues to the lateral side just distal to the tip of lateral malleolus.

**Achilles Tendon**  The subcutaneous soft tissue is dissected with a Mosquito hemostat. The sural nerve at the lateral aspect of Achilles tendon is identified and protected.

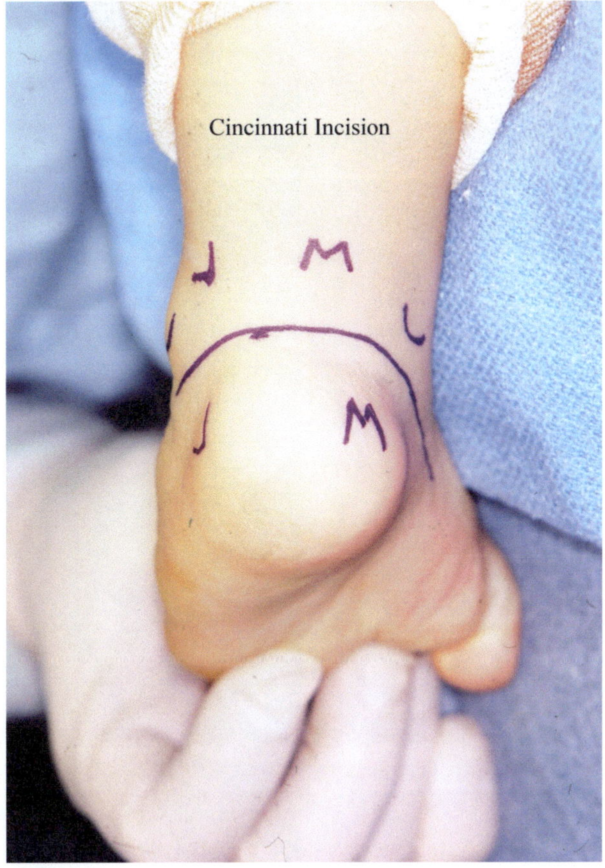


**Fig. 7.1**  Cincinnati incision with patient in prone position. The mark "M" means medial side and "L" lateral side

The Achilles tendon is dissected free from surrounding tissue all the way down to calcaneus. Expose adequate length of Achilles tendon for lengthening. It is possible to expose four centimeters of tendon despite the horizontal skin incision. An Achilles tendon Z-lengthening is carried out with distal horizontal cut at medial side and proximal horizontal cut at lateral side as the foot is in varus deformity (Fig. 7.2). The longitudinal cut is carried out at the center of Achilles tendon. The length of the split would depend on the severity of the equinus deformity.

**Posterior Joint Exposure** The flexor hallucis longus is identified at the posterior medial corner. Blunt dissection is accomplished with a hemostat down to the ankle and subtalar joint. It is important not to accidentally enter the distal tibia epiphysis and cause physeal damage. Usually, it is easier to find the ankle joint. The visible posterior talus is wafer thin as the bone is relatively anterior in this pathological condition, so the subtalar joint is only 2–3 mm below the ankle joint.

**Fig. 7.2** Achilles tendon
Z-lengthening

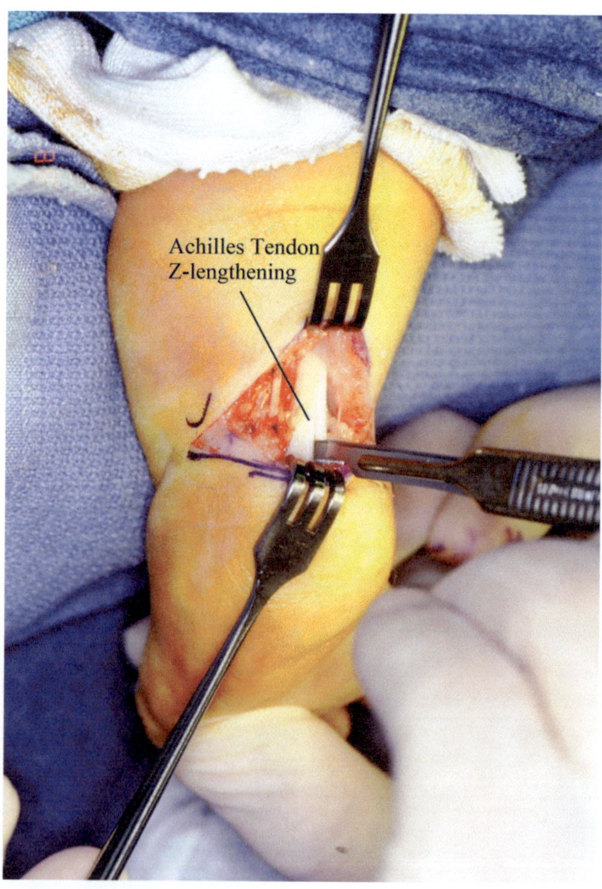

**Lateral Releases** The ankle joint and subtalar joint capsulotomy is performed sharply laterally to the fibula, the posterior talofibular ligament, usually runs in a horizontal direction and should be released longitudinally (Fig. 7.3). The calcaneo-fibular ligament usually is very tight and should be released, so the calcaneus can rotate under talus. It is best to identify both peroneal tendons as they run in the sheath and retract them laterally to visualize this relatively large structure. In older patients with a tight posterior joint, the posterior tibiofibular ligament can be incised to increase the width of the posterior ankle joint.

**Posterior Medial Corner** The incision of the ankle joint and subtalar joint capsule proceeds medially to the flexor hallucis longus tendon sheath, and the tendon sheath is opened (Fig. 7.4). With the neurovascular bundle protected, the capsules can be released to the level of the flexor digitorum longus.

**Neurovascular Structure** At this point, the attention is switched to the medial side of the incision. Palpate the medial malleolus, and immediately posterior to that is the posterior tibial tendon. The laciniate ligament running from medial malleolus to calcaneus over neurovascular structure is released, and the posterior tibial tendon sheath is incised and posterior tibial tendon exposed. The neurovascular bundle behind the tendon is identified and isolated with blunt dissection. The neurovascular bundle along with flexor digitorum longus and flexor hallucis longus can be protected and retracted with a spaghetti vessel loop or umbilical tape passed under (Fig. 7.5).

**Plantar Fasciotomy** If cavus is present, a plantar fasciotomy is performed. Find the interval between the posterior tibial vessels and the calcaneal branch. A mosquito hemostat is used to insert from medial to lateral side of the plantar aspect just in front of calcaneal tuberosity processes. A number 11 knife blade is used to cut the plantar fascia in plantar direction to release the tight structure (Fig. 7.6).

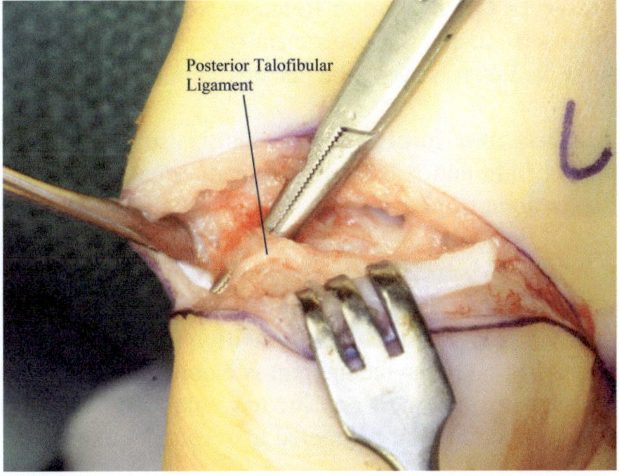


**Fig. 7.3** Posterior talofibular ligament, it runs horizontal direction between posterior talus and fibula

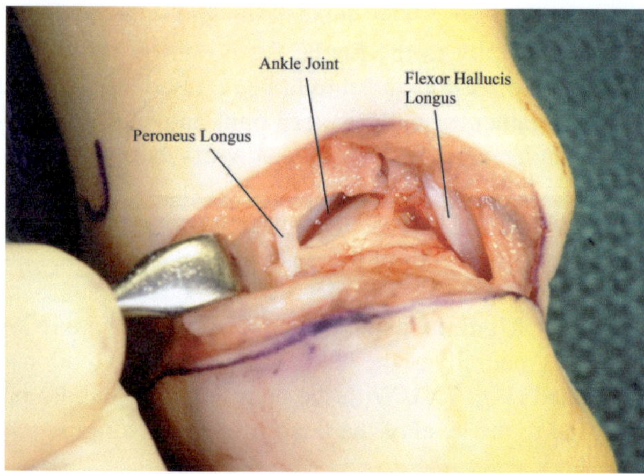



**Fig. 7.4** Posterior ankle joint is opened showing flexor hallucis longus at posterior medial corner and peroneal tendon on the lateral side

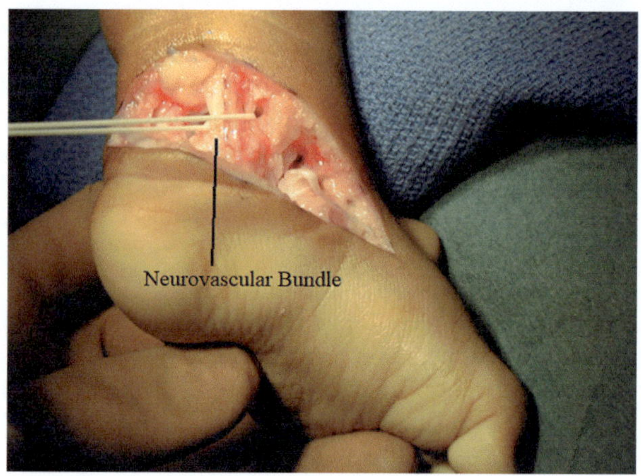



**Fig. 7.5** The neurovascular structure at the posterior medial corner is protected and retracted by a spaghetti vessel loop

**Posterior Tibial Tendon Release** Next, trace the posterior tibial tendon down to the insertion, and dissect it clear (Fig. 7.7). The posterior tibial tendon is detached from the insertion with the distal stump as long as possible for reattachment.

**Talonavicular Joint** The navicular is usually rotated medially to cover the talonavicular joint and is close to the medial malleolus in most cases. Incise the talonavicular joint from the medial side. Carefully divide the junction of the navicular and medial malleolus and excise any redundant soft tissue. In opening the talonavicular joint capsule; one must take care not to cut into the talar neck. The joint capsule should be released from the medial, superior, and inferior sides but not the lateral side to protect the circulation. Caution should be taken not to damage the joint cartilage as the talonavicular joint is a convex–concave shape and is not running perpendicular to the incision. The navicular can be grasped gently with a rake pulling distally and the joint distracted to eventually expose the talar head.

**Fig. 7.6** Plantar fasciotomy using number 11 knife blade

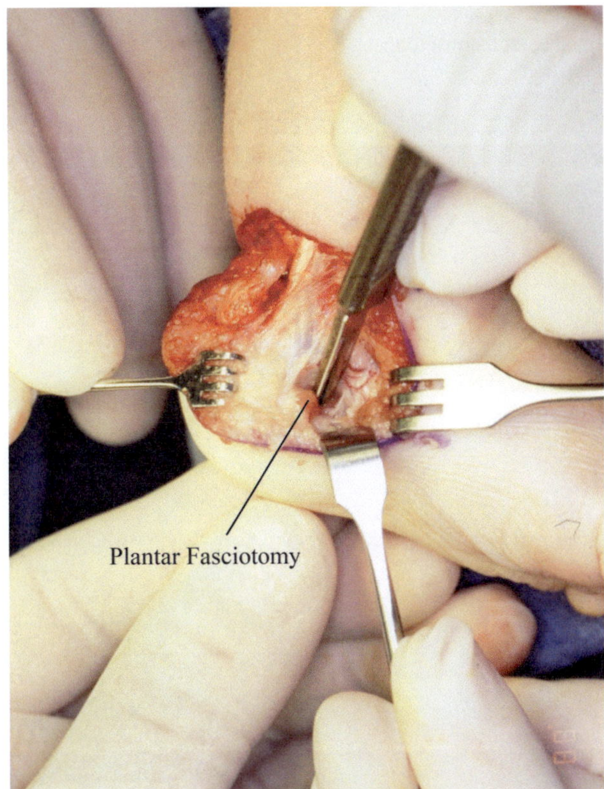



**Knot of Henry**  Find the tendon sheath of the flexor hallucis longus behind the posterior tibial tendon and open the tendon sheath. Trace down distally until the Knot of Henry, which is located below the navicular (Fig. 7.8). After releasing the Knot of Henry, both the flexor hallucis longus and the flexor digitorum longus are free and running together.

**Medial Subtalar Joint**  At this point, the subtalar joint capsule is incised to open the subtalar joint medially. Caution is taken not to damage the deep deltoid ligament of the ankle joint. Watch for contour of medial subtalar joint; take care not to cut into the talus or the calcaneus.

**Plantar Structures**  Now, go plantarly and find the spring ligament (plantar calcaneonavicular ligament), which is a broad, thick band. The release of this ligament is often required to reduce the navicular.

**Calcaneocuboid Joint**  In those patients with medial subluxation of the cuboid on the calcaneus, which is obvious in the anterior–posterior (AP) view of the radiograph, a release of the medial capsule of the calcaneocuboid can be done through

**Fig. 7.7** Trace posterior tibial tendon down to the insertion

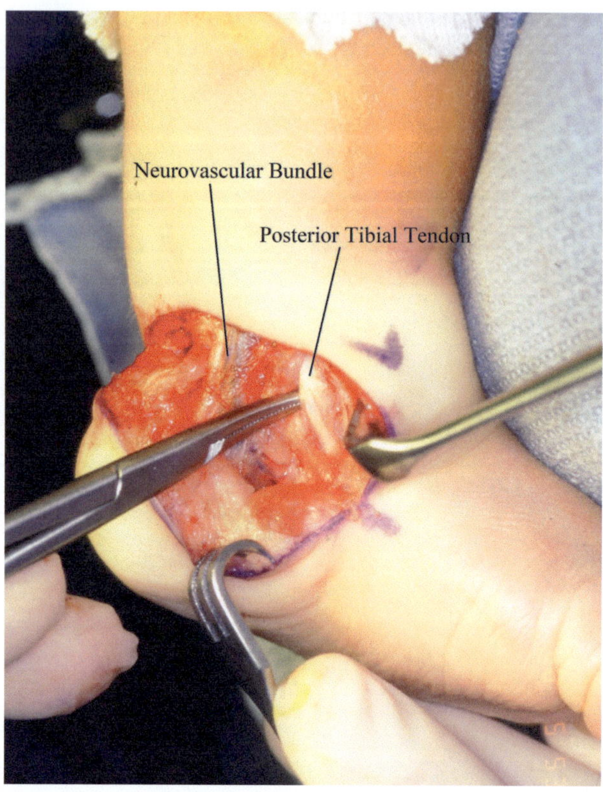


this approach resulting in a reduced cuboid. A Chandler retractor can be placed into the depths of the foot protecting the neurovascular bundle and flexor tendons plantarly. The calcaneal cuboid joint runs obliquely and should release carefully.

K-wire fixation in reduced position: Any varus or inverted attitude of the foot should be resolved. Dorsiflexion at the ankle joint should be improved. Rotate the calcaneal tuberosity medially under the talus, so the distal end of the calcaneus is pointing laterally. Smooth Kirschner wires (K-wire) are used to fix the reduced tarsal bones. The medial column fixation starts from the posterior aspect of talus in the center pointing anteriorly to exit from the center of the talar head. Under direct visualization, the talus is rotated medially with the navicular moved laterally onto the head of talus to reduce the talonavicular joint. The K-wire is then advanced through the navicular to fix the medial column (Fig. 7.9). This pin usually exits the skin on the foot dorsum between the first and the second toes. The posterior part of the K-wire is pulled anteriorly until it is flush with the cartilage surface. Next, if

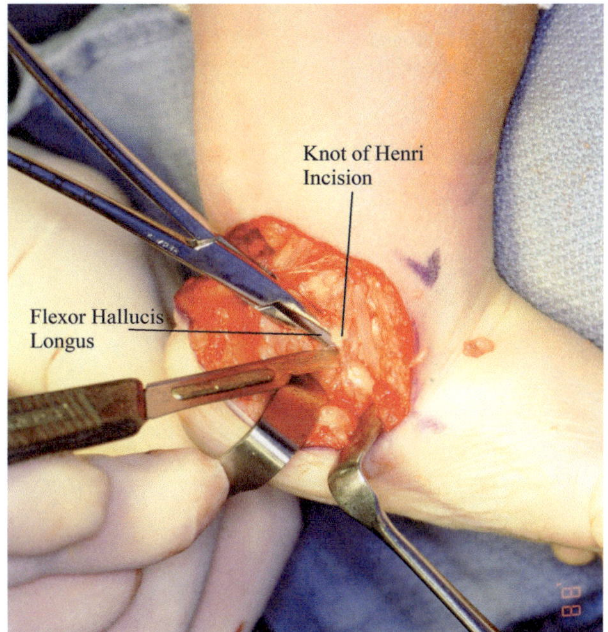


**Fig. 7.8** Trace flexor hallucis longus tendon down to the Knot of Henry

necessary, fix the lateral column. Start distally on the cuboid. With the foot held in the corrected external rotation position, a second K-wire is driven from the cuboid to the calcaneus. The anterior ends of K-wires are cut short and bend outside of the skin.

**Repair of the Tendons** The distal end of the posterior tibial tendon stump is sutured back to the area close to the navicular bone with tension. Next, repair the Z-lengthened Achilles tendon by holding the foot in a neutral dorsiflexion/plantarflexion or, if necessary, in slightly plantar flexed position, and bring both ends of the tendon together under tension. Depending on the length of the tendon, it can be sutured end to end or side to side with interrupted absorbable stitches. The skin is then closed.

**Cast** A long-leg cast is applied with the knee in 90 degrees or less of flexion and the ankle in a neutral position and the foot in external rotation. For those individuals with tight skin posteriorly, less dorsiflexion is applied with cast change in 2 weeks to bring the foot to neutral position. The cast is removed 6 weeks after surgery. At the same time, K-wires are removed, and hinged ankle foot orthosis (AFO) is prescribed.

**Fig. 7.9** Kirschner wire
skewed through talus and
navicular in good position

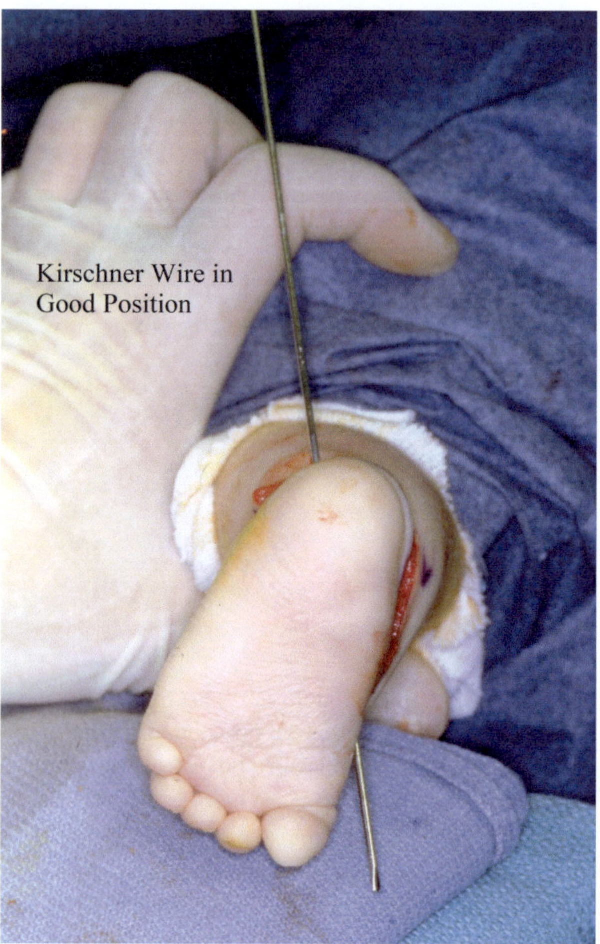


## Pitfalls and Complications

### Intraoperative Complications

1. Nerve damage: The medial plantar nerve is the most common nerve that can be damaged when approaching the plantar area.
2. Vessel damages: In approaching the posterior medial corner, pay attention to the posterior tibial artery. The dorsalis pedis artery is located dorsally. Caution is taken with release of the talonavicular joint.
3. Cartilage damage: The concave–convex relationship of the talonavicular joint is the trap for cutting into the cartilage.

## Immediate Postoperative Complications

1. Infection.
2. Skin slough at posterior aspect of the incision where the tension of the skin can cause skin slough.
3. Loss of reduction occurs with the following conditions:

    (a) Inappropriate cast application
    (b) Poor K-wire fixation or no K-wire fixation

4. Circulatory problems can be caused by pressure and soft-tissue swelling. If the circumferential cast is tight it should be released. Casts can be bivalved and the top half removed in case of severe swelling.

## Late Problems with Clubfoot Posterior Medial Releases

1. Dynamic forefoot supination deformity and adduction deformity: This is one of the most common conditions that require further attention [14]. It is caused by overpowering of the tibialis anterior tendon. The most common treatment is an anterior tibialis tendon transfer. There are two types of transfers, full anterior tibial tendon transfer and split anterior tibial tendon transfer [15]. In a full anterior tibial tendon transfer, the tendon is transferred to the middle or lateral cuneiform, whereas in a split anterior tibial tendon transfer, the split tendon is transferred to the cuboid.
2. Fixed forefoot adduction deformity: In this case, the anterior tibial tendon transfer will not solve the problem [14]. A closing wedge osteotomy of the cuboid and opening wedge osteotomy of the medial cuneiform can be the procedure of choice.
3. Rotatory dorsal subluxation of the navicular: It is caused by the progressive upward rotation of the larger medial end of the navicular that gives an appearance of triangular-shaped dorsal subluxation of the navicular in a lateral radiographic view (Fig. 7.10) [16]. It results in shortening of the medial column, forefoot plantar flexion and adduction and forefoot supination. The foot is usually in a shortened cavovarus deformity. A surgical reduction of the navicular would be necessary to correct the deformity, often combined with an anterior tibialis transfer and lateral column shortening

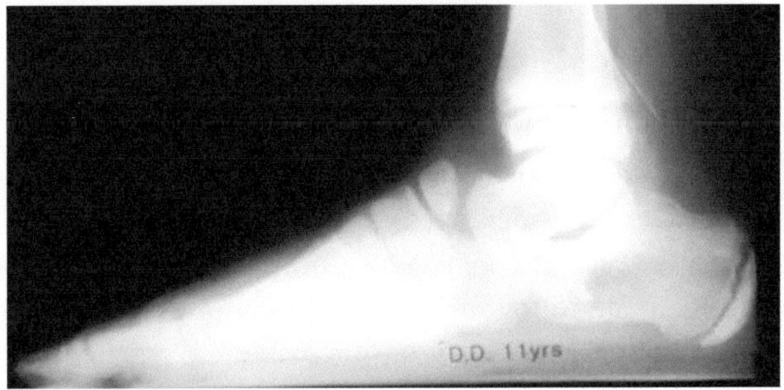

**Fig. 7.10** Rotatory dorsal subluxation of the navicular in this 11-year-old boy who had comprehensive soft-tissue release for clubfoot at age 1. It is an upside-down triangular-shaped navicular

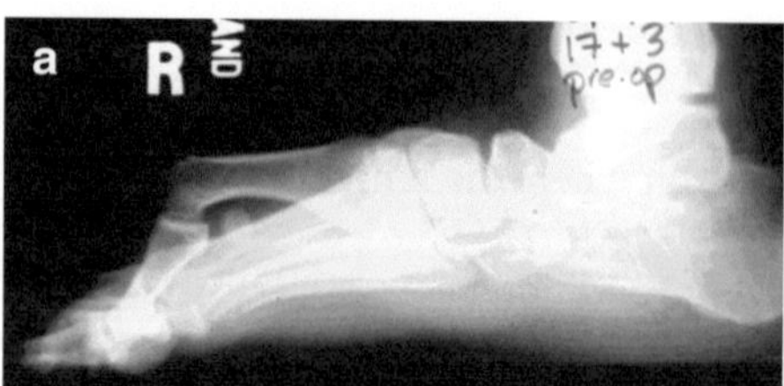
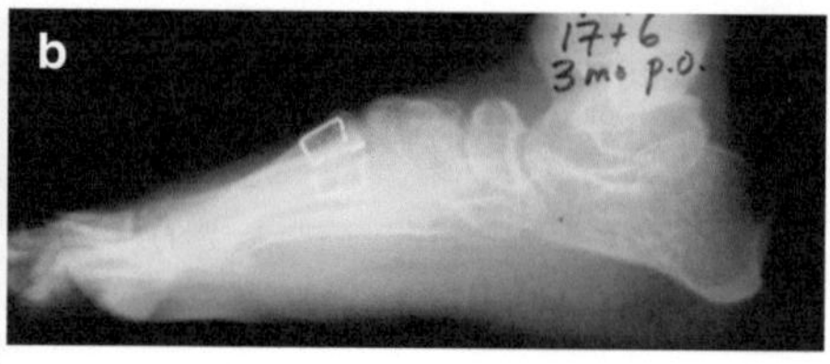


**Fig. 7.11** (**a**) Dorsal bunion in a 17 + 3 half year old boy who had comprehensive soft-tissue release at age 1, and revision later, developed dorsal bunion progressively in this lateral view standing radiograph. (**b**) This is a radiograph 3 months later after reverse Jones procedure, base of first metatarsal base plantar flexion osteotomy and split anterior tibial tendon transfer

4. Dorsal bunion: The dorsal bunion is a progressive deformity (Fig. 7.11a) with a painful and prominent first metatarsal phalangeal joint. It is caused by a combination of factors including a weak Achilles tendon and a substitution of the flexor hallucis longus as a plantarflexor. The strong anterior tibialis and weak peroneus longus contribute to the deformity [17]. The treatment includes a reverse Jones transfer (transfer of flexor hallucis longus to the neck of first metatarsal bone), with a plantarflexion osteotomy of the first metatarsal base and split anterior tibial tendon transfer (Fig. 7.11b).
5. Vascular insult to talus and navicular: With extensive releases, the talar head blood supply may be deprived from medial, lateral, and subtalar routes. The talonavicular joint collapses with a shortened medial column. It usually is associated with a stiff foot. In this case, the triple arthrodesis is one of the choices for the symptomatic foot. A talectomy with a lateral column shortening is another option in those with severe equinus for bringing the foot into plantigrade position.
6. Overcorrection: Overcorrection is one of the most difficult conditions to rescue following clubfoot releases [14]. For those with complete subtalar releases, there is a greater chance of overcorrection. Also, in children with generalized joint laxity, clubfoot surgery can be associated with overcorrection in the long term. Overcorrection may present as simple pronated foot or lateral translation of the calcaneus under the talus. The subtalar joint is rigid and in fixed deformity. In case of symptomatic overcorrection such as pain and difficulty wearing a shoe, a medial calcaneal slide osteotomy is a reasonable salvage procedure. Triple arthrodesis should be reserved as the last resort.

## Introduction of the Clinical Evaluation of Clubfoot Treatment Outcome

Evaluation of individuals with clubfoot treatment is essential to track progress, provide adequate follow-up care, and treat problems in a timely manner. The methods of evaluating outcomes have changed over time from pure radiographic and morphological assessments to functional and patient oriented measures. During adolescence, individuals treated for clubfeet may present with pain, weakness, gait anomalies, and functional deficits. Therefore, evaluations should include morphological assessment, functional assessment, quality of life measures, and clinical and radiographic examination.

Dysfunctional feet may impact a person's activity level and well-being. A comprehensive description of the patient's current condition is useful to show whether the goal of treatment has been successful. Goals typically include plantigrade feet, good shoe fitting, adequate motion, satisfactory morphology, and minimal pain. Dietz et al. explained measurements and described the foot morphology for determining appropriate function [18]. The following section describes useful methods to evaluate individuals with clubfoot in a quantitative comprehensive manner.

## Physical Examination

A good starting point for many clinicians is a comprehensive physical examination, which can quickly provide information about the stiffness, range of motion, and muscle strength of individuals with clubfeet (Table 7.1). Anthropometric measures can be useful to identify asymmetrical anatomy (i.e., foot dimensions, calf circumference, and leg length). Angle-finding tools like a goniometer are commonly used

**Table 7.1** Sample physical exam measures for clubfoot assessment: left clubfoot versus right normal foot

| | Clubfoot | Normal foot |
| --- | --- | --- |
| Measurement | | |
| Calf circumference (cm) | 26 | 30 |
| Leg length (cm) | 91.5 | 90 |
| Foot length (cm) | 24 | 25 |
| Ankle motion | | |
| Dorsiflexion (knee ext) | 0° | 10–15° |
| Dorsiflexion (knee flx) | 0° | 15–20° |
| Plantarflexion (knee ext) | 0° | 45–55° |
| Inversion (knee flx) | 0° | 30–40° |
| Eversion (knee flx) | 0° | 15–25° |
| Thigh-foot angle (knee flx) | 10° internal | 10° external |
| Weight-bearing observations | | |
| Hindfoot | Varus/neutral/valgus | Varus/neutral/valgus |
| | Equinus/neutral/calcaneus | Equinus/neutral/calcaneus |
| Midfoot | Supination/neutral/pronation | Supination/neutral/pronation |
| | Adduction/neutral/abduction | Adduction/neutral/abduction |
| Internal | Internal/neutral/external | Internal/neutral/external |
| | Pes Cavus/neutral/flatfoot | Pes Cavus/neutral/flatfoot |

*ext* extension, *flx* flexion

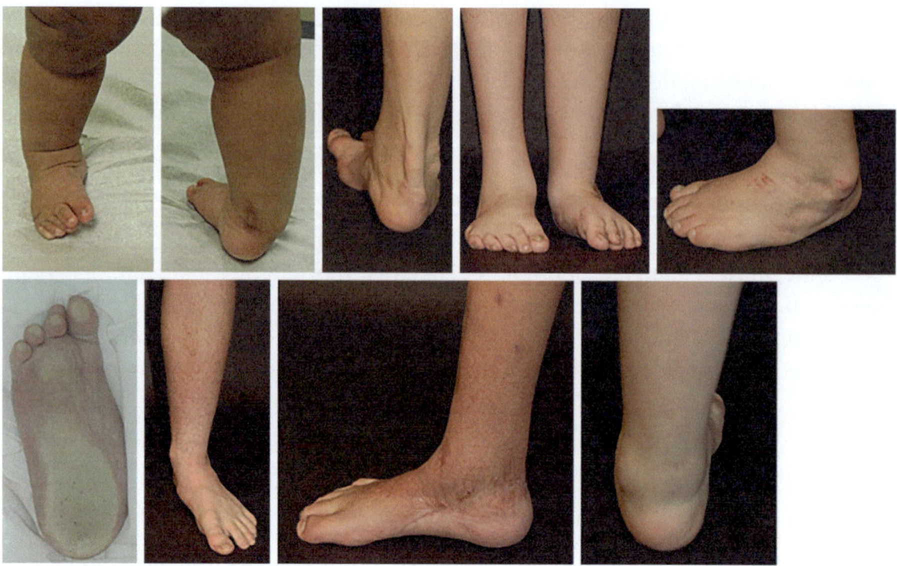

**Fig. 7.12** Documentation of clubfeet using photography from various angles is helpful in tracking the foot's condition and progression

in accordance with the International Clubfoot Study Group (ICFSG) Rating Score to assess ankle dorsiflexion/plantarflexion, hindfoot inversion/eversion, forefoot adduction/abduction, supination/pronation, thigh foot angle, and trans-malleolar axis [19]. Qualitative observations of skin integrity, foot morphology, and static weight bearing alignment are also often noted. Visual assessment can be made immediately in a clinic or lab setting, but it is also recommended to digitally record with video or photographs the patient's current condition for review at a later date. Examples of various photographs of individuals with clubfeet can be seen in Fig. 7.12.

## Radiographic Assessment

Weight bearing radiographs are typically included as standard of care in treatment of the clubfoot. Radiographs help to measure bony alignment and detect osteoarthritis. Views consist of anterior/posterior (A/P) and lateral planes. Some key observations are the following:

- The degrees of talocalcaneal angle in A/P and lateral view: After clubfoot treatment, it is not uncommon to observe residual parallelism of the talus and calcaneus, a reduction of talocalcaneal angle in A/P or lateral view.
- The degree of equinus of the calcaneus relative to the tibia.
- Forefoot abduction/adduction.

- Degree of planus/cavus by measuring the first metatarsal to the talar axis on a lateral view (Meary's angle) [20].
- The dorsal subluxation of the navicular in relation to the talar head.

Kellgren et al. have developed a system of grading joints for osteoarthritis by evaluating specific joints and scoring the degree of osteoarthritis present [21].

## Strength Evaluation

There are a variety of ways to measure muscle/joint strength. Clinicians often utilize the manual muscle test (Jones Classification) and functional strength assessments (heel raises). For quantitative assessments, a dynamometer system can be used to measure inversion/eversion and plantarflexion/dorsiflexion strength for various types of muscle contractions.

## Gait Analysis

Three-dimensional motion analysis provides quantitative data on the motion of joints during gait such as the pelvis, hip, knee, and ankle. This is typically performed on patients over 3 years of age and provides temporal spatial data (walking speed, cadence, step/stride length, etc.), joint kinematics, kinetics, and electromyography. Results can be compared to a typically developing and age-matched controls, and longitudinal data can be used to document changes over time for the same individual (Fig. 7.13).

One limitation in using conventional gait modeling is that the foot is often represented as a single, rigid segment rotating about a revolute joint. To more appropriately examine the dynamics of the human foot, a segmental foot model can be used. Several such models exist [22–24] and provide a more representative model of the segments of the foot affected by clubfoot correction and treatment. The Milwaukee

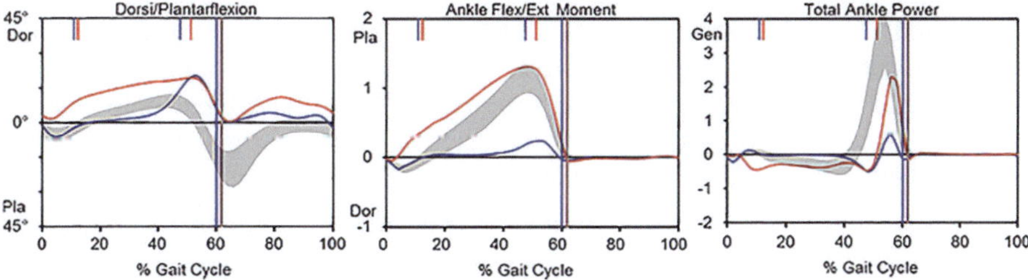


**Fig. 7.13** Kinematic and kinetic gait plots for an individual with a left clubfoot. Blue is the left foot, and red is the right foot

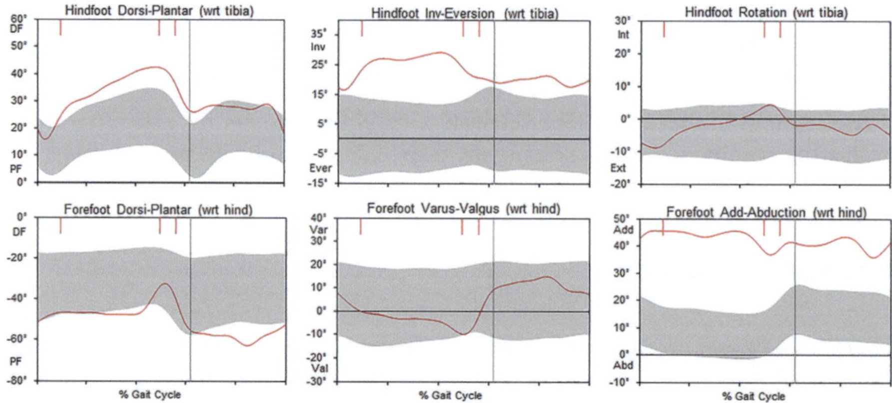

**Fig. 7.14** Segmental foot and ankle kinematics during gait. The segments in this example are the hindfoot and forefoot. The motion is measured relative to a proximal segment (hindfoot relative to tibia (not shown), forefoot relative to hindfoot). The single line plotted is an example of an individual with a clubfoot, and the gray band is a group of normal controls

Foot Model uses weight bearing radiographs to monitor the motion of reflective surface skin markers representing four segments (tibia, hindfoot, forefoot, and hallux) to the underlying bony anatomy [23]. The offsets measured from the radiographs help take into account abnormal bony alignment. The advantages of this type of modeling can be seen in the example from Fig. 7.14 where we can quantify the amount of hindfoot plantarflexion and inversion, as well as forefoot dorsiflexion and adduction.

## Pedobarography

Pedobarography is the study of the pressure distribution across the plantar surface of the foot when in contact with the floor. This can be studied dynamically (during gait) or in quiet standing. This analysis provides a unique perspective on how the foot interacts with the floor and the foot's skeletal alignment. One method of pedobarographic analysis is to trace the center of pressure (COP) or average pressure represented as a single point, throughout the stance phase of gait (Fig. 7.15). Then assess the path the COP takes as it progresses across the plantar surface of the foot during stance phase. This path, or COP Progression (COPP) [25], can help identify characteristics of walking patterns such as excessive calcaneus, equines, varus, valgus, and the condition of the medial longitudinal arch.

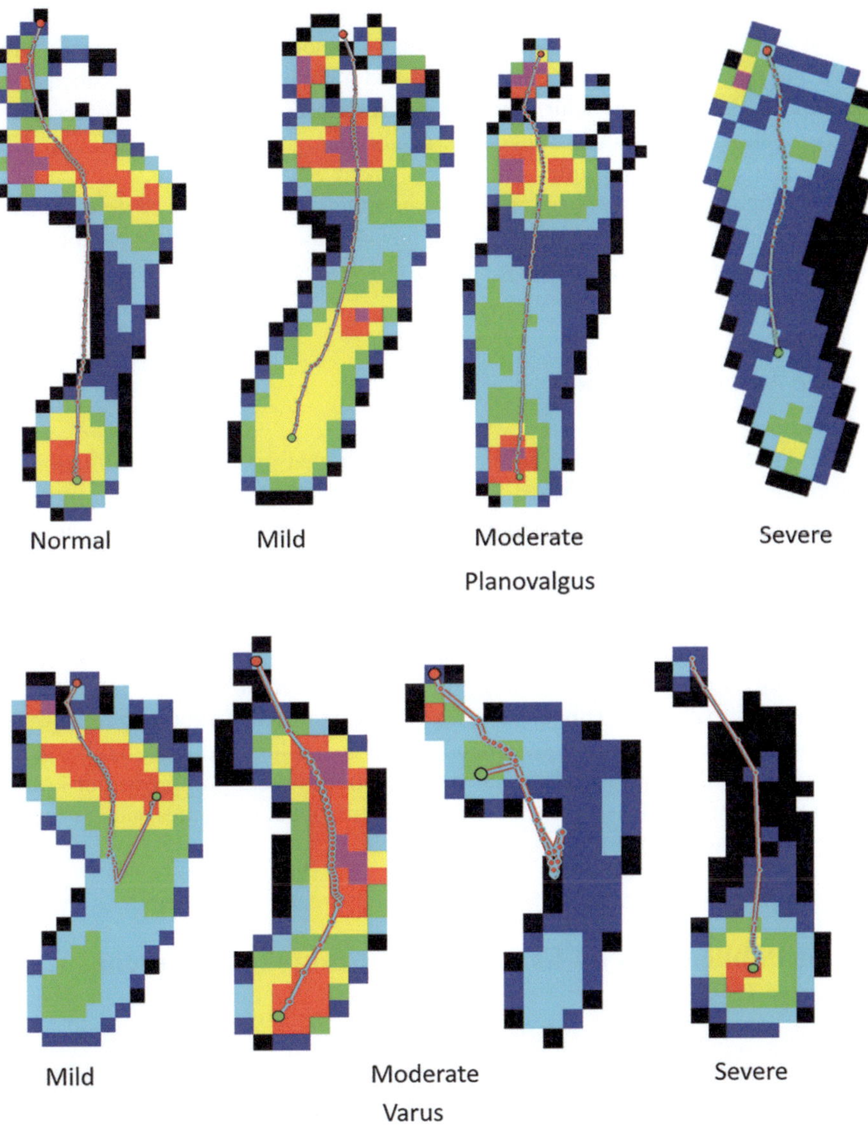



**Fig. 7.15** Pedobarographic images displaying examples of various types of foot deformities and center of pressure (COP)

## Quality of Life Outcomes Self-Assessment

To get a general sense of a patient's quality of life outside of a clinic or laboratory setting, questionnaires can be used. A few tools relevant to clubfoot are the Short Form-36, the Disease Specific Instrument (DSI), and Foot Function Index (FFI).

The SF-36 is a multipurpose, health survey with 36 questions and does not target a specific age. It yields an eight-scale profile of functional health and well-being scores and psychometrically based physical and mental health summary measures. The DSI has 10 questions with four possible responses per question. Topics cover foot pain, shoe wear, social acceptance, disabilities, and person satisfaction. The FFI is a self-administered index that uses a Likert Scale from 0 to 9 to rate pain, level of difficulty, and time spent on various activities. It consists of 23 items divided into three subscales. This was developed to measure the impact of foot pathology on function in terms of pain, disability, and activity restriction.

## Future Assessment Tools

**Kinetic Foot Model** Several future developments that may impact evaluations of the foot and ankle were described by Rankine et al. [26]. A kinetic foot model is described as a tool capable of quantifying forces and moments between multiple segments of the foot. Specialized force platforms will be used to adequately measure the distribution of shear forces on the plantar surface of the foot [27].

**Finite Element Modeling and Simulation Software** Several researchers have begun using finite element modeling to study the internal stresses/strains acting within the foot [28–34]. This is a computerized method of inputting real world effects on a model foot to study the impacts. This technology along with other simulation software like OpenSim [35] has the potential to greatly improve our knowledge of the biomechanics of the foot and predict treatment outcomes such as tendon transfers and osteotomies.

## Recent Publications on Evaluation of Clubfoot Treatment Outcome Research

Recent research by the authors were performed using a variety of assessment tools to assess the long-term outcomes of adults treated surgically for congenital clubfoot as infants [36–38]. These methods were able to detect several measurable differences between a group of patients treated for clubfeet and age-matched controls. The results showed that the clubfoot group ($N = 24$, $21.8 \pm 2.4$ years) was functional in activities of daily living, although foot pain was noticeable during long-distance walking, running, climbing stairs, and exercise. Radiographic analysis revealed bony malalignment compared with controls at the hindfoot and forefoot and early onset of osteoarthritis in 6% of the clubfoot subtalar joints and 11% of the tibiotalar joints. Physical examination revealed reduced range of motion and muscle weakness in ankle plantar flexion, dorsiflexion, inversion, and eversion. Gait parameters were similar to that of age-matched controls except for reductions in sagittal plane ankle plantar flexion during pre-swing phase, ankle push-off power, and walking speed. Pedobarography revealed measures of foot morphology were correlated with pain among a cohort treated for clubfoot. In comparison with the Ponseti method [13], comprehensive surgical release leads to greater long term foot deformity, flatter feet, and greater hindfoot loading time. The surgically treated clubfoot group also scored significantly worse in the hindfoot and midfoot American Orthopaedic Foot and Ankle Society and SF-36 (Physical Function, Bodily Pain, and General Health).

## Conclusion

There are a variety of tools useful in assessing clubfeet. Below is a recommended minimal assessment:

1. Physical Examination: a hands-on examination of foot morphology, foot stiffness, range of motion, and strength. (Age: Infants to adults)
2. Heel Raises: to quantify plantarflexion strength (Age: children–adults)
3. Plain Radiographs: to inspect bony alignment and osteoarthritis (Age: children-adults)
4. Gait Analysis: measure lower extremity kinematics, kinetics, and temporal spatial parameters (Age: children–adults)
5. Photographs/video: documentation of current foot condition (Age: infants–adults)
6. ICFSG: this assessment scores foot morphology, function, and radiographs

## References


1. Brockman EP. Congenital club foot (talipes equinovarus). Bristol: J. Wright and Sons; 1930.
2. Turco VJ. Surgical correction of the resistant clubfoot. One-stage posteromedial release with internal fixation: a preliminary report. J Bone Joint Surg Am. 1971;53(3):477–97.
3. Turco VJ. Resistant congenital club foot–one-stage posteromedial release with internal fixation. A follow-up report of a fifteen-year experience. J Bone Joint Surg Am. 1979;61(6):805–14.
4. Crawford AH, Marxen JL, Osterfeld DL. The Cincinnati incision: a comprehensive approach for surgical procedures of the foot and ankle in childhood. J Bone Joint Surg Am. 1982;64(9):1355–8.
5. McKay DW. New concept of and approach to clubfoot treatment: section I-principles and morbid anatomy. J Pediatr Orthop. 1982;2(4):347–56.
6. McKay DW. New concept of and approach to clubfoot treatment: section III–evaluation and results. J Pediatr Orthop. 1983;3(2):141–8.
7. McKay DW. New concept of and approach to clubfoot treatment: section II–correction of the clubfoot. J Pediatr Orthop. 1983;3(1):10–21.
8. Simons GW. Complete subtalar release in club feet. Part II–comparison with less extensive procedures. J Bone Joint Surg Am. 1985;67(7):1056–65.

9. Simons GW. Complete subtalar release in club feet. Part I–a preliminary report. J Bone Joint Surg Am. 1985;67(7):1044–55.

10. Bensahel H, Csukonyi Z, Desgrippes Y, Chaumien JP. Surgery in residual clubfoot: one-stage medioposterior release "a la carte". J Pediatr Orthop. 1987;7(2):145–8.

11. Ponseti IV, Smoley EN. Congenital club foot: the results of treatment. J Bone Joint Surg. 1963;45:261.

12. Dobbs MB, Nunley R, Schoenecker PL. Long-term follow-up of patients with clubfeet treated with extensive soft-tissue release. J Bone Joint Surg Am. 2006;88(5):986–96.

13. Smith PA, Kuo KN, Graf AN, Krzak J, Flanagan A, Hassani S, Caudill AK, Dietz FR, Morcuende J, Harris JF. Long-term results of comprehensive clubfoot release versus the Ponseti method: which is better? Clin Orthop Relat Res. 2014;472(4):1281–90.

14. Kuo KN, Smith PA. Correcting residual deformity following clubfoot releases. Clin Orthop Relat Res. 2009;467(5):1326–33.

15. Kuo KN, Hennigan SP, Hastings ME. Anterior tibial tendon transfer in residual dynamic clubfoot deformity. J Pediatr Orthop. 2001;21(1):35–41.

16. Kuo KN, Jansen LD. Rotatory dorsal subluxation of the navicular: a complication of clubfoot surgery. J Pediatr Orthop. 1998;18(6):770–4.

17. Yong SM, Smith PA, Kuo KN. Dorsal bunion after clubfoot surgery: outcome of reverse Jones procedure. J Pediatr Orthop. 2007;27(7):814–20.

18. Dietz FR, Tyler MC, Leary KS, Damiano PC. Evaluation of a disease-specific instrument for idiopathic clubfoot outcome. Clin Orthop Relat Res. 2009;467(5):1256–62.

19. Bensahel H, Kuo KN, Duhaime M. Outcome evaluation of the treatment of clubfoot: the international language of clubfoot. J Pediatr Orthop. 2003;12:269.

20. Meary R. On the measurement of the angle between the talus and the first metatarsal: symposium. Rev Chir Orthop. 1967;53:389–467.

21. Kellgren JH, Lawrence JS. Radiological assessment of osteo-arthrosis. Ann Rheum Dis. 1957;16(4):494–502.

22. Theologis TN, Harrington ME, Thompson N, Benson MK. Dynamic foot movement in children treated for congenital talipes equinovarus. J Bone Joint Surg Br. 2003;85(4):572–7.

23. Kidder SM, Abuzzahab FS Jr, Harris GF, Johnson JE. A system for the analysis of foot and ankle kinematics during gait. IEEE Trans Rehabil Eng. 1996;4(1):25–32.

24. Saraswat P, MacWilliams BA, Davis RB. A multi-segment foot model based on anatomically registered technical coordinate systems: method repeatability in pediatric feet. Gait Posture. 2012;35(4):547–55.

25. Jameson EG, Davids JR, Anderson JP, Davis RB 3rd, Blackhurst DW, Christopher LM. Dynamic pedobarography for children: use of the center of pressure progression. J Pediatr Orthop. 2008;28(2):254–8.

26. Rankine L, Long J, Canseco K, Harris GF. Multisegmental foot modeling: a review. Crit Rev Biomed Eng. 2008;36(2-3):127–81.

27. MacWilliams BA, Cowley M, Nicholson DE. Foot kinematics and kinetics during adolescent gait. Gait Posture. 2003;17(3):214–24.

28. Cheung G, Zalzal P, Bhandari M, Spelt JK, Papini M. Finite element analysis of a femoral retrograde intramedullary nail subject to gait loading. Med Eng Phys. 2004;26(2):93–108.

29. Cheung JT, An KN, Zhang M. Consequences of partial and total plantar fascia release: a finite element study. Foot Ankle Int. 2006;27(2):125–32.

30. Cheung JT, Zhang M. A 3-dimensional finite element model of the human foot and ankle for insole design. Arch Phys Med Rehabil. 2005;86(2):353–8.

31. Cheung JT, Zhang M, Leung AK, Fan YB. Three-dimensional finite element analysis of the foot during standing–a material sensitivity study. J Biomech. 2005;38(5):1045–54.

32. Gibbs JC, Giangregorio LM, Wong AKO, Josse RG, Cheung AM. Appendicular and whole body lean mass outcomes are associated with finite element analysis-derived bone strength at the distal radius and tibia in adults aged 40 years and older. Bone. 2017;103:47–54.

33. Yu J, Cheung JT, Fan Y, Zhang Y, Leung AK, Zhang M. Development of a finite element model of female foot for high-heeled shoe design. Clin Biomech. 2008;23(Suppl):31–8.
34. Gefen A, Megido-Ravid M, Itzchak Y, Arcan M. Biomechanical analysis of the three-dimensional foot structure during gait: a basic tool for clinical applications. J Biomech Eng. 2000;122(6):630–9.
35. Delp SL, Anderson FC, Arnold AS, Loan P, Habib A, John CT, et al. OpenSim: open-source software to create and analyze dynamic simulations of movement. IEEE Trans Biomed Eng. 2007;54(11):1940–50.
36. Graf A, Hassani S, Krzak J, Long J, Caudill A, Flanagan A, Eastwood D, Kuo KN, Harris G, Smith P. Long-term outcome evaluation in young adults following clubfoot surgical release. J Pediatr Orthop. 2010;30(4):379–85.
37. Graf A, Wu KW, Smith PA, Kuo KN, Krzak J, Harris G. Comprehensive review of the functional outcome evaluation of clubfoot treatment: a preferred methodology. J Pediatr Orthop B. 2012;21(1):20–7.
38. Graf AN, Kuo KN, Kurapati NT, Krzak JJ, Hassani S, Caudill AK, Flanagan A, Harris GF, Smith PA. A long-term follow-up of young adults with idiopathic clubfoot: does foot morphology relate to pain? J Pediatr Orthop. 2017;39(10):527–33.

# Chapter 8
# Managing Clubfoot Relapses Following Ponseti Method Treatment: Approach Based on Age and Residual Deformity

Steven L. Frick

## Introduction

Managing relapses should be considered a standard part of the Ponseti method for treatment of congenital clubfoot. Multiple studies show that between 11% and up to 50% of children treated with the Ponseti method who have initial excellent correction of their deformity will go on to develop a relapse during early childhood [1, 2]. While much has been written about the methods and results of initial correction using Ponseti principles of manipulation and casting, much less has been written about how to manage relapsed deformities. Ponseti's own textbook on congenital clubfoot devoted only 4 of 140 pages to relapses [3]. Dr. Ponseti believed that relapses were not secondary to incomplete correction but were a consequence of the same pathology that caused the initial deformity. Recent genetic discoveries continue to improve our understanding of congenital clubfoot etiology, with recognition of abnormalities in genes that control early limb bud development. After correction of the clubfoot deformity early in life using the Ponseti method, the same genetic abnormalities remain present in the tissues, and as the foot grows rapidly in the first few years of life, relapses are common. The best way to manage relapses is to avoid them, and that is the purpose of prolonged bracing of the corrected clubfoot in a foot abduction orthosis and follow-up. Multiple studies have shown that adherence to bracing instructions is the number one factor leading to early relapse of deformity [4]. Herzenberg and Noonan have described the initial treatment of

S. L. Frick (✉)
Department of Orthopedic Surgery, School of Medicine, Stanford University, Stanford, CA, USA

Pediatric Orthopedic Surgery, Stanford Children's Health/Lucile Packard Children's Hospital, Stanford, CA, USA
e-mail: sfrick01@stanford.edu



M. B. Dobbs et al. (eds.), *Clubfoot and Vertical Talus*,
https://doi.org/10.1007/978-3-031-34788-7_8

clubfoot using serial casting and manipulation with the Ponseti method as the "doctor phase," and describe the bracing phase of the Ponseti method as the "parent phase" [5].

A key component of the Ponseti method then is to engage, educate, and enlist the parents in the bracing phase of the Ponseti method. During the casting correction phase, each casting session is an opportunity to discuss with the family the risk of relapse, the reasons for relapse of the deformity, and the period of rapid growth of the child's foot in the first 4–5 years of life and explain to them the importance of compliance with the bracing protocol. Some studies focusing on education of the parents during the casting phase have demonstrated lower relapse rates, believed to be affiliated with understanding of the parents about the importance of bracing [6]. Many parents receive information about their child's clubfoot deformity and the Ponseti method of treatment via Internet sources [7]. Unfortunately, some of these sources may lead the parents to believe that the Ponseti method will cure their child's clubfoot and create a normal foot, and many of them do not discuss the high rate of relapse after initial correction. Ponseti himself was noted on some Internet chat rooms to discuss creating a "normal" foot with his method of clubfoot treatment—he likely intended a normal-appearing foot that would function to allow normal childhood activities and shoewear. The casting phase, thus, also offers the opportunity to set appropriate parental expectations and to educate them that since congenital clubfoot is a major developmental deformity that is not possible to create a normal foot. A congenital clubfoot is always somewhat abnormal even after successful correction—typically with a smaller-size foot, smaller leg compartment muscles, and diminished range of motion compared to normal. What has been shown is that the Ponseti method can create a foot that functions normally during childhood and functions well into middle age, with pain levels and functional levels similar to control groups of adults without foot deformity [8]. None of the long-term studies of adult patients with clubfoot demonstrate normal foot range of motion or normalization of the radiographic anatomy of patients successfully treated with the Ponseti method during childhood [8, 9].

Educating the parents and enlisting their assistance both in compliance with brace wear and monitoring for early relapses can be beneficial. Dr. Ponseti believed that the earliest signs of relapse were usually slight equinus and varus, without adduction and cavus, and with weight-bearing laterally on the outer border of the foot [3, 10]. Educating the parents to look for these signs can lead to early recognition and treatment of relapses. It is also very helpful for the parents to be educated and not view a relapse as a failure or a reason to doubt the Ponseti method—instead managing relapses is a continuation of the Ponseti method.

The age at which a relapse occurs changes the way the relapse is treated, as does the anatomical deformity that recurs. The definition of a relapse is the recurrence of one or more component of clubfoot deformity *after* the foot has been completely corrected. Occasionally, the treating physician may believe complete correction has been achieved, when in fact there is some residual deformity. These patients who have an incomplete initial correction will often have difficulty with initial brace wear tolerance. Deformity that becomes an issue within 6 months of treatment has been described as most likely secondary to incomplete correction, whereas relapses were defined as occurring 6 months or longer after initial correction [11]. Whether the deformity is labeled incomplete correction or early relapse, in patients younger than 1 year, the management consists of deformity analysis and restarting manipulation and casting using Ponseti method principles to gain full correction. After correction, foot abduction orthosis wear is reinstituted.

An important consideration when evaluating a clubfoot patient with a relapse is to consider that the patient may not have idiopathic congenital clubfoot. Every patient who presents with clubfoot relapse should be examined carefully for neurologic abnormalities such as the drop toe sign [12] (see Fig. 8.1). Neurologic abnormalities leading to relapses are typically seen in the anterior and lateral compartments, with absent or weak ankle and toe dorsiflexion and weak foot eversion [12, 13]. Another consideration is that infants who appear otherwise healthy and normal in the first few months of life when presenting for initial treatment of clubfoot deformity may be found to have developmental or congenital syndromes over time as they are followed during the first few years of life [14].

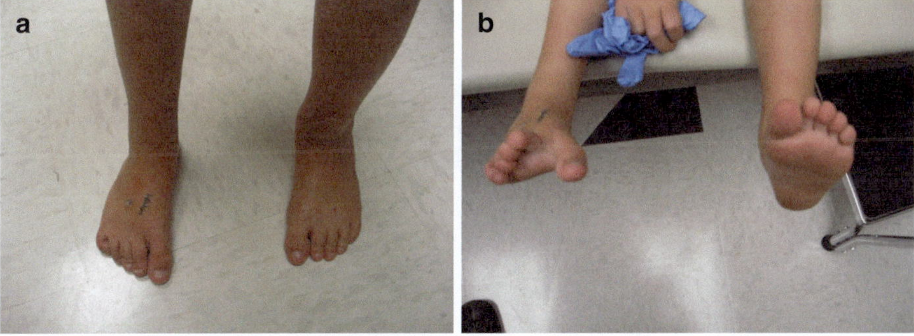


**Fig. 8.1** A 5-year-old with previously well-corrected clubfoot returns for abnormal gait and weight-bearing on the lateral aspect of the foot. Panel (**a**) shows mild relapse of right clubfoot. Panel (**b**) shows drop toe sign when actively dorsiflexing foot and toes. Electrodiagnostic studies revealed a peripheral neuropathy

## Recognition of Relapses

Congenital clubfoot typically has four deformity components—cavus, adduction, varus, and equinus. Which deformity recurs has an impact on the method of management, but in general, relapses are always treated with repeat manipulation and casting using the same principles and manipulation/casting techniques as for the initial correction [1–3]. Cavus deformity infrequently recurs, but when it does can be treated with manipulation and casting to achieve elevation of the first metatarsal and supination of the forefoot to match the hind foot, combined next with abduction of the forefoot and midfoot over the talar head fulcrum laterally. Supination and varus deformities are treated mainly with abduction of the forefoot and midfoot around talar head, with an attempt to outwardly rotate the calcaneopedal block (Calcaneus-cuboid-navicular-cuneiforms-metatarsals) laterally and improve the talocalcaneal relationship. Relapses with cavus, adduction, varus, or supination deformities that occur before 2 1/2 years of age are usually treated only with repeat manipulation and casting, followed by reinstitution of foot abduction orthosis bracing protocols (see Fig. 8.2).

Equinus relapses typically do not respond well to casting alone. Outward rotation of the calcaneopedal block, such that the anterior process of the calcaneus rotates laterally and comes out from underneath the talar head, can improve dorsiflexion. This allows some dorsiflexion of the calcaneus relative to the talus and restoration of a more normal lateral talocalcaneal angle. Often, however, this is not enough correction of equinus, and lengthening of the tendo Achilles is needed to produce a plantigrade foot. Ponseti noted this important determinant for timing of tendo Achilles tenotomy—when one can palpate the anterior process of the calcaneus lateral to the talar head/neck [3, 10]. A surrogate for this direct palpation is outward rotation or abduction of the foot past 60–70°. With this much foot rotation/abduction, the anterior calcaneus should be out from beneath the talus, and Achilles

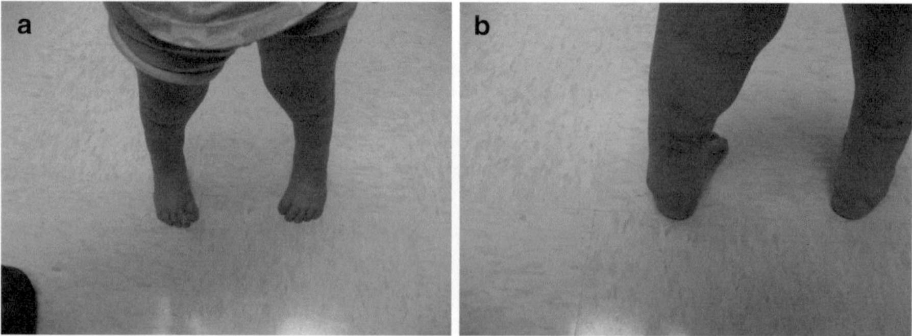



**Fig. 8.2** (**a, b**) Eighteen-month-old female with previously well-corrected clubfeet, now with bilateral relapses. At this age, repeat manipulation and casting should be performed, with possible tendo Achilles lengthening if unable to get dorsiflexion above 15°. Foot abduction bracing should then be reinstituted

tenotomy will allow dorsiflexion of the calcaneus without impingement on the talus and dorsiflexion of the tibiotalar joint.

A recent survey of Pediatric Orthopedic Society of North America members (321 responses) noted that 59% of respondents felt that a tight heel cord was the first sign of relapse, while 30% felt that dynamic supination was the first sign. Treatment of the initial relapse was described as manipulation and casting alone by 55%, and manipulation with casting followed by tendo Achilles tenotomy in 23%. Fourty-three percent responded that posterior capsular release plus tibialis anterior tendon transfer was commonly being performed for relapse [2].

## Principles of Relapse Correction

The fundamental guiding principle of the Ponseti method is to avoid invasive surgery that involves sectioning ligaments and opening up joints to realign them. Long-term studies have shown that using the Ponseti method with manipulation and casting to correct deformity, with extra-articular surgical procedures as needed to address tendon contractures or muscle imbalance, leads to improved range of motion of the ankle and foot and improved patient outcomes at long-term follow-up when compared to surgical realignment using intra-articular procedures [8, 15]. This principle guides decision-making when managing relapses as well. The goal of treatment of congenital clubfoot is to produce a supple, functional foot that allows normal shoe wear and normal activities, while minimizing surgical procedures. Gait analysis studies have shown that children whose clubfoot is corrected with no surgical procedure or minor surgical procedures have improved gait parameters, range of motion, and power when compared to patients with clubfeet treated with traditional open surgical techniques [16, 17]. Any patient with a clubfoot relapse should be treated with serial manipulation and casting to obtain maximum possible correction, prior to undertaking any surgical procedures that involve sectioning ligaments and opening joints [3].

In line with these principles guiding treatment, the management of clubfoot relapses always begins with a return to serial manipulations and casting, again following the principles of manipulation outlined by Dr. Ponseti [3], and typically, these manipulations are successful at correcting the deformity. As is often seen with the initial correction, the final deformity that needs correction is persistent equinus. In older children, once the deformity is corrected, consideration should be given to tendon transfers if it is believed that persistent muscle imbalance across the ankle and foot joints is causing the relapse. It is critical to understand, however, that tendon transfers will not correct deformity [18]. The purpose of the tendon transfer is to maintain the correction that is achieved with serial manipulations and casting, supplemented by extra-articular surgical procedures such as tendo Achilles lengthenings and occasionally plantar fascia lengthenings if there is persistent cavus.

The treating surgeon should have an understanding of the long-term outcomes of congenital clubfoot patients managed with the Ponseti method with regards to the amount of ankle dorsiflexion that is needed for patients to have excellent function, low patient perceptions of pain and limitations, and ability to wear normal shoes without the need for braces or orthotics [8].

Recognition that most of the long-term follow-up studies of successfully treated congenital clubfeet using the Ponseti method will show quite limited ankle dorsiflexion when compared to normal controls will prevent the surgeon from being overly aggressive in performing posterior ankle and subtalar joint releases in an attempt to improve ankle dorsiflexion [8, 19]. Cooper and Dietz found average passive ankle dorsiflexion of only 6° above neutral in clubfoot subjects [8]; thus, the goal should be to achieve at least neutral ankle dorsiflexion to allow plantigrade position of the foot during weight bearing. Some authors have listed 5° as adequate dorsiflexion in childhood [20]. If during childhood treatment of relapse a greater amount of ankle dorsiflexion is able to be achieved, this is desirable as long as it does not require intra-articular surgery [21].

There are some patients, however, that will not have adequate ankle dorsiflexion during treatment for relapses during childhood. These patients occasionally may need a posterior release of the ankle and/or subtalar joints. Dr. Ponseti's colleagues in Iowa have written about this [22], and other practitioners who have studied with Dr. Ponseti have also reported on series of patients treated with serial manipulation in casting for recurrent deformity, followed by posterior releases with or without anterior tibial tendon transfer [23–26]. The risk of intra-articular surgery to release the posterior tibiotalar and subtalar joints is scarring across the joints that may cause stiffness, limited range of motion, and perhaps recurrent deformity and need for further surgeries [19, 26, 27]. Overly aggressive releases may also lead to calcaneus deformity. Multiple studies support the fact that children treated in early childhood with open surgical releases end up having more surgical procedures performed during childhood and adolescence than children managed with the Ponseti method [15, 24]. A recent paper reports limiting the duration of immobilization following posterior release surgery with early physical therapy and maintenance of good ankle plantar flexion range of motion, with adequate ankle dorsiflexion maintained as well [28].

## Specific Relapse Patient Scenarios

### *Recurrent Deformity with Difficulty in Bracewear During the First 6 Months Following Initial Cast Correction (Inadequate Initial Correction Vs. Early Relapse)*

Some patients will have difficulty with the transition from the manipulation and casting phase of care into the bracing protocol. Ponseti method traditional bracing protocol involves 3 months of full-time bracing after the completion of casting. During this initial 3 months, if parents call and complain that the child is not tolerating the brace well, that they are having difficulty keeping the braces on, or they notice redness and skin irritation with brace wear, then the patient should be scheduled for an early clinical reevaluation of the adequacy of deformity correction. At times, the clubfoot has either not been completely corrected with the initial set of casting or has developed an early relapse. The flexibility of the foot should be assessed, and any residual cavus, adduction, varus, or equinus should prompt a return to manipulation and casting. In the vast majority of cases, repeat manipulation and two to three casts will correct the deformity and will result in a well-corrected foot with 60–70 degrees of abduction and 10–20 degrees of ankle dorsiflexion. This should allow comfortable positioning in the foot abduction orthosis. This is also an opportunity to consider the type of foot abduction orthosis ordered and to make sure that the foot abduction orthosis appropriately fits the child's foot. Patients who have recurrent difficulties with keeping the heel down in the brace or skin problems may benefit from switching to a different type of foot abduction orthosis, potentially one that allows some ankle dorsiflexion and plantarflexion instead of being rigid.

Occasionally the cavus, adduction and varus will be corrected, but there will be residual equinus (see Fig. 8.3). This may be in the setting of no prior tendo Achilles tenotomy or may follow a prior tendo Achilles tenotomy. Once the forefoot is abducted 60–70°, further casting seems less effective at correcting the equinus deformity if it has not corrected with forefoot abduction. Later in his career treating clubfoot, Ponseti emphasized overcorrecting the deformity (greater abduction) in the final cast to be certain that the calcaneus is fully abducted, and its anterior joint surface is well out from under the head of the talus [29]. If the patient previously underwent Achilles tenotomy, it is possible that either an incomplete tenotomy was performed or the patient may have healed the Achilles tendon and developed recurrent equinus. Patients will not tolerate bracing if the foot is not completely corrected, and equinus will make it difficult to keep the heel down in the brace, often causing anterior ankle skin problems from the ankle strap, and thus, repeat tendo Achilles tenotomy and casting is indicated.

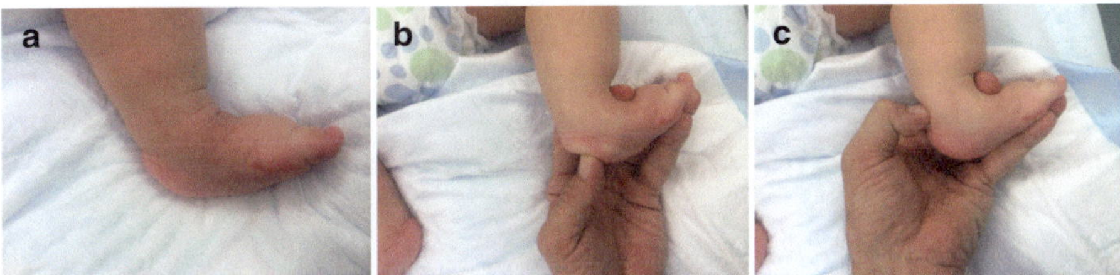


**Fig. 8.3** A 6-month-old boy with bilateral clubfeet corrected with Ponseti method manipulations and casting without tenotomy developed increasing difficulty with brace wear. Examination showed a proximally displaced heel pad (**a**), an empty heel sign (**b**), and a proximally displaced calcaneus marked by thumb (**c**). This is treated with tendo Achilles tenotomy 1.5 cm proximal to the most proximal aspect of the calcaneus, 3 weeks in a dorsiflexion above knee cast, and then foot abduction bracing

There is some controversy as to the number of Achilles tenotomy procedures that can be performed safely and without functional consequences to calf muscle strength and size, but this concern is overridden by the fact that equinus will prevent comfortable brace wear and the development of a plantigrade foot position for standing and walking. Some have advocated for no more than two tendo Achilles lengthening procedures, but good studies defining the timing and consequences of repeated tendo Achilles lengthenings are lacking. It does appear that tendo Achilles tenotomy can be performed safely up to two times in patients less than 2 years of age. Some surgeons prefer an open tendo Achilles lengthening after prior percutaneous tenotomy, while others will repeat the tenotomy. There is no available data to determine the optimal technique.

## *Relapses Before Age 2 1/2 Years*

For patients who are less than 2 1/2 years of age, clubfoot relapses are managed by serial manipulation and casting with possible repeat tendo Achilles tenotomy and then a reinstitution of a vigorous bracing protocol with 3 months of full-time bracing for young patients. In older patients, a minimum of 12 h of brace wear is prescribed. The author uses an above-the-knee cast for patients who are not yet walking but will use a below-the-knee walking cast in patients who are ambulating if the foot is flexible and the subtalar joint complex reduces easily with outward rotation of the foot. This is noted by lateral displacement of the navicular covering the talar head, palpation of the anterior process of the calcaneus laterally out from underneath the talus, and valgus alignment of the calcaneus. If the subtalar joint does not reduce fully, I will use an above-the-knee cast. Ponseti and others use an above the knee cast, although if placed at 90 degrees of knee flexion in an ambulatory child, this can be more difficult for the parents to manage as the child needs to be carried.

In rare patients where this protocol does not result in full correction with easy dorsiflexion above neutral, consideration may be given to the use of a hinged ankle foot orthosis (AFO) brace with a plantarflexion stop at neutral during the daytime and a Ponseti method foot abduction orthosis at night.

## *Early Relapses in Patients Who Are Noncompliant with Bracing*

If patients are noncompliant with bracing, the risk of relapse is known to be much higher in the first 5–6 years of life [4, 25, 30, 31]. If the foot is well corrected and the patient is less than 2 years of age, some authors have advocated early tibialis anterior tendon transfer to prevent relapses in patients at high risk for noncompliance. Whether or not the tendon will heal normally to the unossified cuneiform is not known, and as a result in younger patients, some will transfer the tendon to the cuboid (so-called Garceau transfer). The risk of this more lateral transfer point is overcorrection and perhaps less dorsiflexion strength. These risks have not been well studied and quantified.

## *Dynamic Supination Relapses After Age 2 1/2 Years*

The most common type of relapse in this age group is recurrent adduction and varus related to dynamic supination of the foot during swing phase (see Fig. 8.4). This occurs secondary to muscle imbalance between the muscles that invert the foot and those that evert the foot [3]. Weakness of the lateral compartment musculature has long been recognized as a potential abnormality in congenital clubfoot patients, and recent research utilizing magnetic resonance imaging (MRI) imaging of the anterior lateral compartments has demonstrated that significant abnormalities in the anterior and lateral compartment musculature may indicate treatment resistant clubfoot at higher risk for relapse [32, 33]. Ponseti wrote that the posterior and medial aspects of the lower leg, ankle, and foot are abnormal in congenital clubfoot and that during the period of rapid growth of the foot in the first few years of life, recurrent deformity from" retracting fibrosis" of these posterior and medial structures would cause recurrent deformity unless the feet are splinted in firm external rotation during this period of rapid growth [3, 10]. This period of splinting also allows increasing strength of the anterior and lateral compartment musculature, to balance the muscular forces across the foot and also aid in prevention of relapse of deformity. When those muscular forces do not develop in the young child, dynamic supination may occur, resulting in increased weight bearing along the lateral column of the foot. Initially, this will lead to flexible adduction and varus deformity. This should be

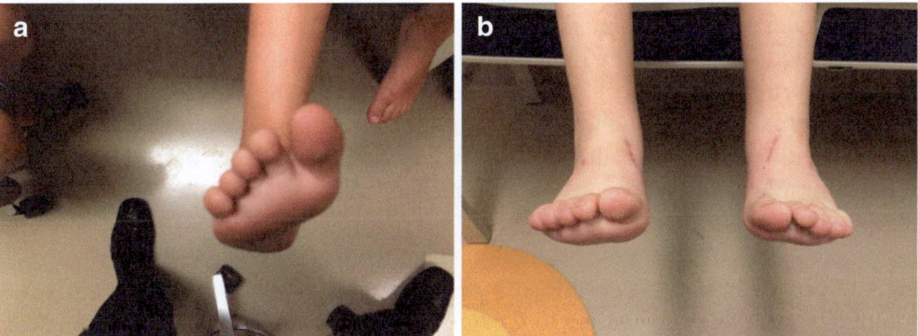

Fig. 8.4 (a, b) Dynamic supination is the most common type of relapse following Ponseti method correction of clubfoot, and leads to a supinated forefoot in the swing phase of gait, followed by initial contact with the lateral border of the foot and overload of the lateral column of the foot during stance. Most children with this will have imbalance of the forefoot with active dorsiflexion as noted in (a). After casting to correct and residual deformity, transfer of the tibialis anterior tendon to the lateral cuneiform will restore balanced dorsiflexion of the forefoot as noted in (b)

recognized and treated with manipulation and casting, followed by tibialis anterior tendon transfer to the third cuneiform as described by Ponseti, as long as the patient is older than 2 1/2 years of age and the lateral cuneiform is ossified [3]. Equinus of the hind foot should also be assessed, and if adequate dorsiflexion is not present, a percutaneous Achilles tenotomy or an open tendo Achilles lengthening can be performed at the same time as the tibialis anterior tendon transfer. Ponseti did not advocate splitting the tibialis anterior tendon, and that has also been the author's practice. In a prospective study of idiopathic clubfoot patients managed with the Ponseti method, Zionts has recently reported that the percentage of patients who need to undergo tibialis anterior tendon transfer is less than 5% at 3 years of age, 15% at 4 years of age, and 29% at 6 years of age [34]. Goldstein reported that 33% of patients initially managed successfully with the Ponseti method needed either anterior tibialis tendon transfer, posterior medial release or both [35]. In a series by Bor on patients followed for 5 years after Ponseti method treatment, 32% had either tibialis tendon transfer, posteromedial release, or external fixation [20]. These studies help inform the parents and surgeon about the potential for relapse and need for surgery in childhood, again allowing for further discussions during early visits about the importance of bracing to avoid relapse, and to discuss with parents that while the Ponseti method can almost always avoid significant surgery in the first year of life, a substantial portion of clubfoot patients successfully treated by the method will eventually need to have tendon transfer surgery. Discussing this possibility with the parents during early childhood, when things are going well, will make it easier to explain and move forward with appropriate treatment if later relapse does occur. A recent long-term follow-up study by Holt et al. of Ponseti's patients treated with tibialis anterior transfer for relapse also provides excellent information for parents that will inform them about long-term prognosis. In a matched comparison with clubfoot patients treated by Ponseti who did not have a relapse, the patients with relapse treated by tibialis anterior transfer had no further need for surgery following the transfer, and at average, 47-year follow-up had results similar to those patients who never relapsed [9]. This is reassuring information to provide parents at the time of relapse, as many may see relapse as a failure of the Ponseti method, rather than a consequence of having a congenital deformity with abnormal growth of medial plantar foot structures and muscle imbalance. Sharing with parents that although in some clubfoot patients more treatment is needed for relapses, the prognosis is for an excellent long-term outcome to alleviate many parental concerns and worries.

Subcutaneous transfer of the tibialis anterior tendon has been well described, and the author performs it as described by Ponseti with fixation using a whip stitch suture in the tibialis anterior tendon pulled through a drill hole in the lateral cuneiform and out the plantar aspect of the foot, sutured down over a sterile piece of felt and a button on the plantar aspect of the foot [3]. The tibialis anterior tendon is passed over the extensor hallucis longus (EHL), while the long-toe extensors and the extensor digitorum brevis are retracted laterally to pass the tibialis anterior subcutaneously into the hole drilled in the lateral cuneiform [1]. A safe corridor for passing the needles exists in the middle of the plantar aspect of the foot as described by Radler et al. to avoid neurologic or tendon injury [36]. Patients are mobilized nonweight-bearing in an above-the-knee cast with the knee-flexed 90° in the foot in maximal abduction of 50–70°, with dorsiflexion of 10–15° above neutral. The cast is worn for 4–6 weeks. Variation to postoperative protocol exists while it is important to remember it takes about 6 weeks for the tendon to incorporate into bone.

Ponseti protocol does not call for any bracing following tibialis anterior tendon transfer. It has been the author's practice to place patients into a pediatric cam walker boot following removal of the long-leg cast and allow weight-bearing as tolerated. A solid ankle foot orthosis with the ankle at 90° is ordered and worn full time for 1 month and then at night for 3 months. This support following cast removal seems to facilitate early return to walking with less limp. Others have reported similar postoperative care protocols following tibialis anterior transfer [1].

## *Equinus Relapses/Inadequate Ankle Dorsiflexion*

Inadequate ankle dorsiflexion is the most difficult problem to manage in the author's clubfoot practice. The typical clubfoot patient will have good passive ankle dorsiflexion during infancy and childhood with successful Ponseti method treatment, but the amount of ankle dorsiflexion decreases with age. It is almost never as much as the normal side in unilateral patients or as much as in age-matched controls for bilateral patients. The average ankle dorsiflexion in the classic Cooper and Dietz long-term follow-up study of Ponseti patients averaged 6°, with a range from −2 to 17° [8]. Dynamic goniometer measurements during walking showed greater ankle dorsiflexion, but it is unclear if that technique was measuring some midfoot motion as well. Other long-term studies also show limited ankle dorsiflexion in older clubfoot patients who are functioning well [21], and thus, the author will not recommend treatment for patients with neutral ankle dorsiflexion and a plantigrade foot.

As noted previously, equinus often does not respond well to manipulation and casting alone, although some benefits can be gained if the calcaneus can be rotated externally beneath the talus to increase talocalcaneal divergence and get the anterior calcaneus out from beneath the talus. This may also increase the distance between the posterior calcaneus and the fibula, stretching the calcaneofibular ligament. The calcaneofibular ligament has been implicated as an important structure limiting ankle dorsiflexion in clubfoot patients [37].

The author's approach to recurrent equinus is as follows:

1. Assess foot abduction and cast to get maximal foot abduction, at least 45–50°, and then try to manipulate into more dorsiflexion.
2. Assess the foot for residual cavus or forefoot plantarflexion and if present cast with modified technique for complex clubfoot.
3. In young patients (less than 2 years), perform repeat tendo Achilles tenotomy and recast for 3 weeks. In any young patient where 10–15° of dorsiflexion is not

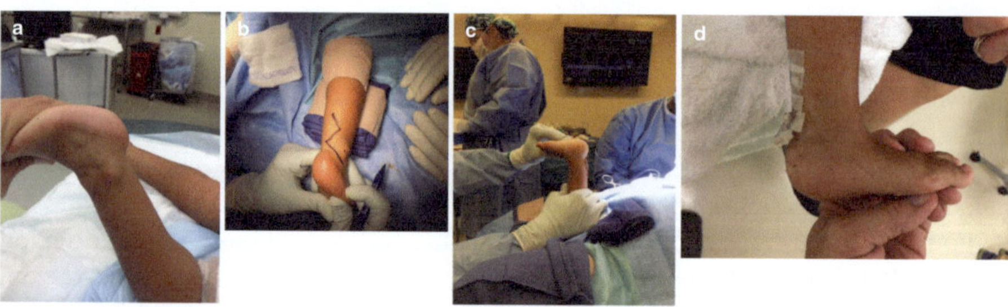

**Fig. 8.5** Residual equinus with a well-corrected midfoot/forefoot does not respond well to casting alone. Typically, a tendo Achilles tenotomy or lengthening is needed, with reassessment of dorsiflexion. If a neutral position is not achieved, then an a la carte approach with judicious posterior subtalar and tibiotalar releases is performed until satisfactory alignment is achieved to allow a plantigrade foot position. In this case of severe bilateral hindfoot equinus and rocker bottom deformity, a posterolateral approach was used to lengthen the Achilles and release the calcaneofibular ligament, posterior talocalcaneal ligaments, and the posterior tibiotalar ligaments. (**a**) Preoperative rocker bottom. (**b**) Posterolateral approach prior tendo Achilles tenotomy (TAT) scar visible. Dot is on tip of distal fibula. (**c**) Intraoperative assessment. Postoperative dorsiflexion to plantigrade position of hindfoot. (**d**) Healed incision

achieved with initial casting and tenotomy, change the cast at 1 week to attempt to increase dorsiflexion with casting.

4. In patients older than 2 years, an open Z-lengthening of the Achilles tendon is done through a posteromedial incision. For severe equinus without varus the author will often use a posterolateral incision (see Fig. 8.5).
5. If open Z lengthening does not improve ankle dorsiflexion to more than 10–15°, a sequential approach is taken. The incision is extended distally, dissection is carried out posterolaterally, and the calcaneofibular ligament is divided. This often provides 5–10° more dorsiflexion. If needed, the rest of the posterior talocalcaneal capsule (subtalar joint) can be divided, with care taken to identify and protect the flexor hallucis longus (FHL). If dorsiflexion still not adequate, the tibiotalar capsule is divided posteriorly as well.
6. A walking cast is applied for 4 weeks; then, a hinged AFO is used with stretching exercises. The amount of dorsiflexion able to be achieved in the operating room is usually quite limited (often only 5–10° above neutral), and thus, the author does not think that early weight-bearing risks failure of the Achilles repair or a calcaneus deformity. In the author's experience, substantial clinical calcaneus deformity (defined as excessive passive ankle dorsiflexion and limited ankle plantarflexion) is rare following Ponseti method treatment, as he has not personally seen it. Calcaneus gait has been described after manipulative clubfoot treatment, but this differs from calcaneus deformity (see Fig. 8.6).

Recurrent equinus following prior posterior capsulotomies is always a difficult problem, well-known to surgeons practicing in the era of extensive early intra-articular surgery for clubfoot. Repeat ankle and subtalar posterior capsulotomies are challenging, as it can be difficult to identify the joints without damaging them, and

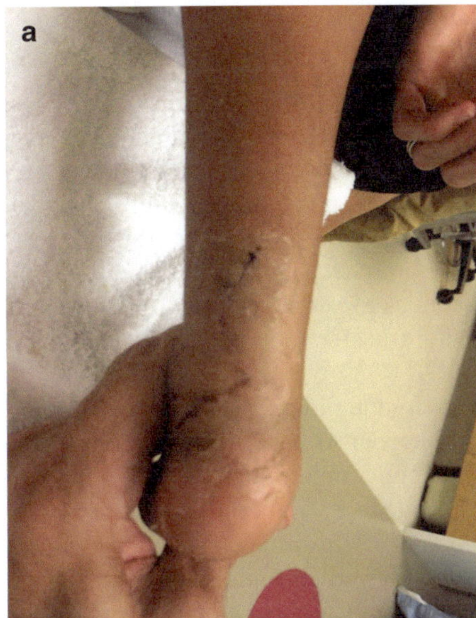
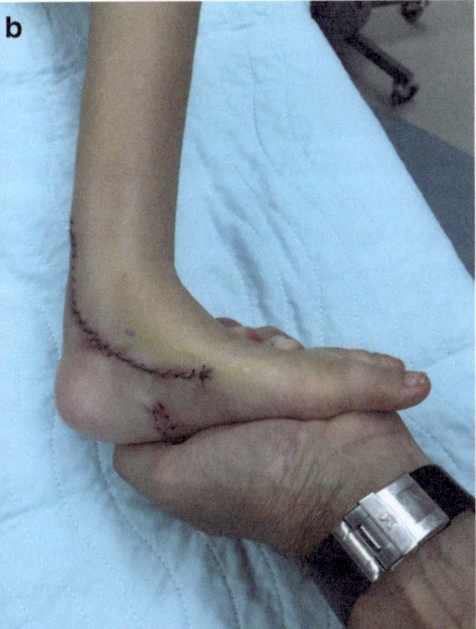

**Fig. 8.6** (**a**, **b**) Equinus can be a combination of ankle, hindfoot, and forefoot equinus (cavus). The patient in panel (**a**) underwent plantar release followed by open tendo Achilles lengthening. The hindfoot still did not get to neutral intraoperatively, so the incision was extended distally to allow identification and protection of the neurovascular bundle, and then the lateral subtalar joint was released (calcaneofibular ligament), and extended medially to the medial malleolus protecting the FHL. Once a plantigrade position is achieved, no further releases are performed. Panel (**b**) shows calcaneus deformity resulting from overly aggressive release posteriorly of the subtalar and ankle joints

often even after extensive release of all posterior soft-tissue structures, ankle dorsiflexion is still limited. Guided growth of the anterior distal tibia has been reported for persistent equinus in older clubfoot patients but has not been able to reliably correct the foot to a plantigrade position. The distal tibia does not grow rapidly, and the maximum correction of lateral distal tibial angulation is small (less than 10°). In addition, the change in lateral distal tibial angulation does not seem to always correlate with improved clinical dorsiflexion [38].

For severe equinus in older patients, anterior distal tibial osteotomy can be considered. Anterior translation of the foot typically occurs and can put tension on the posterior vascular structures in a patient population that may have deficient anterior vasculature plus posterior scarring along the vessels from prior surgeries, so caution is warranted. Use of external fixation can allow posterior translation of the foot. Some authors also use circular external fixation as a "super cast" and can correct all components of recurrent clubfoot using this technique [39]. The end result often is a stiff plantigrade foot following external fixation for residual or recurrent clubfoot deformity. Fortunately, patients treated with the Ponseti method rarely have enough residual equinus for contemplation of external fixation.

### *Relapse Following Prior Tibialis Anterior Tendon Transfer*

There is little written about this, with no reports from Dr. Ponseti himself, but one series out of Iowa detailing management of this problem in 10 patients out of a series of 66 patients with 102 clubfeet [40]. The treatment for relapse following tibialis anterior tendon transfer is individualized to the patient's deformity and may include casting, use of an ankle foot orthosis, physical therapy, or surgical treatment. Surgical treatments named in the paper by Morcuende included cuboid and medial cuneiform osteotomies or peroneus longus to peroneus brevis tendon transfers. Relapse following tibialis anterior tendon transfer should prompt a thorough neurological evaluation.

The author has seen patients who have undergone tibialis anterior tendon transfers and have developed relapse, who do not appear to have any palpable muscle mass or muscle function in the anterior or lateral compartments. In this situation, with recurrent deformity, the approach has been to use serial casting and manipulation to correct the inversion, adduction, and varus deformities; use tendo Achilles lengthening as needed to address equinus; and then use a tibialis posterior tendon transfer through the interosseous membrane to attempt to recreate muscular balance across the foot. These are rare cases, and only one case is reported in Dr. Ponseti's lifetime series out of Iowa [40]. The author has performed this surgery twice for clubfoot patients (see Fig. 8.7).

The lack of anterior tibial tendon function after tendon transfer should prompt the surgeon to assess the integrity of the tibialis anterior tendon insertion. Pullout of the tendon can occur, but is rare, and there is little literature about this complication. If the tendon it is not easily palpable on the dorsum of the foot, exploration of the tendon and intraoperative evaluation of the excursion of the muscle tendon unit is indicated. If a reasonably normal tendon with good excursion is discovered to have pulled out from its insertion point on the lateral cuneiform, a repeat anchoring procedure can be performed. If the tibialis anterior tendon is contracted or has no excursion, then consideration can be given to a tibialis posterior tendon transfer.

### *Late Relapse After Age 4 Years*

Dr. Ponseti noted that relapse was rare after the age of 5 years. This was believed to be because the rate of growth of the foot decreases after the first year of life and diminishes greatly after age 5. Still, late relapses have been reported, even in Dr. Ponseti's practice [41]. The "persistent deforming biology" described by Dr. Ponseti [10] leads to relapsing deformity. In late relapses reported out of Iowa after age 4, 39 patients with 60 club feet were described, and the treatments for these patients included observation, bracing, casting then bracing, casting then tibialis anterior tendon transfer with or without tendo Achilles lengthening, or primary tibialis anterior tendon transfer [22]. Multiple other procedures were performed in these patients

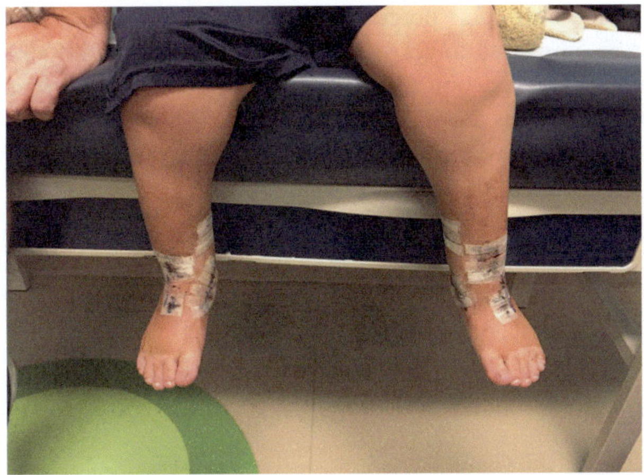

**Fig. 8.7** Tibialis posterior transfer to the dorsum of the foot is rarely needed in the management of idiopathic clubfoot, but is often used in conditions causing weakness or paralysis of the anterior compartment muscles. This 5 years old boy had idiopathic clubfoot that relapsed at age 3 years. He underwent bilateral tibialis anterior transfers but continued to walk on the outside border of both feet. Exploration of his tendon transfers at age 4 found the transfers intact but loose—both sides were reanchored under tension in the lateral cuneiform but gait did not improve. At age 5, he underwent bilateral tibialis posterior tendon transfers to balance his forefoot and allow plantigrade foot positioning in stance

in an à la carte method, with six plantar fascia releases, one extensor halluces longus recession, and limited posterior releases in 5 feet. Five of these patients went on to revision surgery after tibialis anterior tendon transfer and included two eventual triple arthrodeses.

In another Iowa series, 12 of 209 patients with relapse occurring after the seventh birthday led to a finding of a neuromuscular disorder in four of the 12 patients. The diagnoses included myotonic dystrophy, multiple core disease, Charcot-Marie-Tooth type IA, and myasthenia gravis. These patients were treated with tibialis anterior tendon transfers, plantar fascia releases, and peroneus long to peroneus brevis transfers. Subsequently, these patients with neurological disorders were treated with a tibialis posterior tendon transfer in one, triple arthrodesis in one, and a Jones procedure in one [13].

## *Adduction/Varus Relapse in Older Child with Deformities that Do Not Respond to Serial Manipulation and Casting*

Rarely, serial manipulation and casting will not resolve recurrent forefoot adduction and hindfoot varus deformities. If rigid deformities are encountered that do not allow for a good plantigrade position with restoration of the normal plantar tripod weight-bearing surface for the foot, then osteotomies are preferred to reposition the foot rather than intra-articular procedures. This is unusual, and manipulation and casting should be employed to correct as much deformity as possible prior to surgery. Osteotomies preserve joint capsules and should not cause articular injury and thus should preserve joint motion. Closing wedge osteotomy of the cuboid combined with an opening wedge osteotomy of the medial cuneiform is well described as a surgical treatment option for persistent forefoot adduction in clubfoot [42]. Hindfoot varus can also be addressed using the classic Dwyer lateral closing wedge osteotomy or a lateral translation osteotomy of the calcaneus [18]. Fixation of these osteotomies can be performed with Kirschner wires, screws, or staples.

## *Persistent in Toeing Gait Following Congenital Club Treatment*

Published reports of the amount of tibial torsion in clubfoot patients are conflicting [27, 43, 44]. Some studies report no increased incidence of inward tibial torsion in clubfoot patients while some report that persistent inward tibial torsion is present in a higher percentage of clubfoot patients. In principle, it would make sense that clubfoot patients with weak evertors would fail to remodel the inward tibial torsion present at birth. Those authors reporting that clubfoot patients often have excessive external tibial torsion have stated that forceful manipulation attempts create external tibial torsion, particularly if the hindfoot varus is not corrected and the forefoot is still in cavus with midfoot stiffness. The hypothesis is that manipulating the foot with external rotation can cause pressure by the talus on the fibula to rotate it outwardly. The Ponseti principle of applying pressure to the lateral aspect of the talar neck and head with a thumb would prevent abnormal outward pressure on the fibula. Many of the cases used as an example of external tibial torsion are radiographic views only of the ankle, and it is not clear if inappropriate radiographic technique in the setting of persistent forefoot adduction and hindfoot varus leads to an incorrect, improper lateral view of the ankle joint. If the radiology technician lines the X-ray beam up perpendicular to the adducted forefoot instead of perpendicular to the ankle, an oblique view of the hindfoot will be obtained, and the fibula will appear posterior to the tibia.

It is the author's belief that some patients with well-corrected congenital clubfeet have significant persistent intoeing gait (foot progression angle more than 20° inward) that leads to tripping as the swing phase foot strikes the stance phase leg. These patients have an inward thigh foot axis of 20° or more and an abnormally decreased bimalleolar axis. If this persists after the age of 6 years, an outward tibial rotation osteotomy can be offered (see Fig. 8.8).

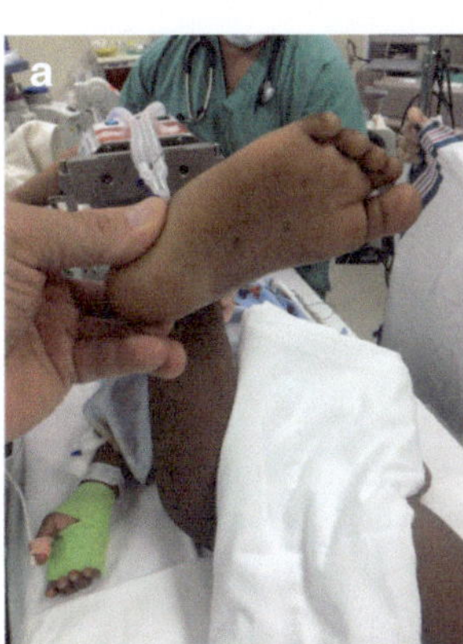
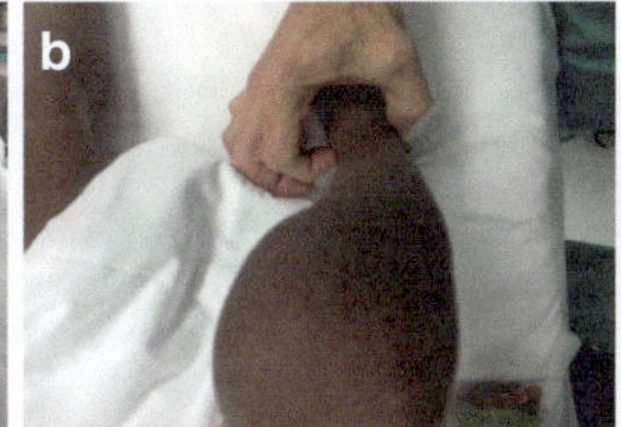
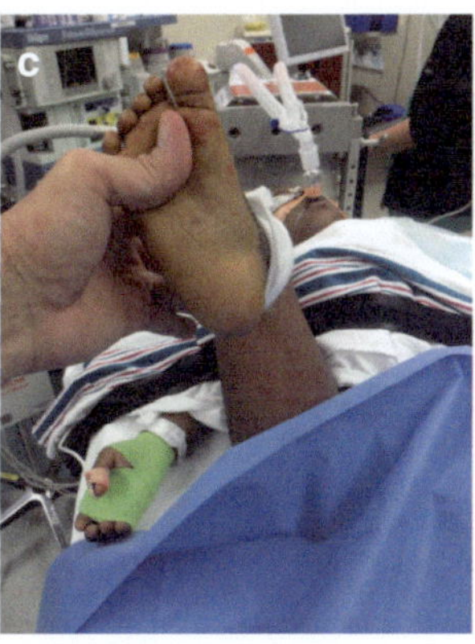

**Fig. 8.8** Residual intoeing gait is common in patients with congenital clubfoot and may be from metatarsus adductus, medial spin of the foot, internal tibial torsion, or femoral anteversion or a combination of factors. Occasionally, severe internal tibial torsion is the cause and can be corrected with a transverse distal tibial osteotomy to correct the rotation. Panels (**a, b**) shows a well corrected foot but substantial internal rotation of the foot by thigh-foot axis and bimalleolar axis. (**a**) Thigh foot axis. (**b**) Bimalleolar axis. (**c**) Postoperative thigh foot axis

## Conclusion

Clubfoot is a major developmental limb deformity, and even after complete correction in infancy or early childhood, the deformity commonly recurs with growth of the leg and foot. Prolonged foot abduction brace wear can markedly lower the incidence of relapse, but the surgeon caring for young clubfoot patients should monitor patients regularly for relapse and should have a thorough approach to the evaluation and management of deformity relapses. The most important consideration is to use manipulation and casting to correct deformity, augmented or supplemented by extra-articular surgical procedures. As much as possible, the surgeon should strive to achieve a corrected, plantigrade foot position without opening joint capsules and dividing ligaments. When intra-articular surgery is needed, the amount of surgery should be limited to achieve an acceptable foot position. Limiting the time of immobilization and promoting early range of motion after intra-articular surgery may improve motion and hopefully long-term outcomes.

# References


1. Hosseinzadeh P, Kelly DM, Zionts LE. Management of the relapsed clubfoot following treatment using the ponseti method. J Am Acad Orthop Surg. 2017;25(3):195–203.
2. Hosseinzadeh P, Kiebzak GM, Dolan L, Zionts LE, Morcuende J. Management of clubfoot relapses with the ponseti method: results of a survey of the POSNA members. J Pediatr Orthop. 2017;39(1):38–41.
3. Ponseti IV. Congenital clubfoot: fundamentals of treatment. New York: Oxford University Press; 1996. p. 140.
4. Dobbs MB, Rudzki JR, Purcell DB, Walton T, Porter KR, Gurnett CA. Factors predictive of outcome after use of the Ponseti method for the treatment of idiopathic clubfeet. J Bone Joint Surg Am. 2004;86(1):22–7.
5. Noonan KJ. Ponseti technique in the treatment of clubfoot. In: Kocher DS, editor. Master techniques in orthopaedic surgery: pediatrics. Philadelphia: Wolter Kluwer; 2016. p. 283–300.
6. Seegmiller L, Burmeister R, Paulsen-Miller M, Morcuende J. Bracing in Ponseti clubfoot treatment: improving parental adherence through an innovative health education intervention. Orthop Nurs. 2016;35(2):92–7; quiz 8-9.
7. Morcuende JA, Egbert M, Ponseti IV. The effect of the internet in the treatment of congenital idiopathic clubfoot. Iowa Orthop J. 2003;23:83–6.
8. Cooper DM, Dietz FR. Treatment of idiopathic clubfoot. A thirty-year follow-up note. J Bone Joint Surg Am. 1995;77(10):1477–89.
9. Holt JB, Oji DE, Yack HJ, Morcuende JA. Long-term results of tibialis anterior tendon transfer for relapsed idiopathic clubfoot treated with the Ponseti method: a follow-up of thirty-seven to fifty-five years. J Bone Joint Surg Am. 2015;97(1):47–55.
10. Ponseti IV. Relapsing clubfoot: causes, prevention, and treatment. Iowa Orthop J. 2002;22:55–6.
11. Halanski MA, Maples DL, Davison JE, Huang JC, Crawford HA. Separating the chicken from the egg: an attempt to discern between clubfoot recurrences and incomplete corrections. Iowa Orthop J. 2010;30:29–34.
12. Edmonds EW, Frick SL. The drop toe sign: an indicator of neurologic impairment in congenital clubfoot. Clin Orthop Relat Res. 2009;467(5):1238–42.
13. Lovell ME, Morcuende JA. Neuromuscular disease as the cause of late clubfoot relapses: report of 4 cases. Iowa Orthop J. 2007;27:82–4.
14. Richards BS, Faulks S. Clubfoot infants initially thought to be idiopathic, but later found not to be. How do they do with nonoperative treatment? J Pediatr Orthop. 2017;39(1):42–5.
15. Dobbs MB, Nunley R, Schoenecker PL. Long-term follow-up of patients with clubfeet treated with extensive soft-tissue release. J Bone Joint Surg Am. 2006;88(5):986–96.
16. El-Hawary R, Karol LA, Jeans KA, Richards BS. Gait analysis of children treated for clubfoot with physical therapy or the Ponseti cast technique. J Bone Joint Surg Am. 2008;90(7):1508–16.
17. Karol LA, Jeans KA, Kaipus KA. The relationship between gait, gross motor function, and parental perceived outcome in children with clubfeet. J Pediatr Orthop. 2016;36(2):145–51.
18. Mosca VS. Principles and management of pediatric foot and ankle deformities and malformations. Philadelphia: Wolters Kluwer Health; 2014. p. 285.
19. Smith PA, Kuo KN, Graf AN, Krzak J, Flanagan A, Hassani S, et al. Long-term results of comprehensive clubfoot release versus the Ponseti method: which is better? Clin Orthop Relat Res. 2014;472(4):1281–90.
20. Bor N, Coplan JA, Herzenberg JE. Ponseti treatment for idiopathic clubfoot: minimum 5-year followup. Clin Orthop Relat Res. 2009;467(5):1263–70.
21. Aronson J, Puskarich CL. Deformity and disability from treated clubfoot. J Pediatr Orthop. 1990;10(1):109–19.
22. McKay SD, Dolan LA, Morcuende JA. Treatment results of late-relapsing idiopathic clubfoot previously treated with the Ponseti method. J Pediatr Orthop. 2012;32(4):406–11.
23. Farsetti P, Caterini R, Mancini F, Potenza V, Ippolito E. Anterior tibial tendon transfer in relapsing congenital clubfoot: long-term follow-up study of two series treated with a different protocol. J Pediatr Orthop. 2006;26(1):83–90.

24. Ippolito E, Farsetti P, Caterini R, Tudisco C. Long-term comparative results in patients with congenital clubfoot treated with two different protocols. J Bone Joint Surg Am. 2003;85(7):1286–94.
25. Haft GF, Walker CG, Crawford HA. Early clubfoot recurrence after use of the Ponseti method in a New Zealand population. J Bone Joint Surg Am. 2007;89(3):487–93.
26. Lykissas MG, Crawford AH, Eismann EA, Tamai J. Ponseti method compared with soft-tissue release for the management of clubfoot: a meta-analysis study. World J Orthop. 2013;4(3):144–53.
27. Kuo KN, Smith PA. Correcting residual deformity following clubfoot releases. Clin Orthop Relat Res. 2009;467(5):1326–33.
28. Jauregui JJ, Zamani S, Abawi HH, Herzenberg JE. Ankle range of motion after posterior subtalar and ankle capsulotomy for relapsed equinus in idiopathic clubfoot. J Pediatr Orthop. 2017;37(3):199–203.
29. Morcuende JA, Abbasi D, Dolan LA, Ponseti IV. Results of an accelerated Ponseti protocol for clubfoot. J Pediatr Orthop. 2005;25(5):623–6.
30. Nogueira MP, Fox M, Miller K, Morcuende J. The Ponseti method of treatment for clubfoot in Brazil: barriers to bracing compliance. Iowa Orthop J. 2013;33:161–6.
31. Dobbs MB, Frick SL, Mosca VS, Raney E, VanBosse HJ, Lerman JA, et al. Design and descriptive data of the randomized clubfoot foot abduction brace length of treatment study (FAB24). J Pediatr Orthop B. 2017;26(2):101–7.
32. Dobbs MB, Gurnett CA. The 2017 ABJS Nicolas Andry Award: advancing personalized medicine for clubfoot through translational research. Clin Orthop Relat Res. 2017;475(6):1716–25.
33. Moon DK, Gurnett CA, Aferol H, Siegel MJ, Commean PK, Dobbs MB. Soft-tissue abnormalities associated with treatment-resistant and treatment-responsive clubfoot: findings of MRI analysis. J Bone Joint Surg Am. 2014;96(15):1249–56.
34. Zionts LE, Jew MH, Bauer KL, Ebramzadeh E. How many patients who have a clubfoot treated using the Ponseti method are likely to undergo a tendon transfer? J Pediatr Orthop. 2016;38(7):382–7.
35. Goldstein RY, Seehausen DA, Chu A, Sala DA, Lehman WB. Predicting the need for surgical intervention in patients with idiopathic clubfoot. J Pediatr Orthop. 2015;35(4):395–402.
36. Radler C, Gourdine-Shaw MC, Herzenberg JE. Nerve structures at risk in the plantar side of the foot during anterior tibial tendon transfer: a cadaver study. J Bone Joint Surg Am. 2012;94(4):349–55.
37. Scott WA, Hosking SW, Catterall A, Club foot. Observations on the surgical anatomy of dorsiflexion. J Bone Joint Surg Br. 1984;66(1):71–6.
38. Al-Aubaidi Z, Lundgaard B, Pedersen NW. Anterior distal tibial epiphysiodesis for the treatment of recurrent equinus deformity after surgical treatment of clubfeet. J Pediatr Orthop. 2011;31(6):716–20.
39. Nakase T, Yasui N, Ohzono K, Shimizu N, Yoshikawa H. Treatment of relapsed idiopathic clubfoot by complete subtalar release combined with the Ilizarov method. J Foot Ankle Surg. 2006;45(5):337–41.
40. Masrouha KZ, Morcuende JA. Relapse after tibialis anterior tendon transfer in idiopathic clubfoot treated by the Ponseti method. J Pediatr Orthop. 2012;32(1):81–4.
41. Dobbs MB, Corley CL, Morcuende JA, Ponseti IV. Late recurrence of clubfoot deformity: a 45-year followup. Clin Orthop Relat Res. 2003;411:188–92.
42. McHale KA, Lenhart MK. Treatment of residual clubfoot deformity–the "bean-shaped" foot–by opening wedge medial cunciform osteotomy and closing wedge cuboid osteotomy. Clinical review and cadaver correlations. J Pediatr Orthop. 1991;11(3):374–81.
43. Bhaskar A, Patni P. Classification of relapse pattern in clubfoot treated with Ponseti technique. Indian J Orthop. 2013;47(4):370–6.
44. Farsetti P, Dragoni M, Ippolito E. Tibiofibular torsion in congenital clubfoot. J Pediatr Orthop B. 2012;21(1):47–51.

# Chapter 9
# Extensive Soft Tissue Release for Congenital Vertical Talus


Ashok N. Johari, Amit S. Nemade, Ratna S. Maheshwari, and Shalin K. Maheshwari


## Evolution of Surgery in Congenital Vertical Talus

Congenital vertical talus (CVT) is a rare deformity of the foot wherein there is a rigid dorsal dislocation of navicular and an equinus deformity of the hindfoot. The first complete description of patho-anatomy was given by Henke in 1914 [1]. If left untreated, it can lead to abnormal gait, shoe wear problems, callosities, pain, and functional limitations [2, 3].

Various authors have tried a spectrum of treatment methods including nonoperative [4] to extensive surgeries. History of CVT surgery dates back to 1939 when Lamy and Weismann recommended astragalectomy [5]. Another surgery not accepted in the current era is naviculectomy recommended by Stone [6].

A two-staged technique was described by Herndon and Heyman [7], Ellis and Scheer [8], Walker et al. [9], and Coleman and colleagues [10] wherein the dorsal structures were released in the first stage followed by a second stage to lengthen the Achilles tendon along with posterior capsulotomy of ankle and subtalar joints. Although performed in a staged manner, these surgeries were not free of wound complications [7, 9–11] and avascular necrosis (AVN) of Talus [12]. Though a single-stage surgery was first described by Osmond-Clarke [13], it was performed by various other authors through different approaches. Recently, several studies have documented the safety and efficacy of a single-stage procedure to address both hindfoot and forefoot deformities [12, 14–17]. Dobbs [18] has introduced a minimally invasive technique for correction of CVT.

This chapter looks at various aspects of extensive soft tissue release in details.


A. N. Johari (✉)
Children's Orthopedic Centre, Mumbai, Maharashtra, India

A. S. Nemade · R. S. Maheshwari · S. K. Maheshwari
ENABLE International Centre for Paediatric Musculoskeletal Care, Mumbai, India




M. B. Dobbs et al. (eds.), *Clubfoot and Vertical Talus*,
https://doi.org/10.1007/978-3-031-34788-7_9

## Surgical Pathology [1, 19, 20]

To understand the concept of extensive release in CVT, it is of paramount importance that we understand its surgical pathology. The etiology of CVT may not be clearly known, but the patho-anatomical changes are constant. The changes can be summarized as follows (Figs. 9.1, 9.2, and 9.3):

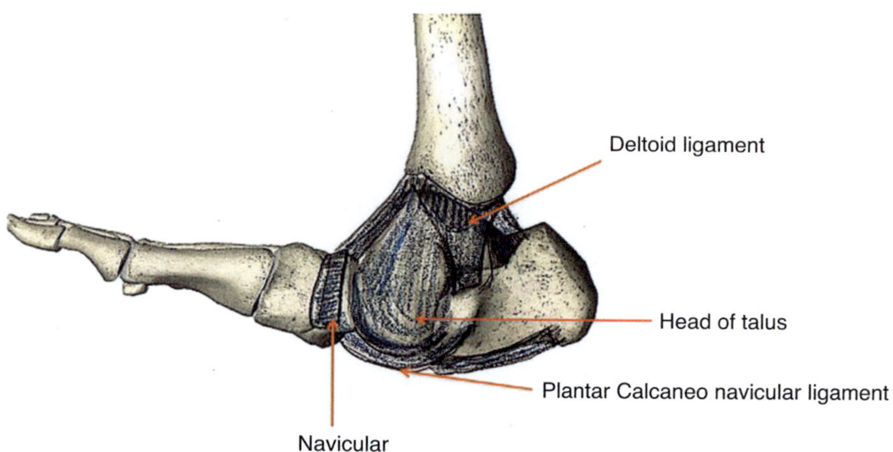


**Fig. 9.1** Osseo-ligamentous structures seen on medial side of foot

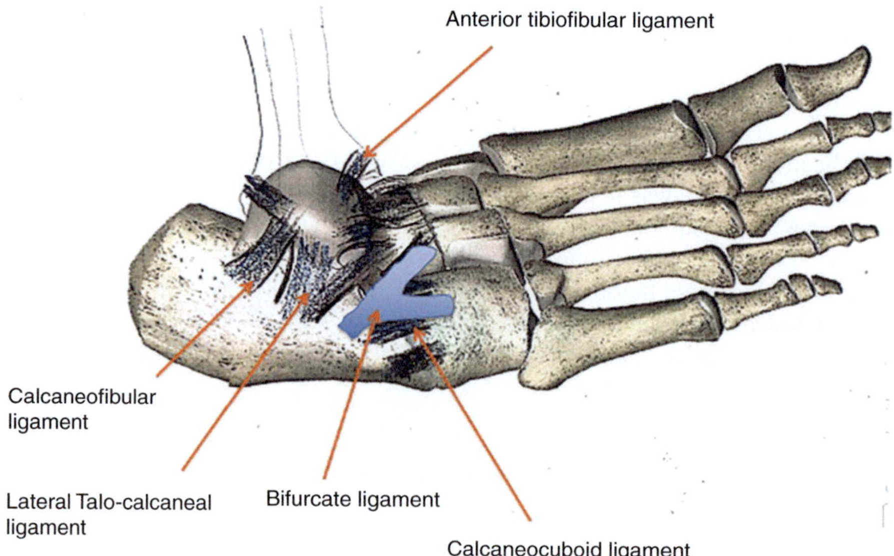


**Fig. 9.2** Osseo-ligamentous structures seen on lateral side of foot

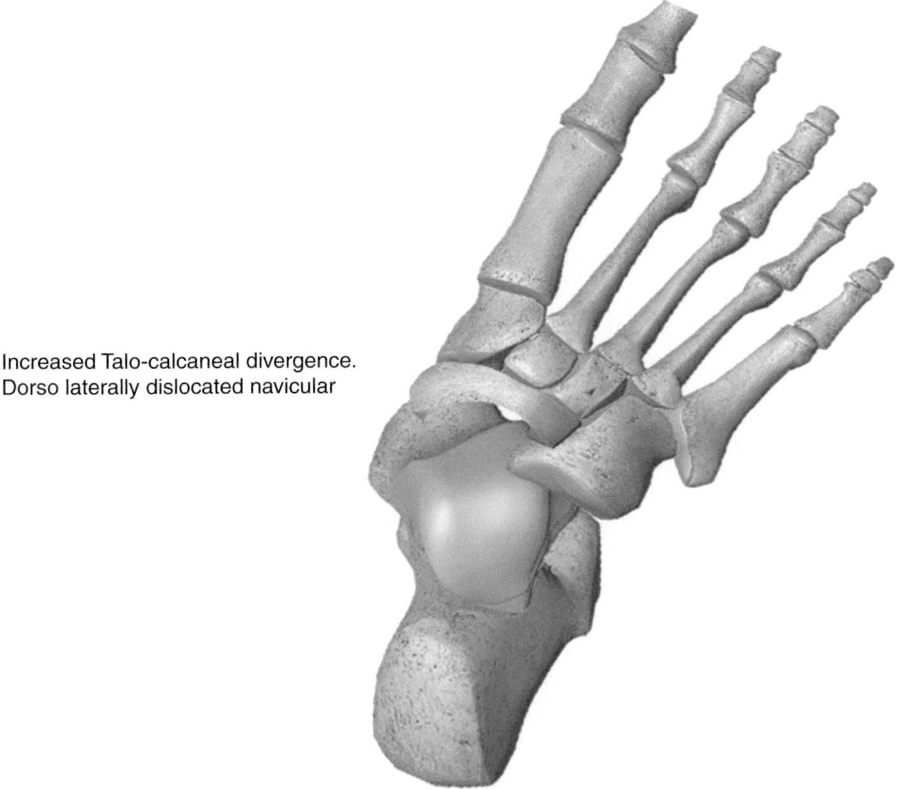


**Fig. 9.3** Osseous alignment seen from dorsal aspect of foot

## *Bone Changes*

### Calcaneum

- Plantar flexed.
- Hypoplastic anterior and middle facets with misshapen posterior facets.
- Hypoplastic sustentaculum tali not supporting the talar head.

### Talus

- Flattened dorsolaterally.
- Articular surface expands to accommodate articular surface of displaced navicular.
- Plantar flexed.
- Only posterior 1/3rd articulates with tibial plafond.

**Navicular**

- Dorsolaterally displaced over talus.
- Wedge shaped.
- Hypoplastic.

**Cuboid**

- Laterally displaced.
- Hypoplastic plantar half in severe cases.

## *Ligament Changes*

- Stretched spring ligament, anterior fibers of deltoid ligament and medial fibers of bifurcate ligament
- Contracture of ligaments
  - Dorsal talonavicular
  - Calcaneo fibular
  - Interosseous talo calcaneal
  - Extensor retinaculum
  - Posterior ankle and subtalar joints

## *Muscle Changes*

- Contracture of Achilles tendon, Extensor (Tibialis anterior, Extensor hallucis longus, Peroneus tertius, Extensor digitorum longus) and lateral compartment musculature (Peroneus longus and brevis)
- Tibialis posterior is subluxated anteriorly so are the peronei now acting as dorsiflexors of foot

## *Joint Changes*

- Capsule of talonavicular is fibrotic and contracted on the dorsolateral aspect
- Dorsal capsule of calcaneocuboid joint also gets contracted
- Contracture of posterior ankle and subtalar joint capsule

## Radiologic Assessment

- Standard set of radiographs are required for radiologic assessment of CVT. The work by Hamanishi [21]and Napiontek [22] is of great importance. Classically anteroposterior and lateral view of the foot (preferably done standing in older children) are advised. The list of radiologic parameters is summarized in Table 9.1.

**Table 9.1** Radiographic parameters for assessment of congenital vertical talus (CVT)

| Radiologic view | Angle | Landmarks | Normal range |
|---|---|---|---|
| Lateral view (Fig. 9.4) | Tibiotalar | Longitudinal axis of tibia and talus | In dorsiflexion—15° to 30° |
| | | | In plantar flexion—15° to 40° |
| | Tibio-calcaneal | Longitudinal axis of tibia and calcaneus | 10–40° |
| | Talocalcaneal | Longitudinal axis of talus and calcaneus | 35–55° |
| | Talus-first metatarsal | Longitudinal axis of talus and first metatarsal | 0–10° |
| | TAMBA[a] | Angle between line 1 and 2 Line 1: Longitudinal axis of talus (between posterior third of trochlea tali and midpoint of anterior curvature of head) | 3.3° ± 6.4° |
| | | Line 2: Joining 2 points: (a) midpoint of anterior curvature of talar head | |
| | | (b) Midpoint of base of ossified metaphysis of first metatarsal | |
| | CAMBA[b] | Angle between line 1 and 2. | −9° ± 4.5° |
| | | Line 1: Longitudinal axis of calcaneus (between the upper end of the apophysis or tuber calcanei and the midpoint of anterior curvature) | |
| | | Line 2: Joining 2 points: (a) midpoint of anterior curvature of calcaneus | |
| | | (b) Midpoint of base of ossified metaphysis of first metatarsal | |
| Antero-posterior view | Talo-calcaneal | Angle between longitudinal axis of talus and calcaneus | 20–40° |
| | Talus–first metatarsal | Longitudinal axis of talus and first metatarsal | 0–20° |

Napiontek has also graded the talonavicular reduction for further assessing the results as Grade 0: reduction, Grade I: first grade of dislocation/subluxation, Grade II: second grade of dislocation (Fig. 9.5)

[a] TAMBA: Talar axis-first metatarsal base angle

[b] CAMBA: Calcaneal axis-first metatarsal base angle

**Fig. 9.4** Radiologic parameters for lateral view. (i) Tibio-talar angle. (ii) TAMBA. (iii) CAMBA. (iv) Talocalcaneal angle

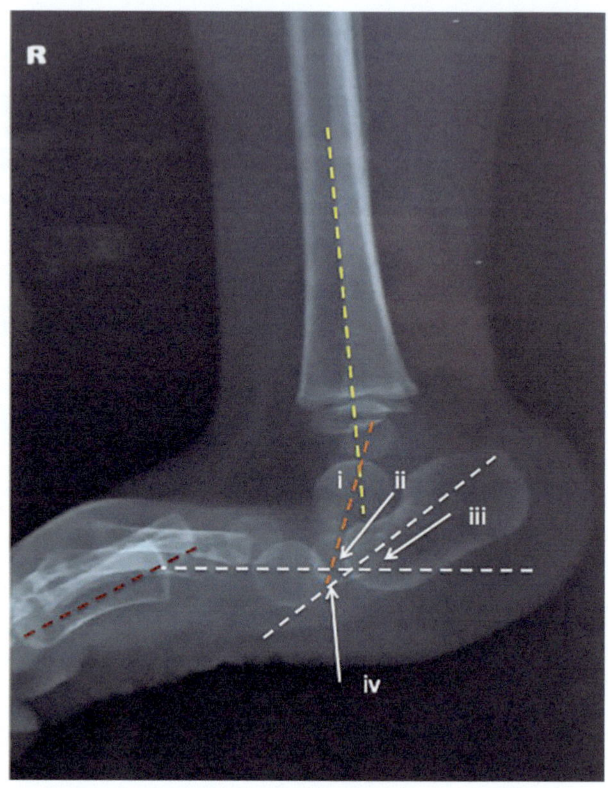

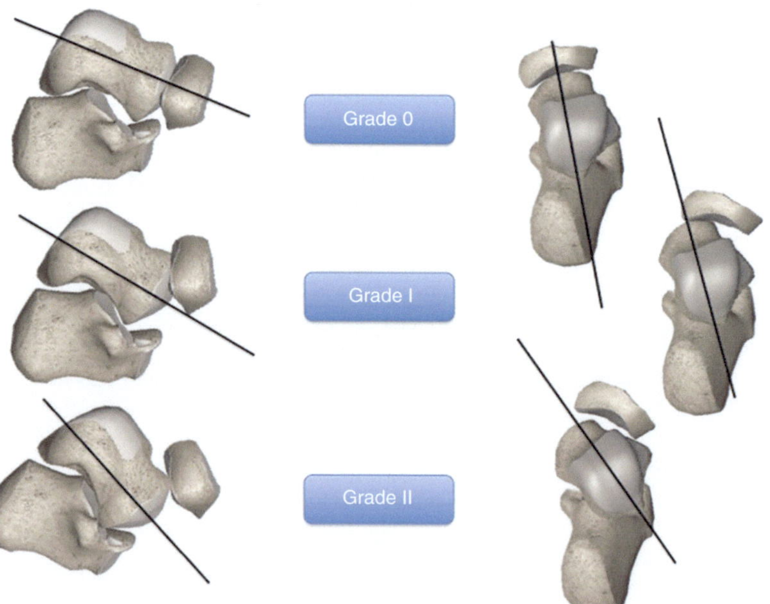


**Fig. 9.5** Grading of talonavicular reduction (Napiontek)

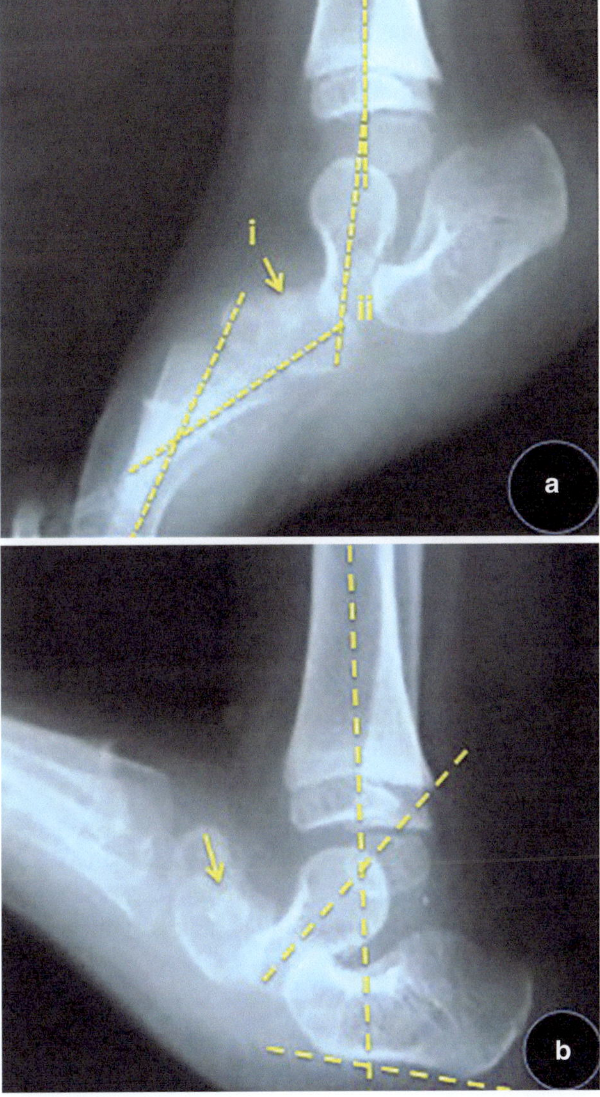

**Fig. 9.6** Radiologic landmarks on stress X-rays: (**a**) Plantarflexion stress view. (i) Dorsally displaced (unreduced) navicular. (ii) Increased TAMBA. (**b**) Dorsiflexion stress view: failure of calcaneum and talus to dorsiflex

In addition, dorsiflexion and plantar flexion stress views are performed to assess the flexibility of deformity (Fig. 9.6).

## Indications for Open Surgery

Considering the extensiveness of the surgical injury to soft tissues in open surgery, soft tissue releases should be considered when less invasive measures have failed to give results in mild to moderate forms of CVT. In moderate to severe varieties including syndromic and neurologic, where open surgery is inevitable, a couple of stretching casts may be helpful. Fear of complications should not prevent the surgeon from early intervention because delay in intervention may lead to loss of valuable time when bone can remodel. Delayed surgeries may lead to permanent deformation of bones and other tissues, which may hamper the final outcomes.

## Aim of Treatment

The primary goal of CVT treatment is to achieve a flexible, plantigrade, and mobile foot in addition to restoration of normal anatomic relations between the bones of the foot to re-establish normal weight bearing capacity of first ray.

## *Incisions*

Various authors have approached the complex patho-anatomy of CVT through different surgical approaches. These incisions can be used independently or in combination as demanded by the clinical scenario. To summarize, the types of surgeries can be grouped as [1].

1. Staged multiple incision technique with extensive soft tissue release
2. Single-stage medial and posterior approach and single-stage dorsal approach
3. Minimal invasive technique

Surgical approaches can be briefly summarized as follows in Table 9.2

Mazzocca [24] felt that a dorsal approach gives excellent exposure to the pathology of CVT. According to the authors, the dorsal approach involved less operative time, less dissection, and similar radiographic improvement, with improved and consistent clinical scores.

**Table 9.2** Various approaches for surgical correction of CVT

| Approach | Reference |
|---|---|
| Anterior/dorsal | Fitton [15] |
| | Seimon [16] |
| | Stricker and Rosen [23] |
| | Mazzocca and colleagues [24] |
| Medial | Ogata [12] |
| Posterior Cincinnati | Crawford [25] |
| | Zorer [2] |
| | Kodros [26] |
| Medial and lateral | Ramanoudjame [27] |
| Posterior + medial + lateral | Duncan and Fixsen [28] |
| | DeRosa and Ahlfeld [14] |

In a publication on surgical correction of CVT, Kodros and Dias [26] state that although Cincinnati incision results in excellent healing of the wound and very good cosmesis, the only limitation of this incision is the difficulty to reach the dorsal anatomic structures. The long-toe extensors can be lengthened through a separate incision over the anterior aspect of the ankle, if need arises. According to the authors, the most important advantage of this incision is the possibility to reach, completely release, and reduce the talocalcaneonavicular joint, which is crucial for correction.

## *Authors' Preferred Technique*

The typical appearance of a foot with CVT is seen in Fig. 9.7. We describe the surgical steps in this same patient.

At our institution, senior author (ANJ) has been following a standard protocol for all cases of CVT. Irrespective of the severity of the deformity, all patients are given weekly serial casts till a plateau in correction is reached (average four to six casts). Standard set of X-rays used are standing anteroposterior and lateral view and stress plantar flexion and dorsiflexion views. A single-stage extensive soft tissue release as mentioned below is then performed. Release of soft tissue is done as an a la carte procedure depending on the difficulties faced intraoperatively.

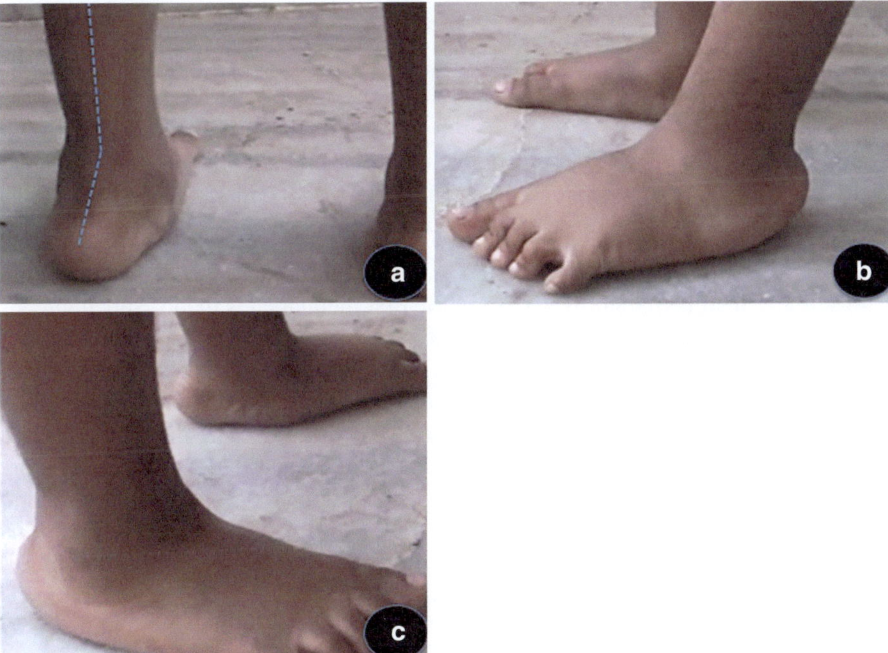

**Fig. 9.7** Preoperative image of a foot with CVT. (**a**) Note heel vagus. (**b**) Note heel equinus and concave lateral border (abduction). (**c**) Medial side shows rocker bottom foot

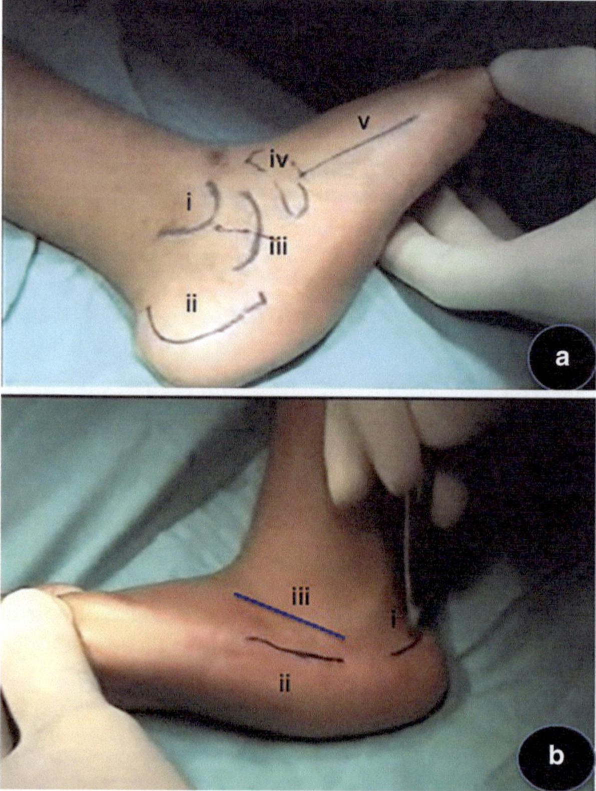

**Fig. 9.8** Preoperative marking of landmarks: (**a**) Medial side. (i) Medial malleolus. (ii) Calcaneum. (iii) Talar head and axis of talus. (iv) Navicular. (v) Axis of first metatarsal. (**b**) Lateral side. (i) Lateral border of calcaneum. (ii) Cuboid and fifth metatarsal plantar border. (iii) Incision centered over sinus tarsi

The procedure is done under tourniquet control with patient under epidural analgesia. We use a three-incision technique (Fig. 9.8). Surface marking for all the bony landmarks is done so as to place accurate surgical incisions.

1. *Medial incision* (Figs. 9.9, 9.10, and 9.11): Longitudinal incision starting from just under medial malleolus to base of the first metatarsal is made. Subcutaneous tissues are dissected to expose the sheath of tibialis posterior (TP), which is then traced to its insertion on navicular. This helps in locating the dorsally dislocated navicular. The TP is then released from its insertion on the navicular for as much length possible and tagged with a suture (3–0 Ethilon). The dissection is then developed dorsally, the talonavicular joint is then identified and an arthrotomy performed to completely release the joint on its dorsal, dorsomedial, and lateral sides. Talar head is seen pointing downwards with navicular articulating on its dorsal aspect. The tendons of Tibialis Anterior (Tib Ant) and Extensor Hallucis Longus (EHL) are then identified and a Z lengthening performed. The cut ends of the tendons are tagged with a suture for later identification and repair.
2. *Dorsolateral incision* (Figs. 9.12, 9.13, and 9.14): The incision starts just distal and anterior to tip of lateral malleolus centering over the sinus tarsi. Extreme

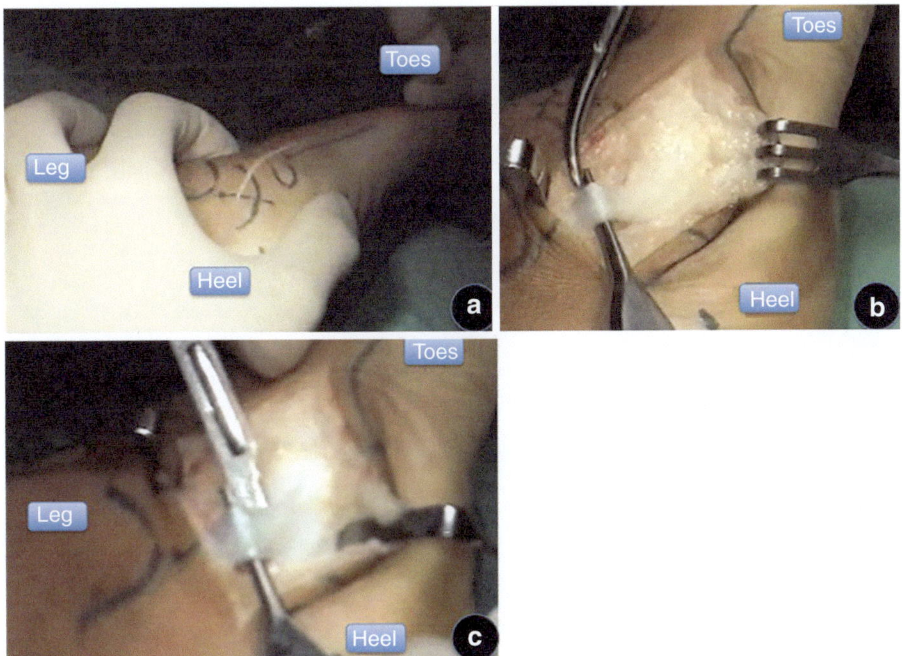


**Fig. 9.9** (**a**) Medial incision. (**b**) Expose tibialis posterior. (**c**) Release it as far as the insertion on navicular

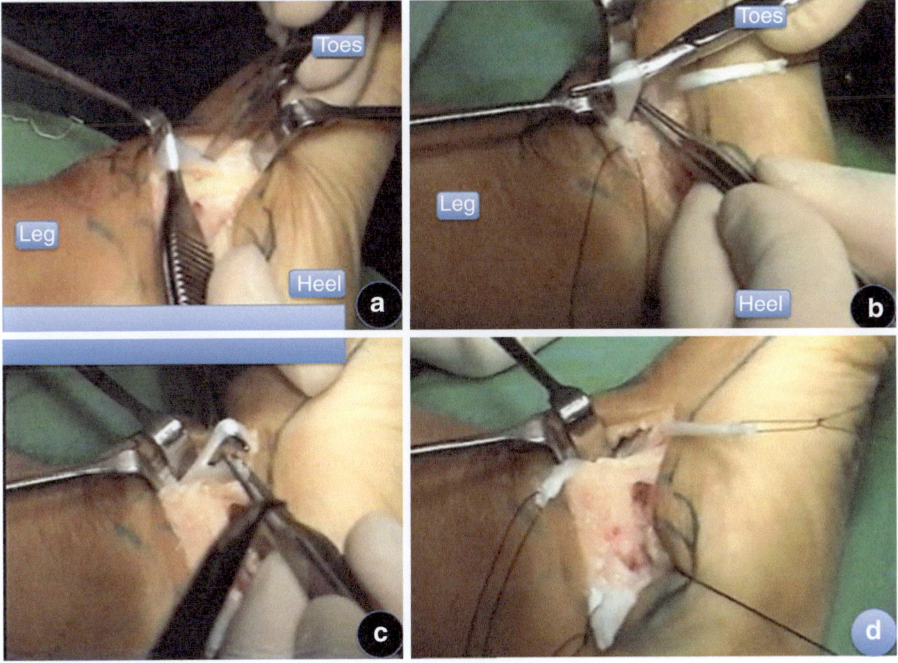


**Fig. 9.10** (**a–d**) Identify tibialis anterior, EHL and perform Z plasty

A. N. Johari et al.

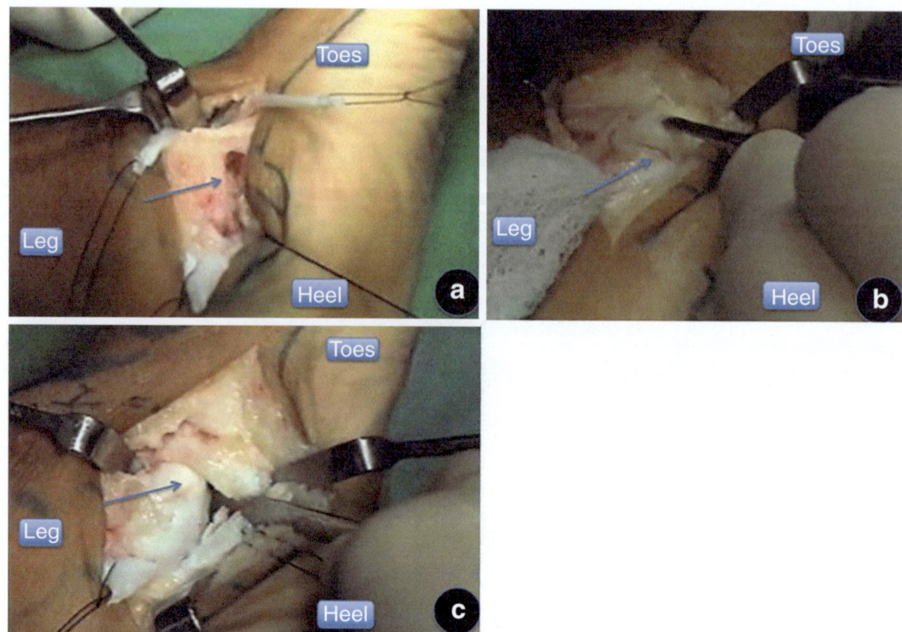

**Fig. 9.11** (**a**) Talonavicular joint identified. (**b**) Capsulotomy done. (**c**) Capsule released from medial and dorsal aspect

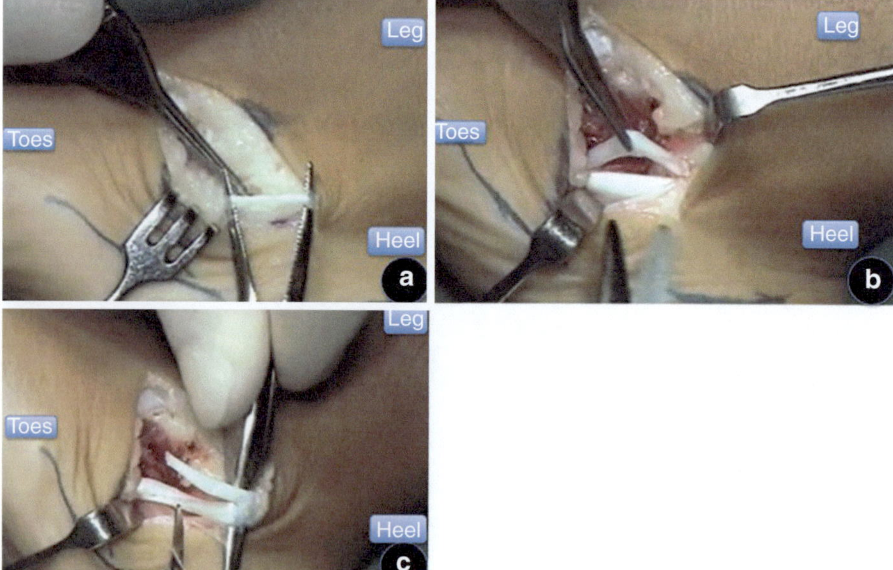

**Fig. 9.12** Lateral aspect. (**a**) Incision taken and sural nerve safeguarded. (**b**) Peroneal tendons identified and (**c**) Z lengthened

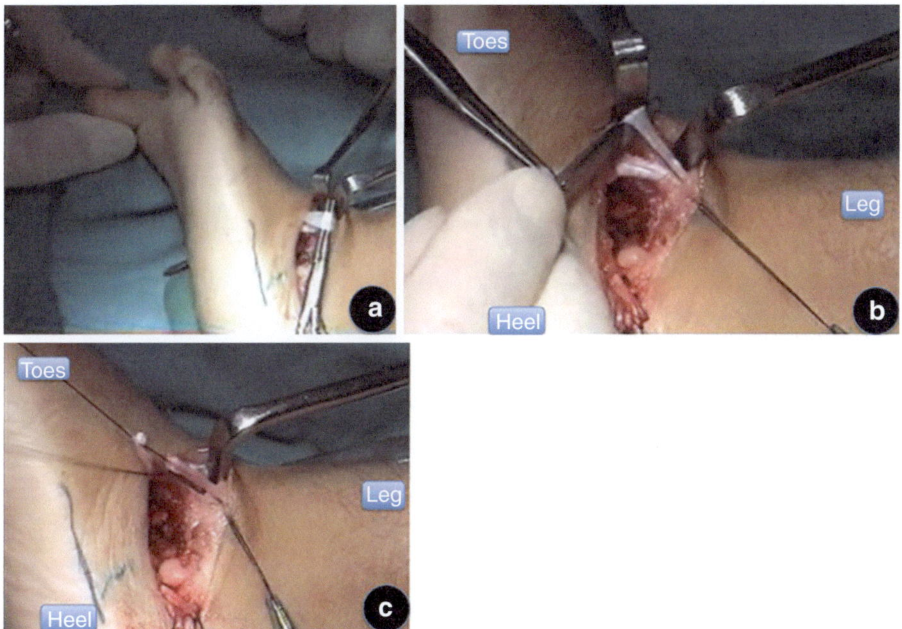

**Fig. 9.13** (**a**) Identify extensor digitorum longus. (**b**, **c**) Z lengthening performed by tying all four tendon slips together proximally and distally and then making cuts proximally and distally

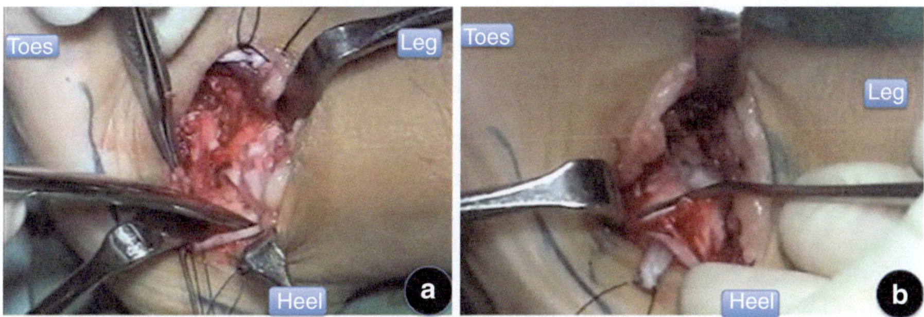

**Fig. 9.14** (**a**) Elevate extensor digitorum brevis. Identify calcaneocuboid (CC) and lateral aspect of talonavicular (TN) joint. (**b**) Capsulotomy of CC and TN joint

care is taken to protect the sural nerve, which lies in the subcutaneous plane. The Extensor Digitorum Brevis (EDB) is elevated from its origin on the calcaneum to expose the sinus tarsi, the subtalar joint and the calcaneocuboid joint. Capsulotomy of the calcaneocuboid joint and lateral aspect of talonavicular joint is performed through this approach. In severe cases, Bifurcate/Y ligament also needs to be released to get a complete reduction. Extensor digitorum longus (EDL) tendon with its four slips are identified and tied to form a single bundle at proximal and distal most visible part. This makes the Z lengthening easy as com-

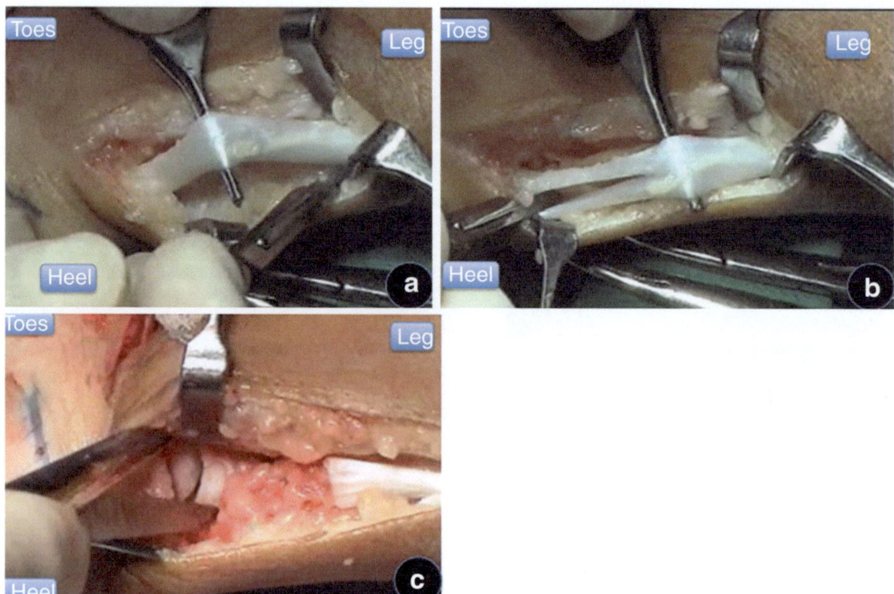

**Fig. 9.15** Postero-lateral aspect. (**a, b**) Postero-lateral incision and expose the Achilles tendon to perform Z lengthening. (**c**) Capsulotomy of posterior ankle capsule (tibio-talar)

pared to lengthening each slip individually. Two slips are cut proximally and two distally and tagged. The peroneal tendons (Peroneus Longus-PL, Peroneus Brevis-PB) are then exposed and Z lengthened. The ends are tagged for later identification. If required tenotomy of peroneus tertius is performed.

3. *Posterolateral/Posteromedial incision* (Fig. 9.15): Either of the incisions can be used as per the surgeon's preference. We prefer to use a posterolateral incision through which Z lengthening of the Achilles Tendon (AT) is performed with a lateral distal cut to correct heel valgus. Adequate care is taken to protect short saphenous vein while using the posterolateral approach. Deep dissection is performed to expose the posterior ankle and subtalar joints. Depending on the need, capsulotomy of one or both joints can be done. Depending on the age of child, a percutaneous tenotomy or a Hoke type of tenotomy can also be performed. Calcaneo-fibular ligament can be released if need arises through this same incision.

Once adequate soft tissue release is done, the talonavicular reduction is achieved under direct vision through the medial incision by elevating the talar head with a blunt dissector and plantar flexing the forefoot (Fig. 9.16). Reduction is stabilized with an antegrade wire passed from posterolateral corner of talus into the navicular. This wire is then withdrawn from anterior aspect so that the posterior tip is just visible under the cartilage of talus at the entry point at posterolateral corner. Another

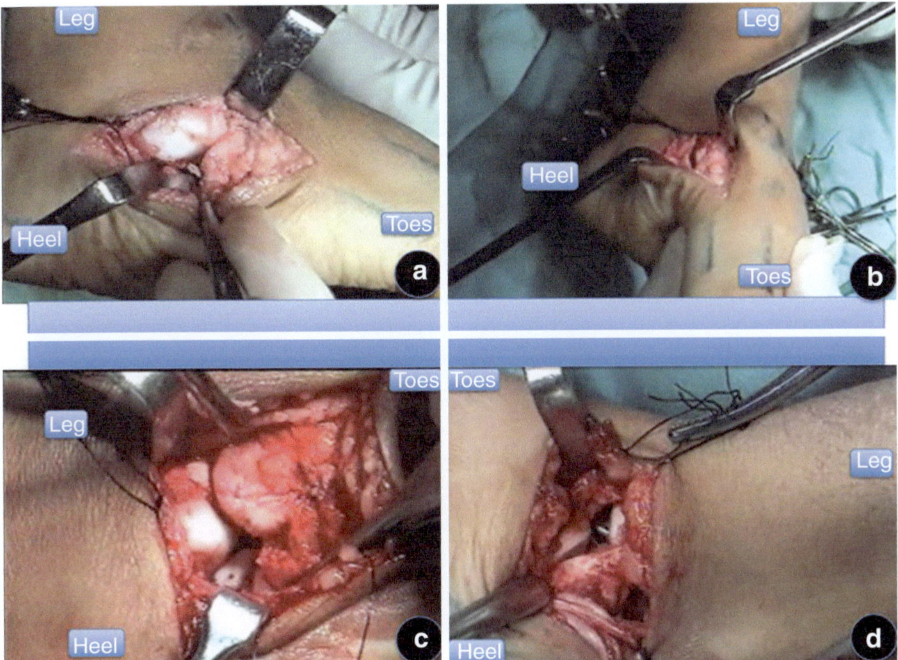


**Fig. 9.16** Medial aspect. (**a**) Reduction of TN joint with help of blunt elevator and (**b**) pressure from plantar aspect. (**c, d**) Lateral aspect: pin the TN and CC joint as described in text

wire is passed retrograde to stabilize the calcaneocuboid joint. Reduction is confirmed under IITV imaging. We do not prefer to pass the vertical wire from the calcaneus in to the talus for the fear of skin complications.

Double breasting of the capsule of talonavicular joint is done on the plantar and medial aspect to give additional support for the reduction (Fig. 9.17). After verifying the reduction, all the lengthened tendons (Tib Ant, EHL, EDL, PL, PB, AT) are repaired. Tibialis posterior is then sutured back on to the navicular with a tight repair (Figs. 9.17 and 9.18). All skin incisions are closed with a subcuticular stitch. Wires are cut and bent with the tip lying outside the skin for ease of removal later. Final check imaging is done to confirm radiologic correction (Fig. 9.19).

An above-knee cast is applied with the foot in relaxed/plantar-flexed position. The cast is changed at 1 week and brought to the neutral position. The wires are removed at the end of 6 weeks and a below-knee cast is given for 4 weeks. The patient needs to use a plastic-molded splint/ankle foot orthosis (AFO) for a period of 9 months.

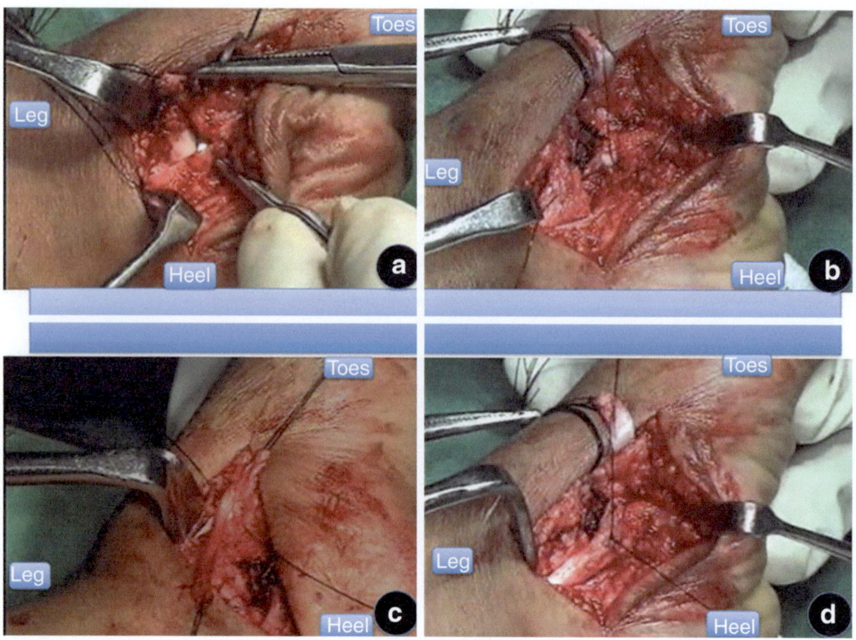



**Fig. 9.17** Medial aspect. (**a**, **b**) Closure of TN capsule and repair of (**c**) tibialis anterior, EHL and (**d**) tibialis posterior

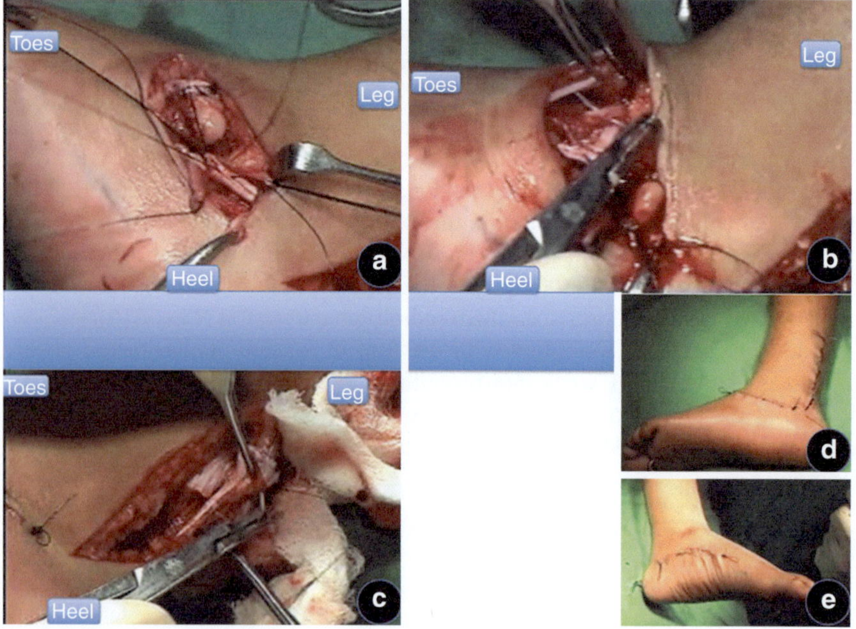



**Fig. 9.18** (**a**) Repair of peroneal tendons. (**b**) Repair of EDL. (**c**) Repair of Achilles tendon. (**d**, **e**) Final picture of scars

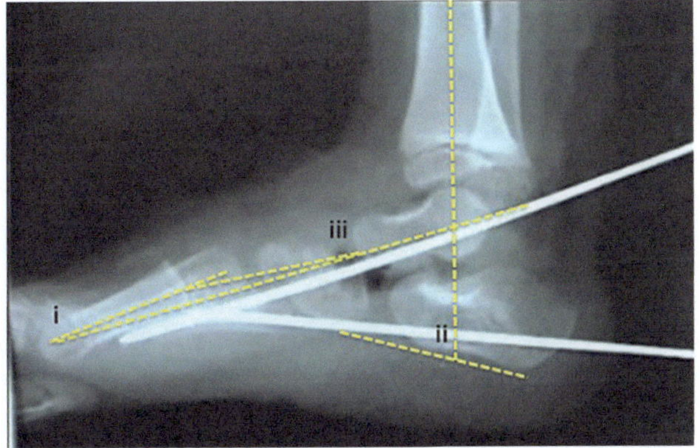

**Fig. 9.19** Restoration of (i) talus-first metatarsal angle, (ii) tibio-calcaneal angle, (iii) TAMBA

## Case Example

A newborn baby with congenital constriction band syndrome presented to our center with a grossly swollen left foot with deformities of hand and foot (Fig. 9.20). He underwent an urgent surgery for release of constriction bands on both feet as they were jeopardizing the vascularity (Fig. 9.21: left foot, Fig. 9.22: right foot). Three days postoperatively, swelling had reduced, and the wound was healing well (Fig. 9.23). At 6 months, the rocker bottom feet was clearly appreciable (Fig. 9.24). Around 4 years of age, he underwent extensive soft tissue release (Fig. 9.25). Figure 9.26 compares the preoperative and postoperative radiologic parameters, confirming an excellent correction. At 1 year (Fig. 9.27) and 3 years (Fig. 9.28) following surgery, correction is well maintained.

## *Assessment of Results*

Surgical results can be assessed by using various tools: Adelaar [29], Kodros modification of Adelaar [26], Mazzocca modification of Adelaar [24], Paediatric Outcome Data Collection Instrument (PODCI) [30], Napiontek [31], and American Orthopedic Foot and Ankle Society (AOFAS) midfoot scale [32]; Laaveg-Ponseti questionnaire was used by Duncan and Fixsen [28].

## *Complications*

### Immediate

- Compartment syndrome.
- Wound dehiscence/necrosis [11].

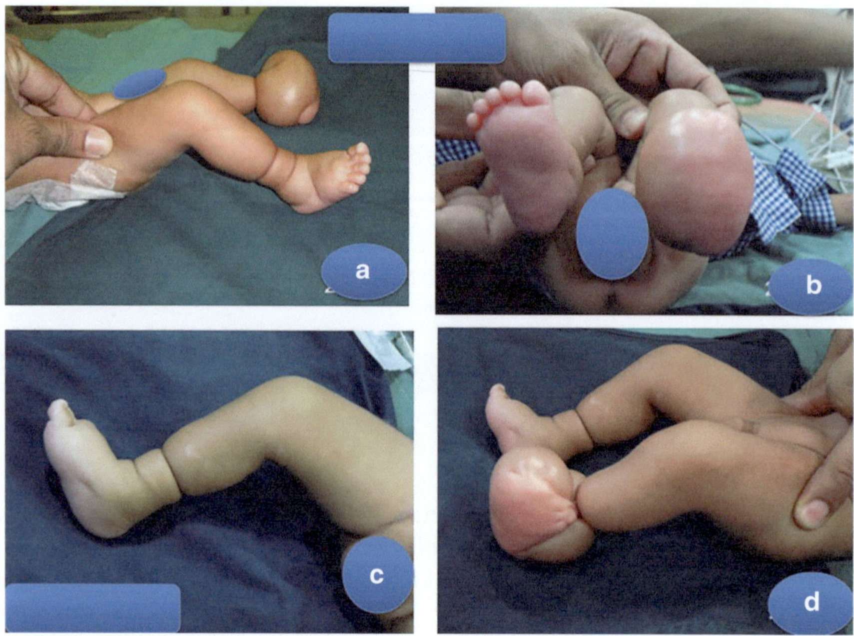

**Fig. 9.20** (**a–d**) Clinical picture of a new born with congenital constriction band syndrome. Severe lymphedema jeopardizing limb vascularity seen on the left foot. Also note adhesion of toes with the dorsum of foot

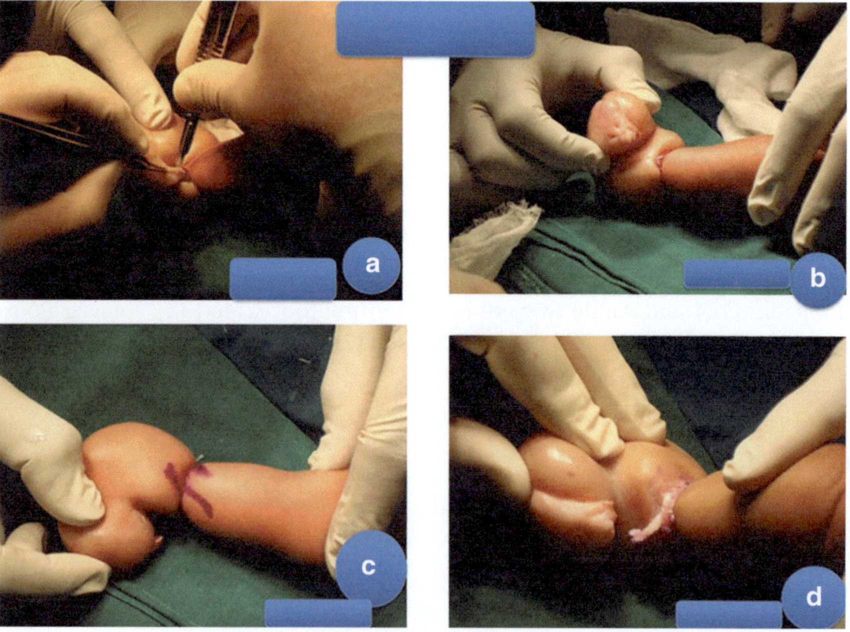

**Fig . 9.21** (**a–d**) Intra op pictures of left showing release of adhesions and Z plasty of the constriction ring. Only half of the circumference was released

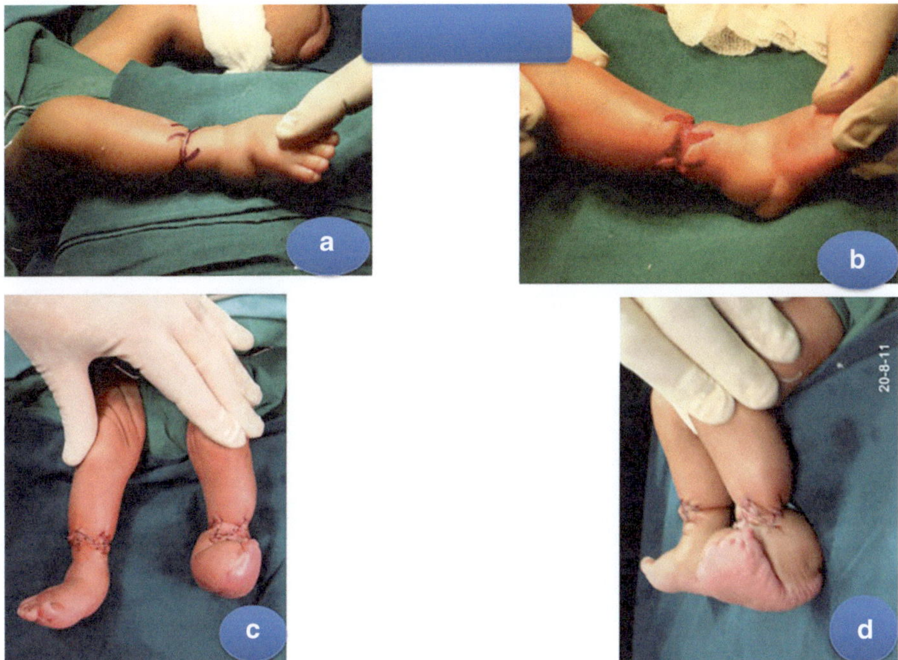

**Fig. 9.22** (**a–d**) Right foot constriction band was also released by multiple z plasties

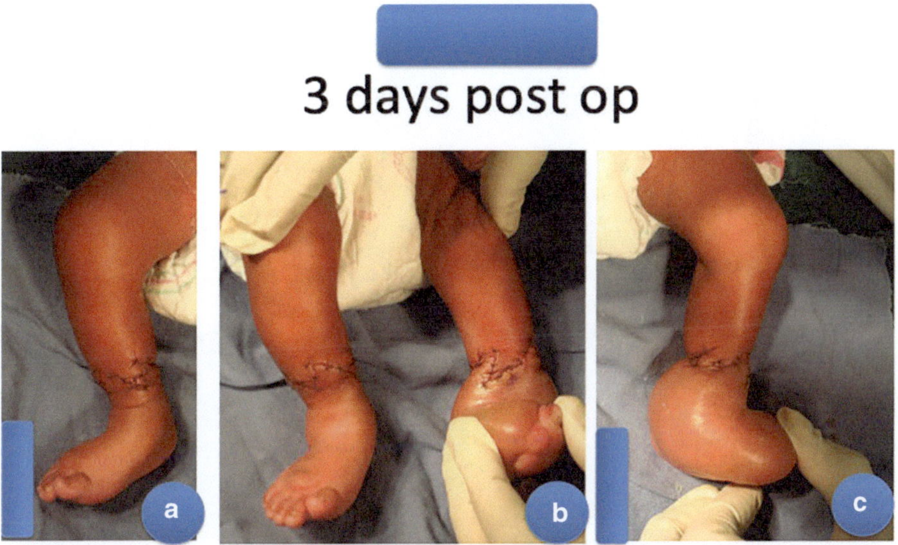


**Fig. 9.23** (**a–c**) Postoperative day 4 picture showing decreased lymphedema and good healing

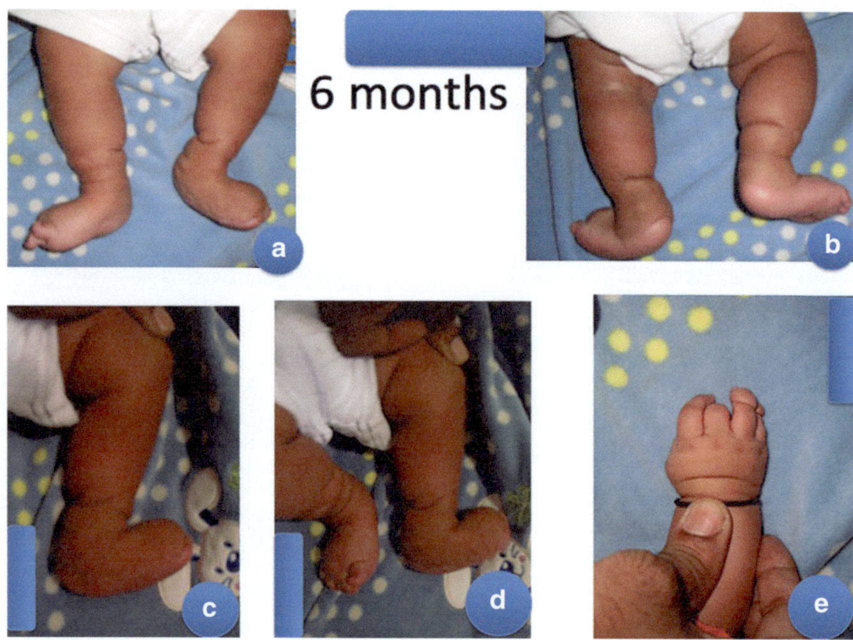



**Fig. 9.24** (**a–e**) Six months postoperative follow-up showing good healing. Rocker bottom foot clearly visible on left

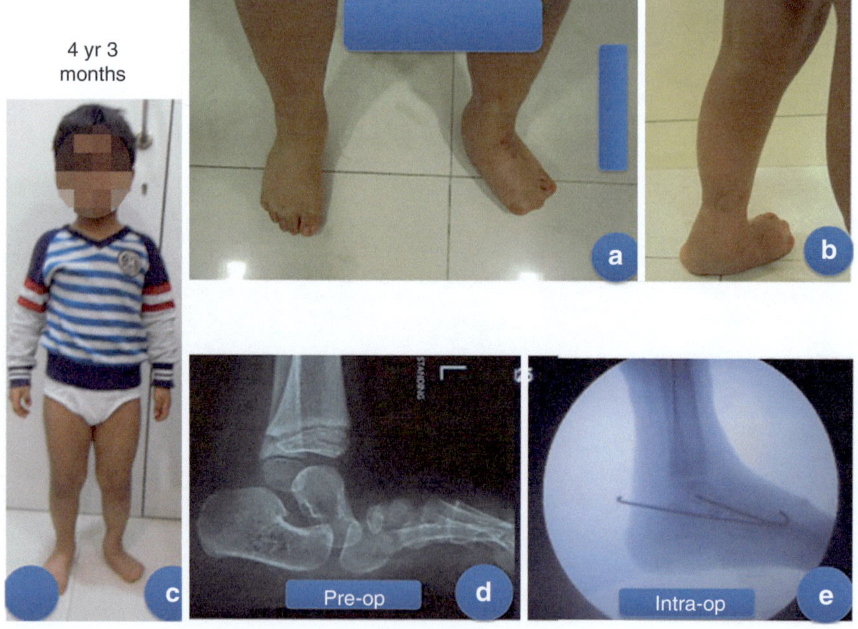



**Fig. 9.25** (**a–c**) At 4 years of age extensive soft tissue release was planned. (**d**) Preoperative X-ray showing vertical talus. (**e**) Intra-operative IITV image showing restoration of anatomy

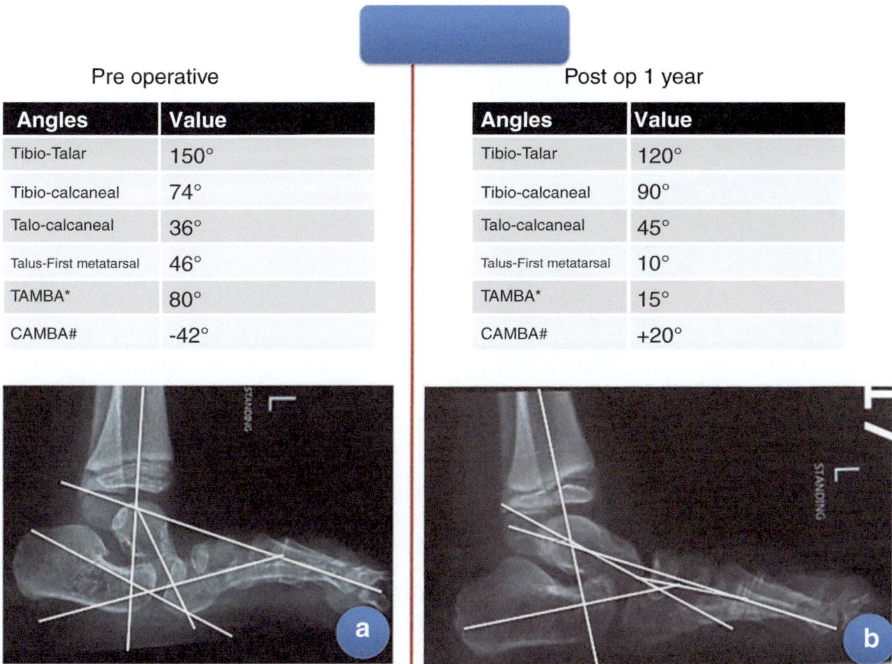



**Fig. 9.26** (**a**) Preoperative radiograph. (**b**) Postoperative radiograph

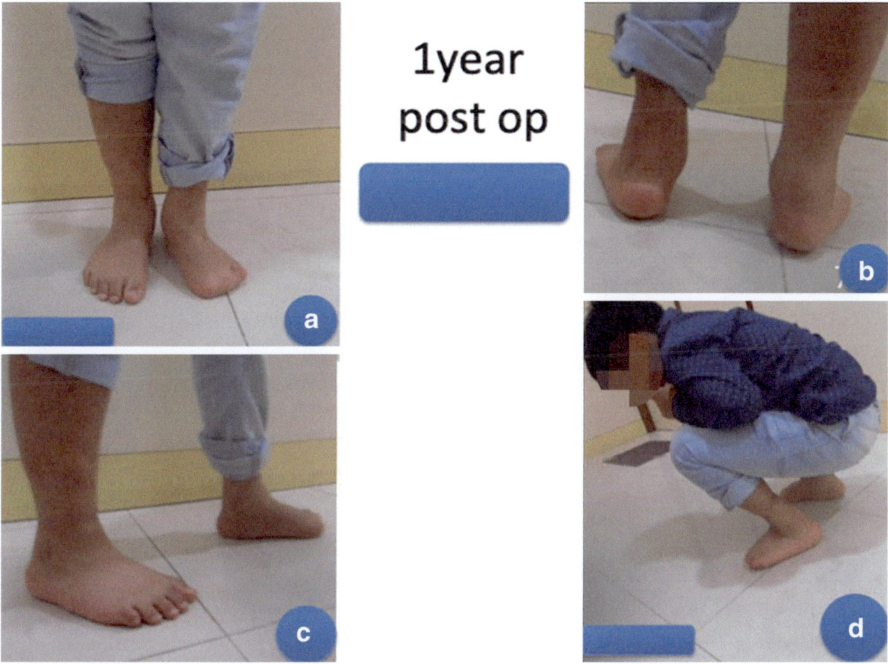



**Fig. 9.27** (**a–d**) Good functional outcome at 1 year

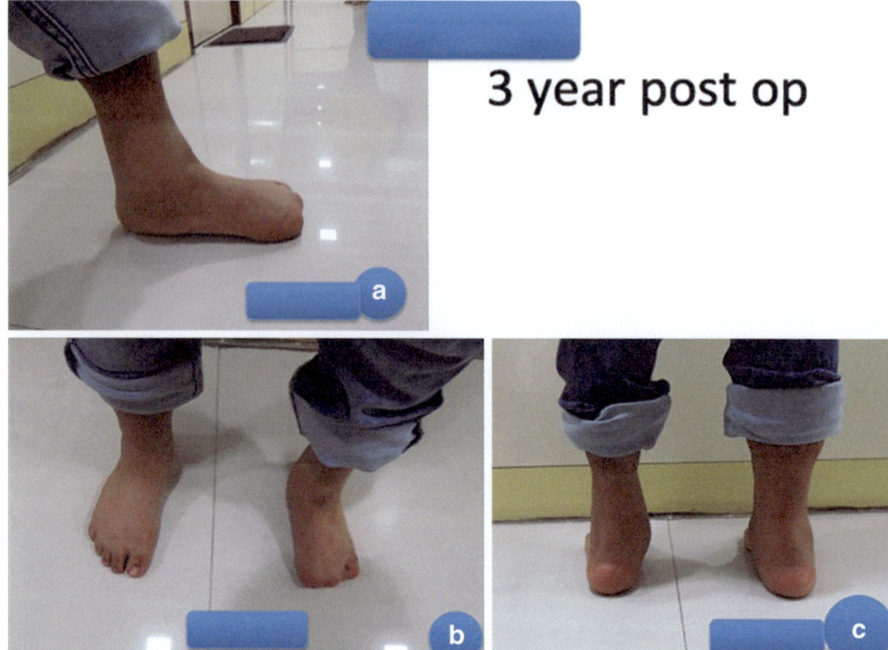



**Fig. 9.28** (**a–c**) Outcome at 3-year follow-up

**Early**

- Infection.
- Pin tract infection.


**Late**

- Under correction/residual deformities [33].
- Recurrence [11, 26, 34].
- Cavus foot [26]: unopposed action of peroneus longus in cases with Tibialis anterior transfer.
- AVN of talus: More common in staged procedures and extensive Soft tissue release (STR) but a single stage approach does have this complication as mentioned by Kodros [26], Seimon [16], Stricker [23], Mazzocca 48% [24], Napiontek 33% [22].
- Stiffness [2, 35–37].
- Arthritis [22] 91%.
- Repeat surgery [22, 24, 27].
- Amputation [38].
- Pseudarthrosis [3].
- Triceps insufficiency.

## *Minimal Invasive Surgery Versus Extensive Release*

Historically minimal invasive procedures have been attempted but failed [4, 39, 40] until Seimon [16] published his results on 10 feet treated by only dorsal release and talonavicular pinning. Achilles tenotomy was performed by percutaneous technique.

Dobbs [18] in 2006 reported his results of a novel minimal invasive technique wherein he applied serial casts followed by a medial approach to achieve talonavicular reduction and pinning followed by a percutaneous Achilles tenotomy. Other authors report good results using his technique [41–43].

Yang and Dobbs [30] compared the minimal invasive technique (24 ft) with the extensive soft tissue release (18 ft). Feet treated with minimal invasive technique had similar radiographic outcome with better long-term ankle range of motion, pain scores, and PODCI normative global function scores.

Chalayon [41] reported few modifications in the original Dobbs technique. A gentle dorsal and lateral pressure was exerted on the plantar aspect of talar head as the foot is brought in to progressively greater plantar flexion and adduction. The laterally directed force corrects the talocalcaneal angle seen on anteroposterior view in addition to the dorsal force that corrects the vertical position of talus. Another modification is the use of a double-ended K wire as a joystick to correct the talus in both anteroposterior and lateral planes. Other modifications are that of use of a bar brace (with specific protocol) and stretching exercises to maintain ankle and foot mobility.

According to the authors, all patients presenting with CVT should undergo serial casting irrespective of severity of deformity. If adequate correction is seen on stress views as objectively measured by Talus first metatarsal angle and TAMBA, minimal invasive surgery should be planned. If the reduction is not satisfactory, extensive soft tissue release should be done.

# References


1. Mckie J, Radomisli T. Congenital vertical talus: a review. Clin Podiatr Med Surg. 2020;27(1):145–56.
2. Zorer G, Bagatur AE, Dogan A. Single stage surgical correction of congenital vertical talus by complete subtalar release and peritalar reduction by using the Cincinnati incision. J Pediatr Orthop Part B. 2002;11(1):60–7.
3. Dodge L, Ashley R, Gilbert RJ. Treatment of the congenital vertical talus: a retrospective review of 36 feet with long-term follow- up. Foot Ankle. 1987;7:326–32.
4. Lloyd-Roberts GC, Spence AJ. Congenital vertical talus. J Bone Joint Surg B. 1958;40(1):33–41.
5. Lamy L, Weissman L. Congenital convex pes planus. J Bone Joint Surg. 1939;21:79–91.
6. Stone KH, Lloyd-Roberts CG. Congenital vertical talus: a new operation. Proc R Soc Med. 1963;56:12–4.
7. Herndon CH, Heyman CH. Problems in the recognition and treatment of congenital pes valgus. J Bone Joint Surg Am. 1963;45:413–29.
8. Ellis J, Scheer G. Congenital convex pes valgus. Clin Orthop. 1974;99:168–74.
9. Walker A, Ghali N, Silk F. Congenital vertical talus. J Bone Joint Surg Am. 1985;67:117–21.

10. Coleman SS, Stelling FH III, Jarrett J. Pathomechanicsand treatment of congenital vertical talus. Clin Orthop Relat Res. 1970;70:62–72.
11. Jacobson S, Crawford A, Jacobson ST. Congenital vertical talus. J Pediatr Orthop. 1983;3:306–10.
12. Ogata K, Schoenecker PL, Sheridan J. Congenital vertical talus and its familial occurrence: an analysis of 36 patients. Clin Orthop Relat Res. 1979;139:128–32.
13. Osmond-Clarke H. Congenital vertical talus. J Bone Joint Surg B. 1956;38(1):334–41.
14. DeRosa G, Ahlfeld S. Congenital vertical talus: the Riley experience. Foot Ankle. 1984;5:118–24.
15. Fitton J, Nevelos A. The treatment of congenital vertical talus. J Bone Joint Surg Br. 1979;61:481–3.
16. Seimon LP. Surgical correction of congenital vertical talus. J Pediatr Orthop. 1987;7(4):405–11.
17. Schrader L, Gilbert R, Skinner S, Ashley RK. Congenital vertical talus: surgical correction by a one-stage medial approach. Orthopaedics. 1990;13:1233–6.
18. Dobbs MB, Purcell DB, Nunley RMJ. Early results of a new method of treatment for idiopathic congenital vertical talus. J Bone Joint Surg Am. 2006;88(6):1192–200.
19. Patterson W, Fitz D, Smith W. The pathologic anatomy of congenital pes valgus: post mortem study of a newborn infant with bilateral involvement. J Bone Joint Surg. 1968;50:458–66.
20. Drennan JCS, Sharrard WJW. The pathological anatomy of convex pes valgus. J Bone Joint Surg. 1971;53:455–61.
21. Hamanishi C. Congenital vertical talus: classification with 69 cases and new measurement system. J Pediatr Orthop. 1984;4:318–26.
22. Napiontek M. Congenital vertical talus: a retrospective and critical review of 32 feet operated on by peritalar reduction. J Pediatr Orthop Part B. 1995;4:179–87.
23. Stricker SJ, Rosen E. Early one-stage reconstruction of congenital vertical talus. Foot Ankle Int. 1997;18(9):535–43.
24. Mazzocca AD, Thomson JD, Deluca PA, Romness MJ. Comparison of the posterior approach versus the dorsal approach in the treatment of congenital vertical talus. J Pediatr Orthop. 2001;21(2):212–7.
25. Crawford AH, Marten JL, Osterfeld DL. The Cincinnati incision: a comprehensive approach for surgical procedures of the foot and ankle in childhood. J Bone Joint Surg Am. 1982;64:1355–88.
26. Kodros SA, Luciano S. Single-stage surgical correction of congenital vertical talus summary. J Pediatr Orthop. 1999;19:42–8.
27. Ramanoudjame M, Loriaut P, Seringe R, Glorion C, Wicart P. The surgical treatment of children with congenital convex foot (vertical talus) evaluation of midtarsal surgical release and open reduction. Bone Joint J. 2014;96(6):837–44.
28. Duncan RD, Fixsen JA. Congenital convex pes valgus. J Bone Joint Surg. 1999;81(2):250–4.
29. Adelaar R, Williams R, Gould JD. Congenital convex pes valgus: results of an early comprehensive release and review of congenital vertical talus at Richmond Crippled Children's Hospital and the University of Alabama in Birmingham. Foot Ankle. 1980;1:62–3.
30. Yang J, Dobbs M. Treatment of congenital vertical talus: comparison. J Bone Joint Surg Am. 2015;97:1354–65.
31. Napiontek M. Value of peritalar reduction in surgical treatment on congenital vertical talus (pes planovalgus taloflexus congenitus) [Thesis]. Poznan: Karol Marcinkowski University of Medical Sciences; 1998.
32. Kitaoka HB, Alexander IJ, Adelaar RS, et al. Clinical rating systems for the ankle-hindfoot, midfoot, hallux and lesser toes. Foot Ankle Int. 1994;15:349–53.
33. Coleman SS, Stelling FH, Jarrett J. Pathomechanics and treatment of congenital vertical talus. Clin Orthop Relat Res. 1970;70:62–72.
34. Lichtblau S. Congenital vertical talus. Bull Hosp Joint Dis. 1978;39:165–79.
35. Harrold A. Congenital vertical talus in infancy. J Bone Joint Surg. 1967;49:634–43.
36. Harrold A. The problem of congenital vertical talus in infancy. Clin Orthop. 1973;97:133–43.

37. Connolly J, Dornenburg P, Holmes C. In: Bateman JE, editor. Congenital convex pes valgus. Foot scien. Philadelphia: WB Saunders Company; 1976. p. 47–66.
38. Hootnick DR, Dutch WM, Crider RJ. Ischemic necrosis leading to amputation following surgical correction of congenital vertical talus. Am J Orthop (Belle Mead NJ). 2005;34(1):35–7.
39. Eyre-Brook AL. Congenital vertical talus. J Bone Joint Surg Br. 1967;49(4):618–27.
40. Hark F. Rocker-foot due to congenital subluxation of the talus. J Bone Joint Surg Am. 1950;32:344.
41. Chalayon O, Adams A, Dobbs MB. Minimally invasive approach for the treatment of non-isolated congenital vertical talus. J Bone Joint Surg Am. 2012;94(11):e73.
42. Bhaskar A. Congenital vertical talus: treatment by reverse Ponseti technique. Indian J Orthop. 2008;42(3):347–50.
43. Eberhardt O, Wirth T, Fernandez F. Minimally invasive treatment of congenital foot deformities in infants: new findings and midterm-results. Orthopade. 2013;42(12):1001–7.

# Chapter 10
# Congenital Vertical Talus (Congenital Convex Pes Valgus)

Mitzi L. Williams and Matthew B. Dobbs

## Introduction

Much like talipes equinovarus (clubfoot) congenital vertical talus (CVT) has undergone an incredible paradigm shift in treatment. Prior to the Dobbs Method, children who presented with CVT underwent large grandiose incisions and surgical releases in the absence of any serial casting. There was often no attempt at serial casting or manipulation for this complex deformity. The deformity was thought to be irreducible without surgery. Children presented with various degrees of rigidity, angulation, and at times spasticity often in the setting of secondary neurologic conditions. An influx of children with CVT sought the expertise of Matthew Dobbs, MD because of genetic studies, and in 2006, the Dobbs Method was published [1]. This less invasive approach focuses on a dorsolateral thrust upon the medial talar head and relocation of the talonavicular joint [1–4]. It remains key to scrutinize reduction in all planes. The foot is stretched serially into a maximal equinovarus position. Essentially, the final cast should mimic a clubfoot position. Following four weekly casts, children undergo a surgical tenotomy of the Achilles tendon and pinning of the talonavicular joint. A fifth cast is then applied keeping the foot in a neutral position. Variations of this approach will be described for children presenting with neurologic conditions and incredible rigidity. Functional outcome scores and maintenance of alignment is noted to be good [4] (Fig. 10.1).

M. L. Williams (✉)
Podiatric Surgery/Orthopedics, Kaiser Permanente Oakland Medical Center,
Oakland, CA, USA
e-mail: mitzi.l.williams@kp.org

M. B. Dobbs
Paley Institute, St. Mary's Medical Center, West Palm Beach, FL, USA
e-mail: mdobbs@paleyinstitute.org



M. B. Dobbs et al. (eds.), *Clubfoot and Vertical Talus*,
https://doi.org/10.1007/978-3-031-34788-7_10

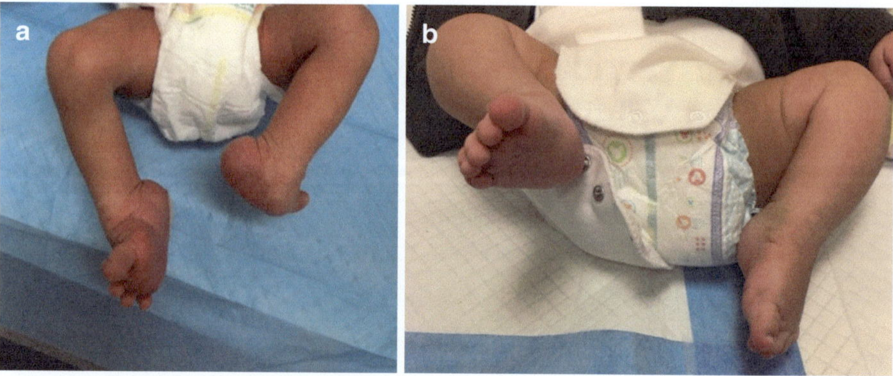

**Fig. 10.1** (**a**) Infant with right-sided clubfoot and left-sided vertical talus. (**b**) Post-Ponseti casting and manipulation right and Dobbs method left

## Etiology

In infancy, this rare deformity often resembles calcaneovalgus or a severe planovalgus foot type. Although the exact incidence of vertical talus is unknown, the estimated prevalence is 1 in 10,000 live births [5]. Due to the hindfoot valgus, equinus, and fixed dorsal dislocation of the navicular on the talus, many have referred to this deformity as a rocker-bottom flatfoot. Despite these findings, it is the rigidity of the deformity and true equinus that distinguishes itself from others such as positional calcaneovalgus or oblique talus. A true congenital vertical talus is generally not easily reduced nor passively corrected. The condition is defined by its inability to reduce, or in essence rigidity, along with equinus. Recognition of this deformity is key, as without treatment vertical talus can lead to significant disability with growth and persistence [3] (Fig. 10.2).

CVT is often diagnosed as clubfoot or classified as a positional foot anomaly by some physicians at birth. Without treatment, vertical talus can lead to pain and disability that hampers daily activities. This foot position can also place some children at greater risk for ulceration or a nonbraceable foot. Traditional surgical management for vertical talus is invasive and fraught with both short-term and long-term complications. These complications include both undercorrection and overcorrection of the deformity, scarring, neurovascular injury, infection, wound dehiscence, and the need for multiple surgical procedures during growth. The scar tissue created with extensive soft tissue releases in a child's foot can lead to both stiffness and pain much like the surgical clubfoot aftermath. A less invasive alternative, the Dobbs method, has proved successful in providing correction while avoiding the need for extensive soft tissue release procedures in many children.

In most cases, the etiology of vertical talus deformity remains unknown. Approximately one half of cases of vertical talus occur in conjunction with neurologic disorders [6] or genetic defects [7]. The remaining children present with further congenital anomalies and are considered idiopathic or isolated cases [3]. The most common neurologic disorders associated with vertical talus are distal

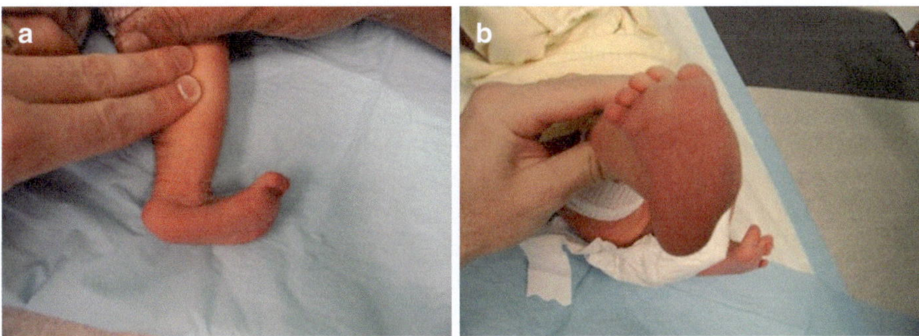

**Fig. 10.2** (**a**, **b**) Infant with vertical talus

arthrogryposis and myelomeningocele [6]. The most common genetic defects include aneuploidy of chromosomes 13, 15, and 18 [8]. Genetic research has gained insight into pathogenesis with the discovery of mutations in the PITX1-TBX4-HOXC transcriptional pathways and their influence in familial clubfoot and vertical talus in a small number of families [9–11]. Subsequent studies continue to be performed [12]. Finally, of the 50% of cases of vertical talus that are isolated, almost 20% have a positive family history of vertical talus (Table 10.1).

**Table 10.1** Etiologies of congenital vertical talus

| *Central nervous system/spinal cord* |
| --- |
| Myelomeningocele |
| Spinal muscular atrophy |
| Diastematomyelia |
| Sacral agenesis |
| *Muscle* |
| Distal arthrogryposis |
| Arthrogryposis multiplex |
| Neurofibromatosis |
| *Chromosomal abnormality* |
| Trisomy 18 |
| Trisomy 15 |
| Trisomy 13 |
| *Genetic syndromes* |
| Neurofibromatosis |
| Prune-Belly syndrome |
| Rasmussen syndrome |
| Split hand and split foot |
| Costello syndrome |
| De Barsy syndrome |
| *Single-gene defects* |
| HOXD10 |
| CDMP1 |

In most of the isolated cases, the condition is inherited in an autosomal dominant fashion [11]. This supports that a significant number of isolated cases have a genetic etiology [13]. Still, while no one single-gene defect has been held accountable of all cases of vertical talus, its etiology is heterogeneous [13]. For example, in patients with myelomeningocele, a weak posterior tibialis muscle with strong ankle dorsi-flexors could contribute to the deformity. Weakness of the foot intrinsics may play a role for other children with neurologic influence. Children with abnormal muscle biopsies such as arthrogryposis may be prone to vertical talus given skeletal muscle abnormalities [7]. Congenital vascular insufficiency of the lower extremities has also been proposed as a potential cause of vertical talus based on magnetic reso-nance angiography findings that demonstrated congenital arterial deficiencies of the lower extremity in a group of patients with vertical talus [14]. Beyond its etiology, early detection is helpful in reduction of deformity and overall outcomes. Correction prior to the age of 12 months is thought to improve functional outcome scores [4].

## Pathoanatomy: Congenital Vertical Talus Deformity

The hindfoot is in equinus and valgus because of contracture of the Achilles tendon, posterolateral ankle, and subtalar joint capsules. The midfoot and forefoot are dor-siflexed and abducted secondary to contractures of the tibialis anterior, extensors, peroneus tertius and brevis, and the dorsolateral aspect of the talonavicular capsule. The navicular is dorsally and laterally dislocated on the head of the talus, resulting in the development of a hypoplastic and wedge-shaped navicular. Both the talar head and the neck are abnormal in shape and orientation. The position of the talus stretches vertically and weakens the plantar soft tissues, including the spring liga-ment, giving the foot a rocker-bottom appearance. The rigid equinus in the hindfoot is often accompanied by either dorsolateral subluxation or frank dorsal dislocation of the calcaneocuboid joint. The posterior tibial tendon and the peroneus longus and brevis are commonly subluxated anteriorly over the medial and lateral malleolus, respectively; the subluxated tendons then function as ankle dorsiflexors rather than plantarflexors (Fig. 10.3).

## *Clinical Features*

Hindfoot equinus, hindfoot valgus, forefoot abduction, and forefoot dorsiflexion are present in all patients with vertical talus. The rigidity of the deformities is the key to differentiating vertical talus from the more common and less severe conditions, such as calcaneovalgus foot, posteromedial bowing of the tibia, and oblique talus (without an equinus contracture). A quick and easy clinical exam finding is testing for tendo-Achilles contracture. This must be done with the subtalar joint inverted. If ankle dorsiflexion is not limited, then the deformity does not meet vertical talus

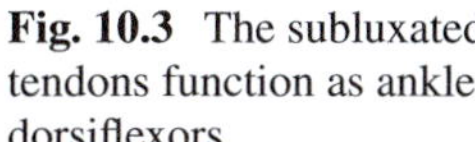

**Fig. 10.3** The subluxated tendons function as ankle dorsiflexors

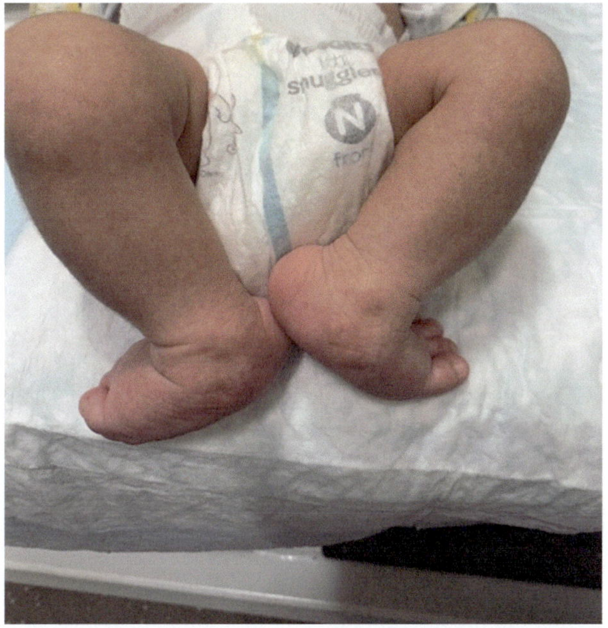

criteria. Because of the frequency of neuromuscular and genetic abnormalities associated with vertical talus, it is important to perform a complete and careful physical examination of the entire patient. The clinician should look for facial dysmorphic features that require a referral to a clinical geneticist or abnormalities suggestive of a neuromuscular etiology, which would require MRI evaluation of the neuroaxis and referral to a pediatric neurologist. The presence of a sacral dimple should alert the examiner to possible central nervous system anomalies.

It is of utmost importance for the examiner to document the ability of the child to dorsiflex and plantarflex the toes. This is done by stimulating the plantar and dorsal aspects of the foot. This should be done on multiple occasions during the early treatment stage because the examination can be difficult, and results from serial examinations are more accurate. The presence of dorsiflexion and plantarflexion of the toes is recorded as absent, slight/subtle, or definitive. This should be recorded for the great toe alone and the lesser toes as a separate group. In our experience, slight or absent ability to move the toes with stimulation correlates with a vertical talus deformity that is more rigid and less responsive to treatment. It may also be indicative of a congenital neurologic or muscular anomaly.

Clinically, a congenital vertical talus foot has a convex plantar surface that results in a rocker-bottom appearance. The skin on the dorsum of the foot has a crease secondary to forefoot and midfoot dorsiflexion. The extreme dorsiflexion of the forefoot creates a gap dorsally where the navicular and talar head would articulate in a normal foot. If the gap reduces with plantar flexion of the forefoot, then the deformity has a degree of flexibility and may fall on the spectrum of oblique talus. This is important to assess because even if the talonavicular joint reduces in plantarflexion indicating an oblique talus, this does not mean that treatment is not needed. In this situation, the examiner must then assess for contracture of the Achilles tendon with the subtalar joint inverted. In our experience, oblique tali in the setting of a contracture of the Achilles tendon needs treatment just like true vertical tali.

## *Imaging*

While X-rays are not indicated routinely in the management of clubfoot, they are useful in the diagnosis of vertical talus. The obliquity of the talus is apparent on X-rays and is almost in line with the longitudinal axis of the tibia in the sagittal plane. A stress plantarflexion lateral radiograph demonstrates the navicular remains dorsally dislocated upon the talar head in vertical talus. It is important to remember that the navicular does not ossify until 2.5–5 years of age. Hence, in vertical talus, the longitudinal axis of the talus fails to align with the longitudinal axis of the first metatarsal in a lateral radiograph when manually plantarflexed. The talus remains vertical as compared to the first metatarsal. On the lateral view of the foot in plantarflexion, the lateral talar axis-first metatarsal base angle (TAMBA) can be used as one criterion to help distinguish vertical talus from oblique talus. Values greater than 35 degrees have been considered diagnostic for vertical talus [15]. However, vertical talus cannot be ruled out with values less than 35°. In such cases, the presence of or absence of hindfoot equinus must be documented to distinguish between vertical talus and oblique talus. It can be difficult to differentiate those oblique tali that need treatment from those that do not based on radiographs alone. In oblique tali, the talonavicular joint reduces in plantarflexion, but this does not necessarily mean treatment is not needed. In these situations, a careful clinical exam must be done to test for the presence or absence of hindfoot equinus by dorsiflexing the ankle with the subtalar joint inverted. If equinus is present, then the deformity benefits from treatment in the same manner as vertical talus. Left alone the oblique tali with tight tendo Achilles often present in adolescence as symptomatic flatfeet with short Achilles tendon (Fig. 10.4).

---

Vertical talus imaging

---

- *Stress plantarflexion X-ray (standard of care)*: In vertical talus the talus fails to align with the first metatarsal. The talus remains vertical when compared to the first metatarsal. In infancy, the navicular is not visible. One focuses on the talus with respect to the first metatarsal. An oblique talus or calcaneovalgus will realign or essentially reduce
- *Neutral lateral X-ray:* in vertical talus the long axis of the talus is vertical when compared to the first metatarsal. The calcaneus is in equinus
- *Stress dorsiflexion X-ray*: Persistent rigid hindfoot equinus is noted with vertical talus

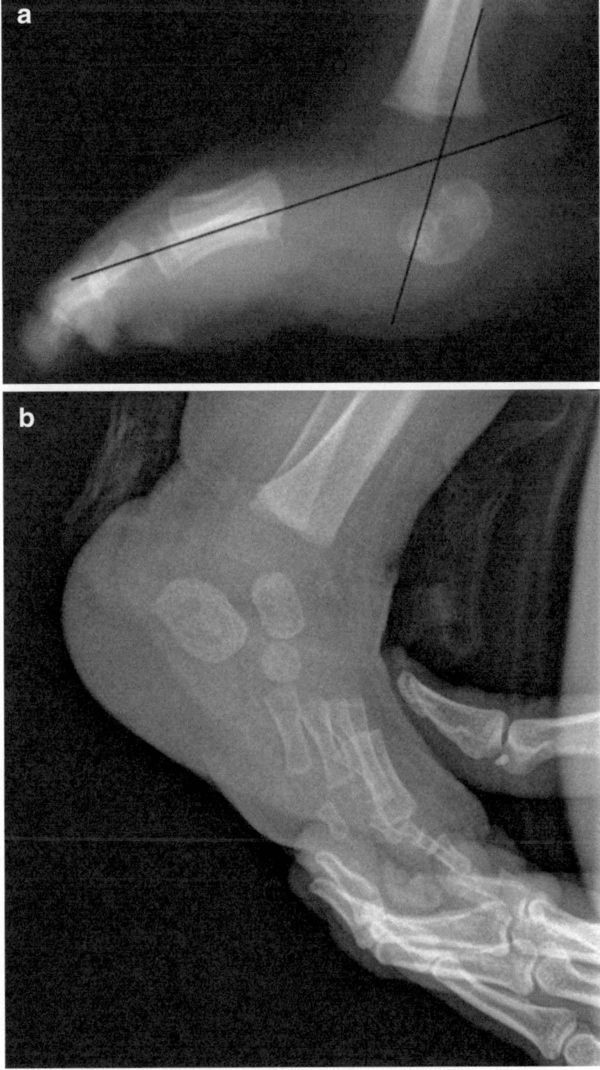

**Fig. 10.4** (**a**) Stress plantarflexion radiograph consistent with vertical talus. (**b**) This lateral radiograph demonstrates the talus aligns well with the first metatarsal excluding vertical talus

## *Classification*

Current classification systems for vertical talus are purely descriptive and not prognostic in nature. The problem with this is that it does not have a dynamic component to account for motor strength in the lower legs. In our experience, weak or absent motor function in the lower leg musculature is predictive of not only poor response to initial treatment but also a risk of relapse. The child's ability to dorsiflex and plantarflex the toes can be evaluated by lightly stimulating the dorsal and plantar aspects of the foot. Movement can be graded as definitive, slight, or absent. This simple examination can be repeated at each clinical visit to improve accuracy. A new classification system that takes this into account is needed because the ability to better predict the response to treatment will allow for the development of an individualized treatment program for patients.

It should also be noted that current classification systems have attempted to define oblique talus as a milder form of vertical talus based on radiographic and clinical examination criteria. However, these attempts at classification have not translated into consistent treatment recommendations because some oblique tali in the setting of equinus do require treatment. In our experience, oblique tali that have an associated Achilles tendon contracture are at risk of becoming symptomatic with time. For this reason, we consider oblique tali and vertical tali to be related entities that occur along a spectrum of severity.

While vertical talus is nonreducible requiring serial casting to manipulate the foot into an improved position, calcaneovalgus remains flexible in nature. Goals of relocating the talonavicular joint and alleviating equinus are key. Over the years many methods of surgical treatment have been discussed while the basic principles of reduction remain the same. The talonavicular dislocation must be reduced and stabilized. The hindfoot equinus must be alleviated to restore a normal talocalcaneal relationship. Lastly, the forefoot which is everted and in calcaneus should be corrected and stabilized upon a corrected hindfoot.

## The Dobbs Method

As Ignacio Ponseti, MD pioneered the method for serial casting and deformity correction for clubfoot without aggressive surgical releases; Matthew B Dobbs, MD has done the same for the treatment of vertical talus. Historically, large releases for this deformity were performed with persistent risks of stiffness, diminished function, and pain. The Dobbs method is a less invasive approach that relies on serial manipulation and casting. Achieving correction without extensive surgery leads to more functional and flexible feet [7]. With the retracting fibrosis and abundance of collagen that forms, it is advantageous to avoid large releases at an early age and approach reduction from a less invasive standpoint. While most of the deformity correction is the result of manipulation and casting, the child does undergo at least an Achilles tenotomy and talonavicular joint pinning upon reduction (Fig. 10.5).

Following tenotomy and talonavicular pinning, the foot is casted and monitored closely over the next 6 weeks following surgery. The wire is then removed, and the child transitions to a boot and bar brace. The foot is held in a straight position. Boot

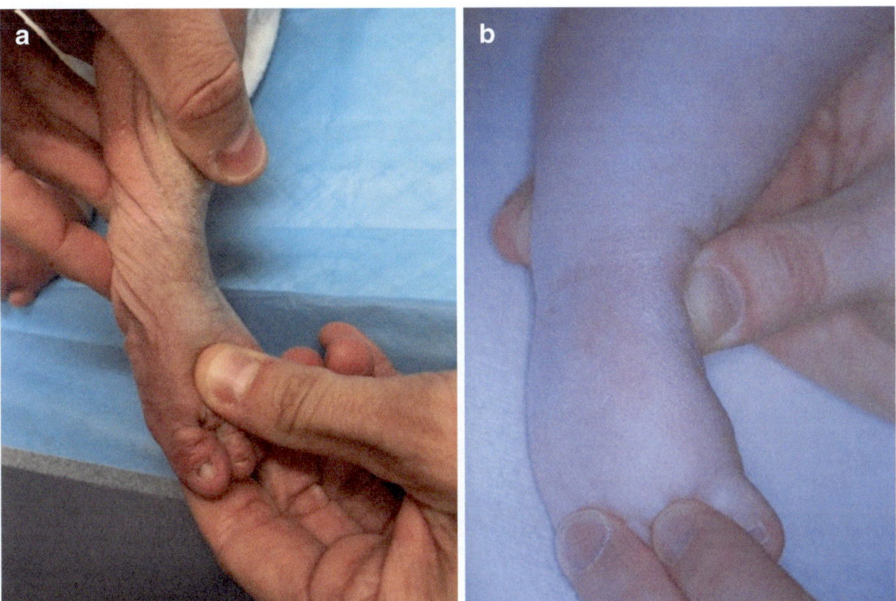

**Fig. 10.5** (**a**) The Dobbs method clinically. (**b**) The Dobbs method demonstrating plantarflexion and inversion with counterpressure on head of the talus

and bar braces are utilized until the child is 2 years of age. The authors use the Easy Click bar, designed by Matthew Dobbs, MD, as there is no dorsiflexion bend in it unlike the other bars. It is important not to brace in dorsiflexion, as the feet are most tight dorsolateral. Since the introduction of the Dobbs Method in 2006 [1], many subsequent studies have demonstrated its efficacy in achieving initial correction in patients with isolated or nonisolated vertical talus [16–23]. The authors lean toward custom ankle foot orthoses that plantar flex and adduct following the boot and bar system until the age of four.

Traditional management involved lengthening the contracted dorsolateral tendons and dorsolateral capsular contractures and reducing both the talonavicular joint and the subtalar joint. Lengthening both the Achilles and the peroneals along with performing a posterolateral capsulotomy followed [24]. Many performed all procedures in a single-stage approach [25–30]. Extensive surgical release is not necessary for most cases of vertical talus, as good results have been achieved with the Dobbs Method [3]. At times other structures do need to be released to obtain full correction.

To perform this manipulation, the treating provider must have knowledge of the subtalar joint and experience in treating clubfoot with manipulation and casting. The ability to accurately locate the talar head is essential. All components of the deformity are corrected simultaneously except for the hindfoot equinus, which is corrected with release of the Achilles in the operating room (Figs. 10.6 and 10.7).

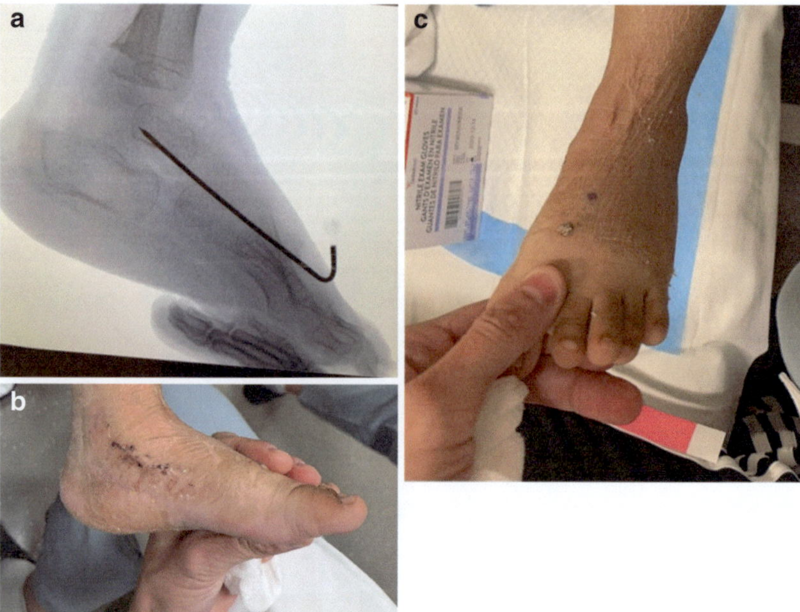

**Fig. 10.6** (**a**) Vertical talus pinning. (**b, c**) post vertical talus pin removal

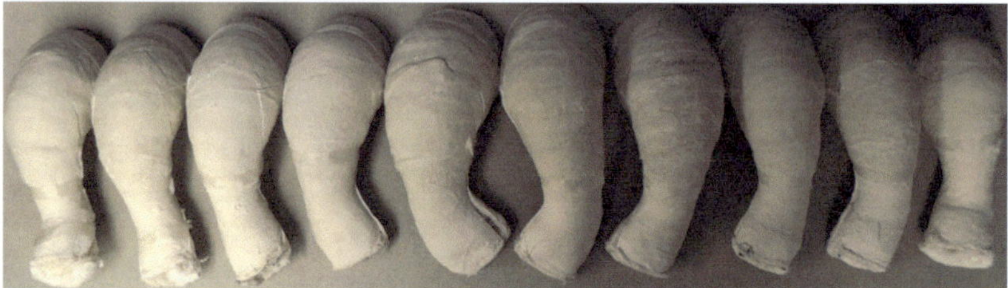

**Fig. 10.7** The Dobbs method casting with final casts in maximum equinovarus

---

Dobbs method for manipulation and casting

- Manipulations are gentle and consist of stretching the foot into plantarflexion with one hand while counterpressure is applied as the thumb of the opposite hand gently pushes the talus dorsally and laterally (from the medial side of foot)
- Do not touch the calcaneus. The calcaneus needs to glide smoothly beneath the talus from its valgus position
- After 1–2 min of manipulation, a long-leg plaster cast is applied to hold the foot into this manipulated position. The cast is applied in two sections, with the short leg portion applied first. This allows for an appropriate mold of the foot
- The foot should be held in position achieved by stretching while an assistant rolls the plaster
- Mold carefully around the talar head, malleoli, and above the calcaneus posteriorly
- Remove excess plaster dorsally to expose the toes
- The cast is then extended above the knee with knee in 90° of flexion
- Weekly casting is advised. An average of five casts is utilized to reduce the deformity. Hindfoot equinus still persists. In the fourth cast, the foot resembles a clubfoot. It is critical to achieve a maximal equinovarus position. This is analogous to achieving 70 degrees of external rotation in a final clubfoot cast
- When reduction of the talonavicular and calcaneocuboid joints is achieved, the child is scheduled for surgery

| Surgical steps: the Dobbs method |
| --- |

- Serial manipulation and casting is performed to improve the talonavicular and hindfoot alignment as described in the Dobbs Method for manipulation and casting
- Surgery is performed in the operating room with full intention of performing a percutaneous Achilles tenotomy and talonavicular joint pinning. In the older ambulatory child, a Hoke procedure can be performed
- A complete Achilles tenotomy is performed. When performed first, this allows for the surgeon to fully stretch the posterior joint capsules. This stretch is maintained for a few minutes prior to any pinning
- When reduction of the medial column is achieved, a small dorsal medial incision is fashioned over the talonavicular joint. The surgeon confirms reduction of talonavicular joint. As the surgeon becomes more familiar with casting and manipulation, this incision may not be needed any further
- If the joint is not completely reduced, a small capsulotomy is made in the talonavicular region to allow an elevator to be placed and visualize the alignment of small cartilaginous structures. At times, some children with syndromes and or neurologic influence may require a vertical incision between the extensor hallucis longus tendon and extensor digitorum longus tendon to perform a sequential release. From this approach, it is an a la carte release of the: talonavicular joint, anterior subtalar joint, peroneus tertius, and the peroneus longus and brevis tendons. One may need to release the calcaneocuboid and tarsometatarsal joints. The extensors may be released in children with functional deficit
- A K-wire is placed from distal to proximal across the talonavicular joint. Central positioning of the 0.062 k wire in younger children and 2.0 pin in older children is utilized
- The pin is distally inserted between the first and the second metatarsal to capture the first metatarsal base, cuneiform, navicular, and talus. One's hand must be dropped down to capture these structures
- The pin is often buried to minimize migration in young children
- A long-leg cast is applied with the ankle and foot in neutral position (foot is perpendicular to the lower leg)
- The cast is changed at a 2-week interval to check skin incisions. Neutral positioning is maintained. This cast is left intact until 6 weeks following surgery
- If buried, the K-wire is removed in the operating room at 6 weeks postsurgery. The child is then transitioned immediately into the boot and bar brace system 23 h/day for 2 months. Stretching is essential, and this is taught in the recovery room along with cast changes prior to initial surgery. The child then wears the boot and bar system at night until 2 years of age. The child is weaned from 23 h/day to 18 h/day to 16 h/day. The boots are pointed straight ahead. Do not place a dorsiflexion bend in the bar
- It is important to stretch the foot into plantarflexion and adduction
- The authors use the Dobbs Easy Click bar. Some research has been performed with other bars
- Not only should the talonavicular joint be reduced on the lateral radiograph but also on the anteroposterior view

| Vertical talus pitfalls |
| --- |

- Given a newborns foot, one may be fooled into thinking the calcaneus is the medial talar head. Pressure on the calcaneus will block reduction of the deformity
- A common error is not achieving maximal equinovarus positioning in the last cast before K-wire placement. This may lead to relapse or inadequate correction of deformity
- Poor compliance with bracing increases risks for relapse

## Calcaneovalgus

Severe calcaneovalgus foot deformity is a deformity in which the foot is hyperdorsiflexed and often abutting the anterior aspect of the tibia. The forefoot is abducted with marked heel valgus. Plantarflexion is often restricted and limited to a neutral position. While parents may be very concerned about the appearance of this deformity, it often improves on its own. Most calcaneovalgus deformities will improve by 6 months of age without intervention. Caregivers can assist with gentle manipulations emphasizing plantarflexion at the level of the ankle. Gentle inversion and adduction can also be helpful based on the deformity.

While calcaneovalgus most typically improves on its own, it is more important to exclude deformities associated with abnormal packing in utero such as hip dysplasia or posteromedial bowing of the tibia. It is important to recognize that the initial infant's hip exam may be normal while there is a greater association of hip dysplasia in children who have calcaneovalgus on one foot and metatarsus adductus on the contralateral foot. Advanced imaging in the form of ultrasound or X-rays, based on the child's age, can be helpful in excluding a silent hip dysplasia.

---

Pearls in evaluating for hip dysplasia

- Document clinical hip exam and any unusual neurologic findings (tone, unusual spasticity for age)
- Ortolani maneuver: posterior dislocation of the hip is reducible
- Barlow maneuver: by adducting the hip and applying pressure on the knee with force directed posteriorly, one can dislocate the hip
- Ultrasound: often utilized to exclude a dislocated hip under the age of 6 months

---

The incidence for calcaneovalgus is 1 in 1000 live births. With intrauterine crowding or packing deformities, the first child was found to be more at risk. Such is found to be the case for hip dysplasia as well.

One will note the calcaneus to be in equinus in vertical talus, whereas the heel is easily palpable, void of equinus, and in a dorsiflexed position with calcaneovalgus. Stress plantarflexion radiographs are most helpful in distinguishing between the two deformities. In congenital vertical talus, the talus will not align with the first metatarsal while the deformity will reduce with calcaneovalgus.

Generally, this deformity will improve by 6 months. Still given the small number of children that have persistent valgus deformities beyond this age group, casting can be utilized to assist with reduction of the deformity during the timeframe in which a child is not ambulatory. Bracing and manipulations for the more severe cases can follow serial casting. The authors have noted some children with persistent deformities in the absence of neurologic conditions, hence, the role of casting in the infant. There is definite variation among clinicians as to casting, treatment modalities, and plan of care. For residual calcaneovalgus deformities that persist beyond 12 months, it is prudent to exclude any neurologic influence.

| Calcaneovalgus pearls |
| --- |

- Educate parents that most children with calcaneovalgus deformities will improve without care
- Severe cases may benefit from serial casting to improve alignment and minimize risks of valgus pediatric foot deformities. This can be complimented by manipulations and ankle foot orthoses for additional months to assist with alignment
- Exclude vertical talus by ordering stress plantarflexion X-rays
- Exclude hip dysplasia

## Oblique Talus

Oblique talus is less understood as compared to vertical talus. Oblique talus is noted by a talus that aligns well with the first metatarsal on a lateral radiograph. Some subsets of such will present with equinus. Equinus is diagnosed by inverting the subtalar joint. An inability to dorsiflex the ankle beyond perpendicular indicates equinus. The authors treat oblique talus with equinus via the Dobbs method. These children often require two to three casts prior to surgical tenotomy of the Achilles and pinning of the talonavicular joint. Recognition of such deformity in infancy may reduce the risks for osseous procedures and symptomatic valgus feet with growth (Fig. 10.8).

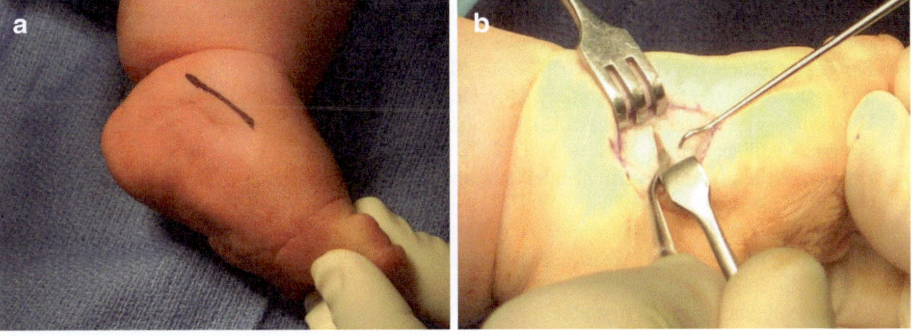


**Fig. 10.8**  (**a, b**) Talonavicular incision for vertical talus or oblique talus in the setting of equinus

# References


1. Dobbs MB, Purcell DB, Nunley R, Morcuende JA. Early results of a new method of treatment for idiopathic congenital vertical talus. J Bone Joint Surg Am. 2006;88(6):1192–200.
2. Alaee F, Boehm S, Dobbs MB. A new approach to treatment of congenital vertical talus. J Child Orthop. 2007;1(3):165–74.
3. Miller M, Dobbs MB. Congenital vertical Talus: etiology and Management. J Am Acad Orthop Surg. 2015;23:604–11.
4. Yang J, Dobbs M. Treatment of congenital vertical talus: comparison of minimally invasive and extensive soft tissue release procedures at minimum five-year follow up. J Bone Joint Surg. 2015;97(16):1354–65.
5. Jacobsen ST, Crawford AH. Congenital vertical talus. J Pediatr Orthop. 1983;3(3):306–10.
6. Sharrard WJ, Grosfield I. The management of deformity and paralysis of the foot in myelomenengocele. J Bone Joint Surg Br. 1968;50(3):456–65.
7. Merrill LJ, Gurnett CA, Connolly AM, Pestronik A, Dobbs MB. Skeletal muscle abnormalities and genetic factors releated to vertical talus. Clin Orthop Relat Res. 2011;469(4):1167–74.
8. Townes PL, Manning JA, Dehart GK Jr. Trisomy 18 (16-18) associated with congenital glaucoma and optic atrophy. J Pedatr. 1962;61:755–8.
9. Dobbs MB, Gurnett CA. The 2017 ABJS Nicolas Andry Award: advancing personalized medicine for clubfoot through translational research. Clin Orthop Relat Res. 2017;475:1716–25.
10. Alvarado D, McCall K, Hecht J, Dobbs M, Gurnett C. Deletion of 5' HOXC genes are associated with lower extremity malformations, including clubfoot and vertical talus. J Med Genet. 2016;53:250–5.
11. Dobbs M, Schoenecker P, Gordon J. Autosomal dominant transmission of isolated congenital vertical talus. Iowa Orthoped J. 2002;22:25–7.
12. Tayebi N, Charng WL, Dickson P, Dobbs M, Gurnett C. Diagnostic yield of exome sequencing in congenital vertical talus. Eur J Med Genet. 2022;65:104514.
13. Dobbs MB, Gurnett CA, Pierce B, et al. HOXD10 M319K mutation in a family with isolated congenital vertical talus. J Orthop Res. 2006;24(3):448–53.
14. Kruse L, Gurnett CA, Hootnick D, Dobbs MB. Magnetic resonance angiography in clubfoot and vertical talus: a feasibility study. Clin Orthop Res. 2009;467(5):1250–5.
15. Hamanishi C. Congenital vertical talus: classification with 69 cases and new measurement system. J Pediatr Orthop. 1984;4(3):318–26.
16. Bhaskar A. Congenital vertical talus: treatment by the reverse ponseti technique. Indian J Orthop. 2008;42(3):347–50.
17. Aydin A, Atmaca H, Muezzinoglu US. Bilateral congenital vertical talus with severe lower extremity external rotational deformity: treated by reverse Ponseti technique. Foot. 2012;22(3):252–4.
18. Khader A, Huntley JS. Congenital vertical talus in Cri du chat syndrome: a case report. BMC Res Notes. 2013;6:270.
19. Eberhardt O, Fernandez FF, Wirth T. The talar axis-first metatarsal base angle in CVT treatment: a comparison of idiopathic and non-idiopathic cases treated with the Dobbs method. J Child Orthop. 2012;6(6):491–6.
20. Eberhardt O, Wirth T, Fernandez FF. Minimally invasive treatment of congenital foot deformities in infants: new findings and midterm-results (German). Orthopade. 2013;42(12):1001–7.
21. Aslani H, Sadigi A, Tabrizi A, Bazavar M, Mousavi M. Primary outcomes of the congenital vertical talus correction using the Dobbs method of serial casting and limited surgery. J Child Orthop. 2012;6(4):307–11.
22. Chalayon O, Adams A, Dobbs MB. Minimally invasive approach for the treatment of nonisolated congenital vertical talus. J Bone Joint Surg Am. 2012;94(11):e73.
23. Eberhardt O, Fernandez FF, Wirth T. Treatment of vertical talus with the Dobbs method (German). Z Orthop Unfall. 2011;149(2):219–24.

24. Walker AP, Ghali NN, Silk FF. Congenital vertical talus: the results of staged operative reduction. J Bone Joint Surg Br. 1985;67(1):117–21.
25. Seimon LP. Surgical correction of congenital vertical talus under the age of 2 years. J Pediatr Orthop. 1987;7(4):405–11.
26. Stricker SJ, Rosen E. Early one-stage reconstruction of congenital vertical talus. Foot Ankle Int. 1997;18(9):535–43.
27. Duncan RD, Fixsen JA. Congenital convex pes valgus. J Bone Joint Surg Br. 1999;81(2):250–4.
28. Kodros SA, Dias LS. Single stage surgical correction vertical talus. J Pediatr Orthop. 1999;19(1):42–8.
29. Oppenheim W, Smith C, Christie W. Congenital vertical talus. Foot Ankle. 1985;5(4):198–204.
30. Mazzocca AD, Thompson JD, Deluca PA, Romness MJ. Comparison of the posterior approach versus the dorsal approach in the treatment of congenital vertical talus. J Pediatr Orthop. 2001;21(2):212–7.

# Index

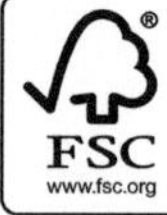



If you have any concerns about our products,
you can contact us on
ProductSafety@springernature.com

In case Publisher is established outside the EU,
the EU authorized representative is:
Springer Nature Customer Service Center GmbH
Europaplatz 3, 69115 Heidelberg, Germany

Printed by Libri Plureos GmbH
in Hamburg, Germany